Infant Depression

Paul V. Trad

Infant Depression

Paradigms and Paradoxes

Springer-Verlag
New York Berlin Heidelberg
London Paris Tokyo

Paul V. Trad, M.D.
Department of Psychiatry
The New York Hospital
Cornell Medical Center
Westchester Division
White Plains, New York 10605
U.S.A.

Library of Congress Cataloging in Publication Data
Trad, Paul V.
Infant depression.
Bibliography: p.
Includes index.
1. Depression in infant.   I. Title.
RJ506.D4T73   1986   618.92'8527   86-6624

Typeset by David E. Seham Associates, Inc., Metuchen, New Jersey.
Printed and bound by R.R. Donnelley & Sons, Harrisonburg, Virginia.
Printed in the United States of America.

9 8 7 6 5 4 3 2 1

ISBN 0-387-96343-X Springer-Verlag New York Berlin Heidelberg
ISBN 3-540-96343-X Springer-Verlag Berlin Heidelberg New York

Preface

For me, the word "infant" has always had a strange and compelling fascination. This book, in essence, represents the first step of what I hope will be a long and fruitful journey into the mysteries of the infant psyche, with special emphasis on the phenomenon of early-life depressive symptomatology.

From the outset of my medical training, I was particularly attracted to the field of psychiatry. As a resident exposed to adult patients in a psychiatric ward, I can vividly recall, even these many years later, the deep sense of poignancy and distress while in the presence of minds gone awry. It is my belief that psychiatry, more than any other branch of medicine, presents the physician with the ultimate paradox—the elusive diagnosis. By this I mean that while the symptomatology of psychiatry may be classified and analyzed, while diagnoses, prognoses, and treatment schedules can be devised, within psychiatry the unique configuration of each individual patient emerges with a clarity and distinction unparalleled in any other medical field. Before any psychiatric diagnosis can be formulated, the therapist must first delve deeply into the ultimate singularity of the patient. As a consequence, psychiatry is, in the final analysis, concerned with the dignity of each patient, and the psychiatrist is continually challenged to explore the most formidable and elaborate aspect of each person—the human mind.

That said, I need to express the reasons for my dedication to child psychiatry. During my years of treating adult patients, I grew increasingly more convinced that the aberrant behavioral manifestations encountered in adults were merely the sequelae or residue of earlier experiences of childhood and infancy. Indeed, the accuracy of the notion that "the child is father to the man" became more apparent with each patient I treated. Nevertheless, my motivation for conducting child and infant psychiatric research was not merely fueled by scientific curiosity or a desire to delineate the etiology of psychopathology. I was stimulated, additionally, by a desire to identify precise pressure points and to formulate more finely-honed instruments for determining when vulnerability to depression occurs, in order that the anguish of later psychopathology be averted. If the goal of the adult psychiatrist is to mend the damaged psyche, then the ambition of the child and infant psychiatrist is, for me, to prevent later psychopathology by developing a keen awareness of the vulnerabilities to depression encountered by young patients.

Infant Depression: Paradigms and Paradoxes strives to present child psychiatrists, child psychologists, social workers and psychiatric nurses with a new perspective for viewing the infant's psyche. As I became increasingly more immersed in this book, the data accumulated confirmed my previous impressions, derived from therapeutic experience, that infants—from the first weeks of life—are endowed with an apparatus of infinite delicacy and complexity, enabling them to develop and represent themselves in the world. Moreover, my research also confirmed that embedded within this rich potential are inherent vulnerabilities to psychopathology, including depressive-like phenomena. The allegation that even infants may be "at risk" for developing psychopathology may be disheartening for some, but it is my sincere hope that through honest investigation the susceptibilities of the infant to psychiatric disorder will be understood and such disorders will eventually be conquered. This book is offered in the spirit of achieving that goal.

Now that a completed manuscript has been delivered to the publisher, the task remains to express my deepest thanks to all those whose unflagging support and encouragement helped to make the work possible. Whenever I think of the word "infant," my thoughts turn to Professor Daniel N. Stern, M.D. During my years at Cornell University Medical Center, where Dr. Stern conducts both his academic and research activities, he has stimulated my imagination and enabled me to recognize how profound the myriad of questions and challenges surrounding infant-depression research can be. In addition, in all of my exchanges with Dr. Stern, he has always conveyed the compassion and insights of a fine teacher, as well as the friendship of a colleague. In pursuing a certificate of psychoanalysis at the William Alanson White Institute from 1980 through 1985, I had the good fortune to meet and work with Earl Witenberg, M.D., who is currently the director of the institute. I wish to express my sincere gratitude to him for instilling me with the confidence and inspiration to continue laboring over this book, especially during those times when my own enthusiasm waned. During the past several years, as a child psychiatry fellow at Cornell University Medical Center, Paulina F. Kernberg, M.D. has provided me with a strong sense of fortitude, encouraging me to exercise my capacities to their fullest potential within the therapeutic setting. My thanks are also extended to Donald McKnew, M.D., of the Child Development Unit at the National Institute of Mental Health. Two and one half years ago Dr. McKnew graciously reviewed a draft of a paper entitled, "Infant Depression: The Affect in Search of the Syndrome." His considered critique of the paper resulted in substantial improvements in the text. Further, Dr. McKnew was ever willing to discuss his insights during numerous conversations. This paper was subsequently awarded the Elise Kraft Ledman Prize for Psychiatric Research at Cornell University Medical Center in 1984, and represents the earliest articulation of some of the theories discussed in these pages.

This book was also made possible by the skill of several talented research assistants, whose enduring patience facilitated my assemblage of the data into a coherent framework. Among these were Morton Milder, Madeleine Robins, Vernon Bruete, Brian Steller, and Flora Lazar. To each of these individuals who gave generously of their time, intelligence, and critical insight, I express my warmest thanks. Special thanks are also accorded to Wendy J. Luftig, for helping me to articulate my thoughts and formulate my perceptions, and for having faith in me. To Richard H. White of Seattle, Washington, warmest acknowledgment for allowing me to transform some of my academic wishes into realities.

Ultimately, the rewarding relationships I have been able to experience were made possible by the affection and thoughtful concern that my parents, Blanche and Jorge Trad, who have consistently shared with me throughout my life.

Finally, this book is dedicated to every infant born during its genesis, from the early summer of 1982 through the late fall of 1985—especially those named Paul.

Paul V. Trad, M.D.
New York, New York

Contents

CHAPTER 1

Developmental Psychopathology

Investigations of many types of psychiatric disorders in infants and children begin with the convenient assumption that the condition under scrutiny exists as a distinct clinical phenomenon. The study of depression in infants and children enjoys no such position. As its relatively brief history attests, childhood depression has almost constantly found itself in the throes of a debate about whether or not it exists as a clinical syndrome at all, and if it does, how it relates to depression in adulthood.

The classical psychoanalytic literature postulated that certain preconditions for depression can develop even in the first year. Spitz and Wolf (1946) viewed their findings on anaclitic depression as clinical confirmation of these theories. In a landmark paper, they described over 10% of 123 institutionalized infants as severely depressed, and another roughly 20% as mildly depressed. Subsequent research, however, has failed to replicate Spitz and Wolf's findings in young infants.

As late as the 1960s, it was assumed that depression, as a syndrome analogous to that in adults, did not exist in childhood. Depressive symptoms were viewed merely as nonpathological manifestations of a specific developmental stage. Opinion then shifted to the "depressive equivalents" or "masked depression" argument, in which childhood depression was accepted as a discrete entity whose manifestations differed from those of adult depressives. Researchers and clinicians interpreted behaviors such as aggression, hyperactivity and enuresis, as well as sleeping and eating disturbances, as signs of an underlying but "masked depression."

There is still no consensus about the prevalence of depression in infancy and childhood. For example, Rutter and Garmezy (1983) consider depression prior to adolescence comparatively rare. A recent study by Kashani, Ray, and Carlson (1984) corroborates this view, at least within the preschool age group. In sharp contrast, Chess, Thomas, and Hassibi (1983) contend that the phenomenon is far more widespread than heretofore recognized, and, in fact, is not uncommon.

The debate concerning infant and childhood depression has been continued, at least in part, because of the difficulties that researchers and clinicians have confronted in defining and identifying depression among the very young who have not yet developed the facility to express subjective emotional states. Measurement, after all, requires a certain degree of definitional clarity. The currently prevailing approach relies on adult–based criteria, such as *DSM–III* (*Diagnostic and Statistical Manual of Mental Disorders,* 3rd Ed.) (American Psychiatric Association, 1980) to diagnose depression in children. This most recent approach starts with the known—the understanding of adult depression—and posits that childhood depression is analogous to adult depression and can be studied in the same way by means of a multifactorial approach. According to this model, measures of depression in adults should provide adequate measures of depression in children.

In fact, use of *DSM–III* criteria for diagnosing depression in young children has had only questionable success. The first prospective study using *DSM–III* to examine depressive disorders in preschoolers (Kashani, et al., 1984) found the condition far less common among younger than among older children. Taken at face value, such a finding could mean that depression in this population occurs only rarely. Alternatively, as the authors note, such findings may raise questions about the adequacy of *DSM–III* for diagnosing affective disorders in the very young. These questions have been posed before, with respect to depression and with respect to the suitability of *DSM–III* for diagnosing other disorders (Garber, 1984; Poznanski, Makros, Grossman, and Freeman 1985; Tanguay, 1984).

This book evolves from a similar set of beliefs: the notion that depression in infancy and childhood is probably more common than heretofore recognized, and that its ostensibly low prevalence rates may serve more as a condemnation of our diagnostic methods than as an accurate reflection of an epidemiological trend. Infancy and childhood are periods of rapid change—more rapid, perhaps, than at any other point in development. It should not be surprising that symptoms of depression might also fluctuate rapidly during this chronological period. The concept of infant and childhood depression embodied by *DSM–III* provides researchers and clinicians with important fundamental criteria for detecting childhood depression. Nevertheless, *DSM–III* fails to capture the dynamic dimensions of depression occurring in early life. This book turns to the field of developmental psychopathology to correct some of these deficiencies.

The Perspective of Developmental Psychopathology

Developmental psychopathology is not only the newest, but it is also one of the most ambitious approaches to understanding the parameters of childhood depression. Although the discipline is barely 10 years old, it has recently attracted an increasing amount of attention and has produced a growing volume of research in such areas as maternal deprivation, autism, schizophrenia, and retardation. Its primary objectives are the establishment of lines of predictive validity from childhood to adult mental disorders and demonstration of the evolving nature of such disorders. As the goals of this book are to show: 1) that depression can occur in infancy; 2) that it can alter with development; and 3) that it can predispose a child to further deficits, the developmental framework offers a particularly useful approach for identifying and tracing the etiologies of childhood depression. This framework has yet to be applied in a truly comprehensive fashion to the study of depression in both infancy and childhood.

Before applying this model to the specific issue of infant and childhood depression, it is helpful to articulate the general theoretical foundations of developmental psychopathology. In seeking to understand and predict maladaptation, developmental psychopathologists probe beyond specific behaviors to broader challenges facing individuals at different developmental periods. According to two of the pioneers in the field, Sroufe and Rutter (1984), developmental psychopathology focuses on the "ontological process whereby early patterns of individual adaptation evolve into later patterns of adaptation" (p. 27). The paradigm is based on the premise that the competence with which individuals confront developmental challenges in the course of their lives will create differing patterns of adaptation and maladaptation that interact throughout their lives, coloring their ability to resolve subsequent interpersonal confrontations successfully.

Central to the developmental perspective is the proposition that both normal and disordered individuals undergo a common course of development in which functioning at one level has predictable implications for subsequent functioning. This developmental viewpoint has often been misconstrued as a belief in behavioral stability. Coherence, however, should not be confused with stability, as Sroufe and Rutter (1984) emphatically note. Developmental psychopathologists expect that growth will result in behavioral changes as well as behavioral continuities. They thus abandon a belief in linear development, favoring instead a model that allows for behavioral transformations, as well as regressions. In contrast to clinical professionals (child psychologists and psychiatrists), developmental psychopathologists' efforts are devoted to tracing the origins and evolution of disorders and describing their manifestations over time— both before and after these disorders emerge in clinical form. While the former focus on pathology that actually manifests itself in childhood, the latter also devote attention to nondisordered childhood behavior in the context of child pathology, and to disordered childhood behavior that does not result in pathology until later in life. As Sroufe and Rutter note, developmental psychopathologists are as interested in the precursors of a disorder as they are in its sequelae.

Clearly, this model recognizes the significance of growth and maturity in childhood, and attempts to frame both normal and abnormal development within this context (Garber, 1984). Although a concern for the relationship between childhood and adult disorders is central to the developmental perspective, the model specifically avoids "adultmorphism," the tendency to focus on the similarities and overlook the differences between the child and adult forms of a disorder.

Developmental psychopathologists recognize that individuals meet developmental challenges with different biological and temperamental constitutions and that both inborn characteristics as well as environment will influence development. Their model advocates neither the "nature" nor the "nurture" side in the heredity versus environment controversy that, if anything, has tended to overly simplify a complex interaction between individuals and the external world.

Tyson (1984) summarizes the developmental approach well. She writes that it is:

. . . based on an epigenetic view of psychic structure formation resulting from successive interactions between the infant's biologically and genetically determined maturational sequences, on the one hand, and experiential influences, on the other. The outcome of each developmental phase is understood to depend on the outcome of all previous previous phases as well as on the interactions among a variety of development lines . . . Changes over time involve a number of dynamic interactions, continuities and discontinuities . . . At each new stage, the system, while maintaining a degree of integrity . . . differs qualitatively from the preceding stage. Each new stage . . . should be understood more in terms of spirals; analogous developmental issues are worked and reworked at successive developmental levels. (p. 123)

Focusing on a multi–dimensional array of variables, developmental psychopathology broadens the medical model that clinicians, until recently, have applied in their search for the diagnostic criteria of psychopathology, i.e., that psychopathology must be traced to an isolated, unresolved conflict from early life (Cicchetti, 1984). Tyson identifies only some of the many facets of development charted by the paradigm: the interactions of psychic structures, conscious and unconscious motivations, object relationships, self–esteem, sense of identity, and physical maturation. Biological factors, encompassing a broad range of variables (including genetic, endocrinological and perinatal factors), also receive significant consideration by developmental psychopathology. Because of its breadth, the discipline draws upon numerous branches of medical science, including neurophysiology, embryology, physiological psychology, and developmental neurobiology (Cicchetti, 1984).

A Developmental Perspective on Depression

The multi–dimensional and evolutionary approach of the developmental model is essential for understanding how depression can unfold in infants and children. Recognition of this approach has become evident to researchers in the field. For example, the "masked depression" theory described by Cytryn and McKnew (1974) was one of the first to acknowledge an evolving set of symptoms for depression in early life. Other research on depressive states in early life documents the developmental nature of symptomatology, as well. Older children, capable of some degree of self–reflection and verbalization, often express feelings of guilt, self–blame, a sense of rejection, and a negative self–image, according to a review of the literature performed by Rutter and Garmezy (1983). Identifying depressive symptoms in infants, however, presents a greater challenge, since researchers have to rely exclusively on behavioral indices rather than verbal clues. Spitz and Wolf (1946) enumerated a number of depressive symptoms (such as weeping, withdrawal, apathy, weight loss, sleep disturbance, and decrease in developmental quotient) among the infants they studied, and traced these behaviors to the second half of the first year. In addition, after six months, and as late as four years, loss of the major caregiver will cause children to react first with protest, then with despair, and finally with detachment (Bowlby, 1969). Prior to six months, however, infants display no grief reaction following the kinds of losses that Bowlby links to depression in the last half of the first year. Thus, it has proven difficult to isolate psychopathological manifestations during the first few months of life.

Nevertheless, the traceable sequence of events that occurs following caregiver loss may be replicated by other phenomena occurring prior to the sixth month. Despite Spitz and Wolf's findings that infants under six months will not display depressive patterns, various researchers have shown that presentation of extreme discrepancies or presentation of disrupted contingencies can evoke a facsimile of the Learned Helplessness Paradigm response described in adults by Seligman (1972) and can eventually produce the kind of despair, followed by detachment, that Bowlby describes. The implication, then, is that although a full–blown grief reaction linked to depression may not manifest itself until after six months of age, the developmental process whereby the infant integrates these behavioral patterns may be "learned" much before six months of age. In a related vein, infants' seemingly intrinsic capacity for empathy may, if they are exposed continually to distress—for example, parental depression—predispose even a young infant to depression.

Consistent with the developmental approach, this book examines a multiplicity of factors that may contribute to depression in early life. By applying the developmental framework, the milestones discussed reveal the mechanisms by which learned helplessness, which has been described and validated in adults, can occur in incipient stages during early infancy. This book also uses the developmental framework to trace the contribution of temperamental predisposition, attachment behaviors, self–object representation, and empathic development to infant and childhood depression. Particular emphasis is placed on how aberrant behavioral manifestations may emerge from these developmental milestones. Such manifestations may represent expression of depressive symptomatology in infants and young children.

Depression clearly represents the outgrowth of a complex set of interactions involving constitutional elements, such as neuroendocrine and temperamental endowment, as well as the products of affective and cognitive development. This book posits that depression in early life is a function of the dynamic interplay of these variables and begins its analysis with a concentrated discussion of temperament and three developmental milestones: attachment, self, and object–representation. These variables have been pinpointed for a number of reasons. First, disorder in each, independently, has a well documented relationship to adult depressive symptomatology as an interpretive reading of *DSM–III* reveals. Lack of self–esteem, for example, is enumerated as a *DSM–III* symptom of adult depression. Second, empirical studies have shown that, within certain parameters, these variables have strong temporal predictability and they correlate with patterns of adaptation or maladaptation in later life. Finally, the developmental milestones are mutually reinforcing. For instance, a "difficult" temperament may exacerbate strained parent–child interactions, generating insecure attachment and ultimately resulting in negative self–referencing.

Given the limited behavioral repertoire of infants, it is often difficult to rely exclusively on behavioral information as a key to emotional states. Therefore this book also includes a discussion of the neuroendocrine correlates of depression. Such a discussion serves two purposes relevant to the developmental framework. First, it provides a bridge between the infant's natural endowment as expressed via temperament dimensions and early affective development as manifested in attachment behavior. Second, the neuroendocrine analysis draws parallels between biochemical models for adult depression and analogous processes in infants and children. This latter objective sheds light on whether depressed infants and children can respond to the types of biochemical interventions that have proven effective in adults.

Predictive Validity

Needless to say, theories achieve credibility in many ways. In the sciences, predictive power is weighted heavily in determining theoretical validity. Evaluating a theory requires, therefore, an evaluation of its predictive ability. Developmental psychopathology is still a relatively new approach, wrestling with numerous unresolved theoretical and methodological issues concerning its ability to predict adaptation and maladaptation from early functioning. Indeed, in the course of its early refinement, developmental psychopathology has, not surprisingly, encountered a number of challenges to predictive validity.

Longitudinal studies, which attempt to follow individuals over time, have served an important validating role for developmental theory. One of the most ambitious early longitudinal investigations, conducted by the Fels Research Institute, casts doubt on the ability of infant behavior to predict through childhood and beyond (Kagan & Moss, 1962). The Fels study found few correlations between adolescent behavior and anxiety due to loss of an early attachment figure. It should be noted that this study predated the development and widespread use of modern instruments, such as Ainsworth's Strange Situation Procedure, for measuring attachment security. Additionally, several studies have sought to isolate specific biological factors that impede development or actually bring about a developmental deficit. Attempts to find significant and enduring developmental consequences for such early crises as prematurity and anoxia have not generated conclusive results (Drillien, 1964; Sameroff & Chandler, 1984; Weiner, Rowland, Oppel, Fischer, & Harper, 1965).

Most explanations for the seeming lack of continuity in development rely on the unpredictability of environmental factors. Environmentalists, such as Kagan, assert that many psychological states are products of the vagaries of the environment that impact on the individual, causing discontinuities rather than continuities. Taking this proposition a step further, Kagan (1984) implies that behaviors at one developmental stage, whether pathological or not, do not lead inexorably to similar behaviors at later stages. Conversely, characteristics of a later age are not dependent upon, nor derivative of, experiences of an earlier stage. If environment, rather than early patterns of functioning, governs the course of development, this hypothesis suggests that deviance can not only appear, but can also disappear abruptly. Indeed, research has demonstrated that environmental factors can trigger a disorder (Garmezy, Masten, & Tellegen, 1984; Sameroff, 1975; Sameroff & Chandler, 1984). According to this line of thought, environment operates in conjunction with the body's own homeostatic tendencies and can reverse the impact of early deficits, thereby creating discontinuities in development.

In elevating environmental factors to greater stature throughout the course of development, several researchers, such as Kagan, have added an important dimension to developmental theory. While the implications of their argument have frequently been construed as antagonistic to developmental theory—and hence to the assumption of continuity and predictability—the two concepts need not be mutually exclusive. The fact that environment can change and prove to be a source of instability rather than stability does not mean that it necessarily *does* change with respect to an individual's life. In fact, it has been shown that disordered individuals often actively seek environments that reinforce, rather than correct, their disorders.

Challenges, in any case, are healthy for the evolution and application of a theory. They force researchers to articulate its assumptions and implications more clearly, as well as to assess its strengths and weaknesses. Indeed, in attempting to correlate findings on many of the environmental risk factors cited to refute developmental theory, developmental psycho-pathologists have modified certain theoretical points to reflect new evidence on the relationships between intra–psychic experience and different risk factors, and the implications of these relationships for predictability.

It is crucial to keep in mind that environmental influences, anatomic equipment, and intra–psychic experience all coalesce in the infant. These variables are the separate analytic components of a unitary, interactional process in the organism. The dichotomy between nature and nurture is useful for identifying developmental influences, but does not reveal the increasing capacity of the infant to integrate the forces of each element. The correlations between these forces and the manner in which each modifies the others should be the focal point of developmental psychology.

Rutter's (1977) interpretation of changes occurring at puberty serves as a good illustration of the way in which developmental psychopathology incorporates factors causing apparent behavioral discontinuities into a model of continuity and predictability. He concedes that many ostensibly abrupt changes occur during adolescence, seeming to correspond with the onset of puberty. However, he argues, these changes are not simply a product of puberty, but are a conditioned response to the new set of demands and stresses that accompany the change. The relevant factor is not the inevitability of change with puberty, but differential capacities for negotiating through these changes. These adaptive patterns grow from successes in early adaptation. Conversely, early failures in specific developmental tasks, such as attachment formation or self–representation, accumulate to shape later behaviors. Knowledge of early developmental deficits should, therefore, enable us to predict subsequent developmental outcome.

In this mode, individuals enter into reciprocal relationships with their environments. They are not merely passive products, but full participants, from the earliest moments of life, in shaping the contours of their interactions with the external world. Sameroff (1975) coined the term *transactional* to describe this relationship, implicitly suggesting a form of continuity based on evolving interactions between individuals and their environments. Deviance in this framework occurs not because of any innate characteristic of the child or because of random events, but because individuals continually malfunction in organizing and integrating their experiences (Sameroff, 1975).

Empirical Support for Developmental Model in Study of Depression

No theoretical construct predicts all phenomena equally well. This is certainly true of the developmental model. Even though many of the theorists most enthusiastic about the breadth of its explanatory power have narrowed their focus somewhat, developmental psychopathology has weathered the initial criticism well.

When discussing predictability, it is important to bear in mind that we are concerned with two basic dimensions of predictability—inter–variable and temporal—and, more importantly, the relationship between them. *Temporal stability* refers to the stability of a variable, e.g., attachment behavior, from one point to another. *Inter–variable predictability* denotes consistency in the influence of one variable upon another. The relationship between temperament and attachment might be one example of this kind of predictability. Early attempts to apply developmental theory to the prediction of various disorders have tended to focus narrowly on one dimension or the other. As this book demonstrates, in the context of depression, stability inheres not as much in any single factor in isolation from the others, but in the system of interactions. Relationships between two variables can "borrow" stability from predictable relationships to other variables. What remains stable is the overall adaptiveness or maladaptiveness of the individual. This is the implication of the transactional model described by Sameroff (1975). It is part of the researcher's job to identify the dimensions of predictability that "glue" the separate variables together into a continuously operative, predictable system. In fact, research on many facets of affective development reveals a comparatively high level of predictability.

In a review of the literature, Rutter (1977) claims there is growing evidence that early development of skills for coping with adversity will affect later success in coping with environmental stress. Other studies also support the notion of continuities in affective development. In a longitudinal study of three to five year olds, Lerner, Inui, Trupin, and Douglas (1985) found that the 20 children with the greatest overall affective disturbance as preschoolers had the greatest risk of developing psychiatric disorders by the time they were teenagers. Early behavioral disorders such as aggressiveness, withdrawal, and hyperactivity predicted many affective disorders. Interestingly, however, these disorders did not predict psychotic disorders (Lerner et al., 1985).

Attachment behavior, in particular, reveals a great deal of stability over time (Antonucci & Levitt, 1984; Waters, 1978). Moreover, attachment appears to predict other types of behavioral manifestations, such as self–esteem, positive affect, ego–control, resiliency, and autonomous functioning (Arend, Gove & Sroufe, 1978; Matas, Arend, & Sroufe, 1978; Schneider–Rosen & Cicchetti, 1984; Sroufe, 1983; Waters, 1978; Waters, Wippman, & Sroufe, 1979). This record of predictability is particularly significant in light of findings of some degree of stability in early attachment behavior. From a developmental perspective, the significance of these relationships lies in the translation of competence and adaptiveness in attaining one developmental milestone—attachment security—into success in reaching another.

Temperamental predictability—both over time and in relation to depression—has been the focus of more heated debate among researchers. Thirty years of longitudinal research in the New York Longitudinal Study

(NYLS), reported by Thomas and Chess in 1984, suggests that *specific* categories of temperament show little long–term predictability. However, Thomas and Chess, the pioneers of this study, did feel that there was considerable continuity in *clusters* of traits followed through childhood. They found that the nine dimensions of temperament on which infants were evaluated tended to cluster into three distinctly identifiable groups— difficult, easy, and slow to warm up temperaments   and that these broad dimensions showed greater stability than the individual measures of which they were comprised (Thomas, Chess, & Birch, 1970), (see Chapter 2). Other researchers have demonstrated that broad temperamental profiles remain stable in early life (Peters–Martin & Wachs, 1984). These findings on temperamental stability in early life, when natural endowment may exercise greater influence than environment, appear consistent with the prevailing belief that temperament has a strong genetic component (Gold- smith, 1983; Goldsmith & Gottesman, 1981; Matheny, 1980; Plomin & Rowe, 1979; Shields, 1981; Thomas & Chess, 1977). (See also Chapter 2).

Not surprisingly, therefore, individual temperamental categories, which themselves are less stable over time than composite profiles, do not predict behavioral outcome as reliably as do composite temperamental profiles. Plomin (1983) observes in a review of the literature that composite tem- perament profiles have succeeded in predicting a variety of behaviors both concurrently and later in life, among them mother–child interaction, school achievement, and adjustment disorders. Research using temperament profiles to predict long–term behavioral outcomes is still limited, however, and the study of depression suffers from this shortage. We can make strong inferences from studies using other indices such as conduct (Puig–Antich, 1982) to predict depression. Puig–Antich found that over one third of the 43 pre–pubertal boys treated for major depression at the Child Depression Clinic of New York State Psychiatric Institute met *DSM–III* criteria for conduct disorder. Although only long–term study can establish the long- term predictiveness of pre–pubertal conduct disorders for other disorders (be they depression, antisocial personality, or other disorders), Puig–An- tich expects that a substantial proportion of these young boys will suffer from one of the depressive spectrum disorders.

Predictability: Time–Frame Issues

In tracing developmental continuities, researchers have sought answers to two particular questions: first, is there a particular developmental period at which stability emerges; and second, how long can the stability endure? Researchers disagree on the earliest point from which long–term pre- dictability in behaviors and attitudes can be discerned in any facet of func- tioning. Although Kagan (1980) argues that continuities do not verifiably appear before age six, several studies indicate that they may appear during preschool years (Matheny, Wilson, & Nuss, 1984).

Many areas of affective development appear to exhibit stability earlier (Lewis, Feiring, Mcguffog, & Jaskir, 1984). Among the attachment theorists, a stable pattern of attachment is usually thought to have been established by the age of 9–12 months as measured by Ainsworth's Strange Situation Procedure (see Chapter 3 for a description of this procedure and its uses). In addition, these early attachment patterns can predict other behavior with significant reliability. Temperament patterns may appear even earlier and sustain themselves longer according to the NYLS. Thomas & Chess (1977) initially evaluated subjects at three months and found that almost three quarters of those classified as "difficult" during this evaluation developed behavior disorders by age seven years. Plomin (1983) took a more limited view, tracing stability in temperament to childhood rather than infancy. One of his findings was that difficult temperaments, in particular, have significant predictive power beginning in early childhood.

Other theorists argue, however, that the rapid pace of development during infancy makes prediction before the age of two years unreliable. The temperament study of Peters–Martin and Wachs (1984), for example, suggests an inverse relationship between predictability and measurement interval, at least in the first year. This study discloses temperamental continuity in six month intervals, but not continuity spanning over one year. By the age of two, however, the development of ego may enhance predictability. Around that time, children learn to interpret experience and develop a belief system about interaction with the environment. Provided this belief system finds continued reaffirmation in the environment, it may create the basis for stability (Kagan, 1980).

Given the plethora of unanswered questions about how frequently depression occurs at different ages and what constitutes depressive symptomatology over the course of time, it is not surprising that research to date offers only limited help in determining whether depression in early life predicts depression in adulthood. Rutter and Garmezy (1983) present several seemingly contradictory pieces of evidence in their review of the literature. On the one hand, they observe that most adults with depression who were studied longitudinally did not exhibit depression as children. On the other hand, depression seems to show stronger continuity than all other disorders except obsessive–compulsive disorders. Among the most depressed children who continued to have psychiatric conditions in adulthood, depression constituted part of their clinical picture. Notably, however, the depression was one component in a broader constellation of symptoms and rarely represented the primary diagnosis.

These data seem to suggest that we direct our investigations not toward diagnostic categories such as depression, but toward the variety of age–specific maladaptive variables that evolve and interact over time—ultimately determining an individual's vulnerability to depression. Biochemical/neuroendocrinological investigations into the nature of depression have followed a similar course, culminating in the Permissive Amine Hypothesis.

This theory postulates that abnormally low levels of brain serotonin increase an individual's vulnerability to depression.

If links between affective symptoms from infancy to adulthood demonstrate more stability than do clinical diagnoses, then there is great merit in the recommendation of Sroufe and Rutter (1984) that we adopt a different level of analysis and focus on adaptational failures such as poor peer relations, as well as both conduct and affect disturbances. Consideration of both is critical in formulating a comprehensive diagnosis. As Sroufe and Rutter note, ". . . it is unlikely that the specific affect aberration, in the absence of the broader adaptational failure, would predict adult depression. Rather, presence of both the general, age–related adaptational failure and the particular pattern of maladaptation are required for predicting adult disorder" (p. 27).

The prediction of adult depression from childhood depression is thus subject to the same potential pitfalls as predictions of other disorders. Reliability inheres not only in the method used to measure continuity, but more importantly in the criteria used to identify child and adult depressives. Since depressive behaviors are clearly not isomorphic over time, researchers will have to examine the interaction of different processes, such as reactions to separations and the control/expression of feelings, to know whether childhood depression evolves into adult depression.

Future Directions: Need for Improved Research and Classification Methods

As developmental psychopathology progresses, it will face two major challenges. First, it will need to develop a classification scheme better able to distinguish between normal and abnormal behaviors at different developmental periods. Second, it will need to refine current research methods to capture the effects of a broader range of variables—affective, cognitive, sociological, physiological and biochemical—encompassed in the developmental model. Clearly progress in each area is essential; progress in one without the other will leave questions unanswered. Without improved research methods *and* a better classification scheme, researchers will continue to ask themselves whether certain conditions such as childhood depression rarely exist or whether they exist but go undetected by current methods.

Paradoxically, the developmental psychopathologist's perspective arises from, and is most hampered by, the lack of a classification scheme capable of accounting for the many factors that may make pathological conditions express themselves differently at different points in development. By ignoring developmental considerations, most classification schemes have, without modification, applied criteria derived from experience with adults directly to children. However, with the particularly rapid pace of change that occurs during childhood, the search for static adult traits in diagnosing childhood disorders such as depression may provide misleading evidence. Certain types of cognitive, physiological, and affective maturity are pre-requisites for the emergence of particular types of symptoms (Tanguay, 1984). Therefore, some symptoms characterizing the adult form of a dis-order may not be manifested in the childhood disorder. The absence of the adult symptom should not lead to the conclusion, as it often has, that psychopathology does not exist in the child. Researchers have, however, often fallen into this trap. Failure to find the adult characteristics in children has led them to conclude that continuity does not exist; the difficulty in assessing adult–like qualities at an early age has led many researchers to the specious conclusion that adult pathology has no childhood antecedents. On the opposite end of the spectrum, many apparent later–life adjustments from early psychopathology may not represent adjustments at all, but rather failures of existing methods to detect pathology as it evolves through developmental periods.

These theoretical problems have heightened interest in refining clas-sification methods to address developmental considerations. Although some authors have rejected classification of childhood disorders altogether because of the constant changes that occur during childhood, Tanguay (1984) and Garber (1984) still maintain that, for children, a developmentally oriented classification scheme would provide greater insight into the causes of psychopathology than does the symptomatic approach of *DSM–III*. Garber contends that a classification scheme focusing on methods of ad-aptation is essential for identifying and treating psychopathology in chil-dren. She argues that:

. . . the natural course and prognosis of a disorder in childhood should be assessed independently of its continuity with adult psychopathology . . . and classification of developmental psychopathology should have a way of capturing the process of change and development that children undergo. It should not be limited to the classification of isolated and static behaviors and attributes. Rather, some notion of the coherence of the individual in terms of his or her manner of organizing and integrating information and experiences needs to be included in a developmental system of classification. (p.35)

Garber's scheme is necessarily multidimensional, and incorporates ex-pectations for age, sex, developmental phase, level of functioning, and environmental, familial, and cultural influences. A gradual adoption of Garber's stance is reflected in the incremental steps toward defining infant and childhood depression, from the early concept that depression, as a syndrome analogous to that in adults, does not exist in childhood, to the currently widespread view that starts with an understanding of adult depression and posits a similar childhood phenomenon that can be studied in the same way by means of a multifactorial approach. Using *DSM–III* as a framework, researchers hope to incorporate the specific symptom-atology for infant and childhood depression and depressive–like phenomena. Their aim is to provide a more precise developmental framework for the phenotypic changes that coincide with the development of depression. There is also a need to define more clearly whether these milestones are co–occurring with depression or only with some subtypes of depression.

The urgency for developing such a classification scheme for childhood depression is underscored in a recent study by Poznanski et al. (1985), who compared the results of four different sets of diagnostic criteria in detecting depression among children six to 12 years old. Although the four sets of criteria—Research Diagnostic Criteria (RDC), *DSM–III*, Poznanski, and Weinberg—concurred in most instances about the diagnosis, in cases of disagreement, the differences lay in essential rather than qualifying criteria. Moreover, the particular criterion—the determination of dysphoric mood—that accounted for most of the variance has a significant developmental dimension, as recognized in *DSM–III*'s acceptance of nonverbal ratings of affect in children under six years old.

Organization of Book

This book begins by tracing each of the variables—temperament, attachment, object relations, self–representation, and empathy—independently as they relate to depression. In the interactive section that follows, the discussion focuses on how these variables operate in conjunction with one another and suggests ways in which disorder in one variable may reverberate through other facets of development, leading to frustration, interruption, or arrest, and ultimately to depressive symptomatology. This interactive section first discusses depressive phenomena in the context of face–to–face mother–infant interaction studies. It then turns to a developmental analysis of the Learned Helplessness Model of infants and children, tracing means by which infants develop contingency and discrepancy awareness that may lie at the foundation of depression in early life. A review of the latest neuroendocrinological studies follows. The closing chapter addresses the various transitions that the concept of infant and childhood depression has undergone in the last four decades. The purpose of this chapter is to identify the limitations of using adult models for diagnosis and to suggest innovations that take into consideration incipient symptomatology currently omitted from *DSM–III* guidelines.

CHAPTER 2

Correlates of Temperament to Depressive Phenomena

Attempts to identify precisely the phenomenon of infant depression have been hindered by a lack of consensus concerning what constitutes depression in general. Currently, no universally reliable and valid definition of depression exists. Indeed, perceiving depression per se as a common clinical phenomenon appears to be the only reliable point of agreement among investigators.

Nevertheless, the precept that the nature of personality changes with maturation has been one of the few points about which there has been some small degree of agreement (Bell, Weller, & Waldrop, 1971; Birns, Barten, & Bridger, 1969; Buss & Plomin, 1975; Escalona, 1963; Fries, 1944; Goldsmith & Campos, 1982; Kagan, 1971; Korner, Hutchinson, Koperski, Kraemer, & Schneider, 1981; Lewis & Starr, 1979; Rothbart & Derryberry, 1982; Shirley, 1933; Sroufe & Waters, 1977; Thomas, Chess, & Birch, 1963). Dispute remains about whether depression in infants is a legitimate clinical entity and whether the occurrence of depression and depressive–like phenomena in infants and adults is similar. In addition, researchers have been intrigued with the developmental nature of personality and this has provoked continued explorations of whether depressive manifestations in infants and in adults are similar.

This chapter explores the premise that infant and adult depression share a common origin. It does so by embarking on an examination of temperament, one of the key developmental milestones traced through the book. Temperament, as such, has been considered a milestone precisely because it provides a mechanism, vocabulary, and set of instruments for measuring and tapping into affective states at a relatively early age. That is, the various traits or dimensions that have been isolated by temperament researchers (for example, quality of mood, intensity, and distractibility) have enabled researchers to identify the subtle nuances of affect displayed by very young infants. In turn, affective states have classically been used as signposts to depressive symptomatology. Indeed, the parameters of childhood depression outlined in *DSM–III* rely almost entirely on affective states.

By grouping temperamental traits or dimensions into constellations often referred to as clusters—in essence, syndromes of temperament—researchers have been able to correlate temperamental types with affective profiles. These temperamental clusters provide an identifiable connection to affective disposition, which in turn may be used to predict and diagnose the constellation of symptoms that comprise depression as a syndrome. Temperament may then be viewed as a tool facilitating access to affective states that correlate with depressive symptomatology.

It is the contention of this chapter that the affective states that correlate with temperament dimensions and clusters are the identical affective states used to measure and diagnose depression. That is, temperament dimensions and clusters are the parameters for isolating the affective proclivities of each individual infant. These affective proclivities, in turn, serve as key indicators for diagnosing depression.

Throughout the chapter, as the reader gains familiarity with the basic definitions of temperament, the instruments used in temperament research, and the conclusions of the seminal studies that have explored temperament in infants and children, three basic questions should be asked. First, how may discrete temperament dimensions, as evidenced in the affective patterns revealed in temperament studies, be used to trace the risk of developing depression and depressive–like phenomena? Second, how can temperament clusters or constellations, which tap affective profiles, be used to identify depression as a syndrome composed of affective symptoms? Finally and most crucially, how may current data gleaned from studies of infant temperament be used to enhance prevailing definitions of infant and childhood depression.

Case Report

Brad was one of the 133 middle–class subjects followed from infancy through adulthood in the New York Longitudinal Study. He was temperamentally difficult as an infant, characterized by withdrawing from new stimuli, low adaptability, negative mood, and irregularity. Fortunately, his parents were patient and flexible and were able to deal with his temperamental idiosyncrasies in infancy. There was no family history of mental illness.

When Brad was 12, his parents were divorced. He chose to stay with his father. However, there were frequent fights between father and son. His relations with his mother were also hostile and difficult. During this time, Brad recognized that his sexual orientation was leaning toward the homosexual. This stressful entry into adolescence led to a clinical diagnosis of depression at age 13. He suffered from sleep disorders, had poor school performance, and began to use marijuana frequently. At 15, he also began to drink heavily. Brad underwent two unsuccessful attempts at psychotherapy. He was rediagnosed as suffering from a depressive disorder that met *DSM–III* criteria for adjustment disorder with depressed mood. Brad was sent to a boarding school at 15. There he received treatment through Gestalt therapy. He continued to use drugs, but gradually improved both social and scholastic performance. His substance abuse gradually decreased. At age 18, there were no signs of depression, but there was still some disturbance in functioning. He was diagnosed at that time as demonstrating narcissistic personality disorder (Chess & Thomas, 1984).

Individual Differences and Importance of Stability Over Time

Beginning in 1935, Fries and her colleagues (Fries, 1937, 1941a, 1941b; Fries & Lewi, 1938; Fries & Woolf, 1953) examined differences between newborn infants in their congenital modes of adjustment. Categorizing the infants by what was referred to as their "Congenital Activity Type," a term describing the amount of reactivity the newborn exhibits when presented with various stimuli, and following the infants through several years of development, Fries and her coinvestigators drew inferences about which modes of adjustment might predispose an infant to eventual psychopathology. Fries gave as an example of what she called an "overactive newborn," a three-month "colicky infant". This is a pediatric term used for infants, who after crying excessively and suffering from colic, quiet down at three months (Fries & Woolf, 1953). At the other end of the scale, she identified an autistic child as developing probably from the "extremely pathologically quiet type" (Fries and Woolf, 1953). Fries stressed the interactive relationship between the child's congenital activity type and parental attitude (Fries & Woolf, 1953). Fries observed that one infant whose congenital activity type she described as "especially quiet," and who as a newborn had suffered partial facial paralysis, developed recognizable schizoid traits by age six years. Her observations of this and other infants led her to suspect that "the pathologically quiet child, in a sick environment, was . . . more apt to develop schizophrenia" than others (Fries & Lewi, 1938; cited in Fries & Woolf, 1953, p. 57). Fries's early findings are important because they suggest that newborn infants exhibit unique temperamental characteristics that remain stable over a period of years and significantly affect early development.

In another study investigating individual differences in activity, Fries (1944) found enough intra–individual stability in the activity patterns of neonates to group infants as either quiet, moderately active, or active. Later investigators, such as Thomas and Chess, have expanded on this tripartite classification, and by incorporating other dimensions of temperament, have identified three categories of infant based on temperamental classification: the easy, difficult, and slow-to-warm-up.

More recent studies support Fries' suggestion that newborn infants can exhibit stable temperamental tendencies. Clifton and Graham (1968) investigated the stability of individual differences in heart rate activity during the newborn period. They followed a sample of 16 neonates for three days and a subsample of 10 neonates for five days, and found that "thirteen of the measures showed some significant stability although they differed in the size of correlations and in the degree of concordance" (Clifton & Graham, 1968, p. 38). Kagan (1971) found temporal stability in smiling and certain observed correlates of smiling, including relatively long periods of sustained attentiveness in play and considerable inhibition in conflict situations. His findings suggest that significant differences in affective behavior relate to temperamental predispositions.

The formal study of temperament originated with investigations to determine if characteristic tendencies in infants predict later developments in personality. Over the years, various studies revealed not only that certain traits found in neonates exhibit stability over time (Birns, 1965; Birns et al. 1969; Shirley, 1933; Thomas et al., 1963), but that they may also relate to personality characteristics exhibited in childhood and even later in life (Chess & Thomas, 1984; Shirley, 1933). Other investigators accepted this proposition, but cautioned that although early tendencies may predict personality development, the relationship between early and later tendencies may not always be readily apparent (Bell et al., 1971; Kagan, 1971; Lewis & Starr, 1979).

Most researchers concurred that temperament was a precursor to personality. However, possibly because they began their studies from different operational perspectives, investigators disagreed about what factors comprise or contribute to temperament. Since neonates seemed to possess identifiable temperamental characteristics, some investigators examined birth history, biomedical status, or genetic factors (e.g., Cohen, Dibble, & Grawe, 1977; Goldsmith & Gottesman, 1981; Matheny, 1980; Scarr, 1969; Torgensen & Kringen, 1978; Willerman, 1973). Indeed, temperamental characteristics that appeared to be genetic in origin proved to demonstrate significant stability across ages and methods (Buss & Plomin, 1975; Vandenberg, 1966).

The earliest definitions of temperament were an outgrowth of research into the nature of personality. Temperament was conceived of primarily by exclusion. It was not cognition, nor emotion, but instead that innate part of the infant's nature that was demonstrated by characteristic affective response. This response, the existence of which was generally recognized, was thought to govern the way an infant modulated his or her social relations. Allport (1937) formulated the definition of temperament that anticipated the modern operational definitions:

Temperament refers to the characteristic phenomena of an individual's emotional nature, including his susceptibility to emotional stimulation, his customary strength and speed of response, the quality of his prevailing mood . . .; these phenomena being regarded as dependent upon constitutional make-up, and therefore largely hereditary in origin. (Allport, 1937, p. 54)

Like Allport, Buss and Plomin (1975) emphasized the hereditary determinants of temperament. Whereas Allport merely referred to the general component "emotional nature," Buss and Plomin filled in the contours of emotional nature by arguing that emotional nature specifically consisted of emotionality, activity, sociability, and impulsivity. In a manner similar to Allport and Buss and Plomin, Goldsmith and Campos (1982) were concerned with the emotional aspects of temperament, equating temperament with the behavioral expressions of emotionality and arousal. During this century, empirical evidence gradually accumulated for the existence of this temperamental factor, even in the absence of a clearly defined construct (Allport, 1937; Cattell, 1965; Fries, 1937, 1941a, 1941b; Gesell & Ames, 1937; Pavlov, 1935). Because various researchers failed to agree on a precise definition of temperament, a broad array of characteristics was examined, all of them loosely defined as "temperamental." This chapter examines four prominent operational definitions of temperament, those of Thomas and Chess, Buss and Plomin, Goldsmith and Campos, and Rothbart and Derryberry.

Buss and Plomin

These behavioral geneticists' operational definition of temperament has been widely applied, and is a prime example of an operational definition based on Allport's formulation. Buss and Plomin defined Allport's "emotional nature" as consisting of the specific dimensions of emotionality, activity, sociability, and impulsivity. Furthermore, they stipulated that dimensions of temperament must be inheritable, stable, predictive of adult personality, and adaptive in the evolutionary sense. Their model attempts to assess the degree to which temperament is attributable to genetic differences and/or to differences in experience (Buss & Plomin, 1975; Buss, Plomin, & Willerman, 1973; Plomin, 1981, 1983; Plomin & Rowe, 1979; Rowe & Plomin, 1977). Plomin (1983) warns:

In order to assess the main effects of temperament and environment, as well as their possible interactions, a conservative attempt should be made to measure temperamental behaviors as independently as possible from the environment and to measure the environment as independently as possible from temperament. (p. 54)

Summing up, he notes that these combined measures "become the operational definition of temperament" (p. 72). (See Table 2.1.)

Buss and Plomin found the strongest evidence for genetic effects on the dimension of sociability and relatively strong evidence for genetic effects on emotionality and activity. In order to consider the etiology of individual differences, Plomin and Rowe (1979) compared behavioral observations of both fraternal and identical twins (25 and 21 pairs, respec-

TABLE 2.1. Dimensions of affect and arousal related to temperament.

Affect/arousal	Dimensions of temperament (Buss & Plomin, 1975)
Mood	
Personal	
Fear, anger, & distress	Emotionality
Latency of expression of either affect or activity	Impulsivity
Interpersonal	
Interest/positive affect toward others	Sociability
Arousal energy level	
Psychomotor	
Psychomotor arousal activity	Activity
Attentional	
Latency of expression of either affect or activity	Impulsivity

Note. Adapted from Campos et al. (1983, p. 835).

tively). The average age of the twins was 22.2 months. Among various behavioral measures, the authors were able to identify certain social behaviors for which the identical twins showed greater correlations than the fraternal twins. Of these, the most notable was the social responding behavior toward strangers. This study demonstrated one manner in which heredity affects individual differences.

In another study, Buss, Block, and Block (1980) conducted a longitudinal study of 129 children from age three years to age seven, to determine the correlates for activity level. In this study, it was found that children with high levels of activity were independently described by their teachers as being less inhibited, less physically cautious, less compliant, and more aggressive. The authors concluded that activity level had well–definable correlates.

This model outlines temperament dimensions that are highly replicable and capable of being used jointly with other methodologies of temperament dimensions (e.g., NYLS dimensions) in multi–method research strategies (Plomin, 1983; Rowe & Plomin, 1977). Moreover, the model's measures outline a coherent operational definition of temperament.

Rothbart and Derryberry

Rothbart and Derryberry defined temperament as follows:

. . . [We] will define temperament as constitutional differences in reactivity and self–regulation, with 'constitutional' seen as the relatively enduring biological makeup of the organism influenced over time by heredity, maturation, and experience. By 'reactivity' we refer to the characteristics of the individual's reaction to changes in the environment, as reflected in somatic, endocrine, and autonomic nervous systems. By 'self–regulation' we mean the processes functioning to modulate this reactivity, e.g. attentional and behavioral patterns of approach and avoidance. (Rothbart & Derryberry, 1981, p. 37)

The theoretical model of Rothbart and Derryberry (1981, 1982) offers an approach for studying the developmental influences that temperament exerts. Their model proposes that the organization of temperament involves a complex integration of two mutually interacting systems. The first system consists of response components. The patterns of response overlap structurally and temporally. This system reflects the "reactive" nature of the infant. By 1984, Derryberry and Rothbart had expanded their view of temperament to include the central nervous system among the physiological systems involved in reactivity. Rothbart and Derryberry approached reactivity in terms of its central, autonomic, and somatic manifestations, measuring each of these three categories of manifestations separately, according to conceptually distinct scales. Across all response systems, they employ a number of parameters in measuring temperamental traits. They refer to response threshold, latency, intensity, rise time, and recovery time parameters.

The second system devised by these investigators concerns the infant's experience and "self–regulatory" abilities. This system reflects the "active" nature of the infant. Regulation occurs by structuring the infant's reactivity; "that is, they [the self–regulatory processes] influence the intensive and temporal aspects of response" (Rothbart & Derryberry, 1981, p.54). Dynamically, it is the affective tone that accompanies the infant's experience of his or her own reactivity that sets in motion the self–regulatory mechanisms.

For Rothbart and Derryberry, temperament develops over time and is influenced by maturational processes in the context of experience. It operates within a larger social system that involves the caregiver. Both reactivity and self–regulation have identifiable developmental changes. These changes provide the context for Rothbart and Derryberry's progressive and hierarchic elaboration of more sophisticated and more refined "levels of control." Behaviors through which self–regulation takes place include: approach, avoidance, self–soothing, and attentional behaviors. As a result of these behavioral potentials, the impact of stimulation can be maintained, dampened, and/or enhanced.

In order to understand regulatory systems, Rothbart and Derryberry investigated the relationship between arousal, emotion, and self–regulation. To do so, they dissected the general concepts of emotionality and self–regulation and devised scales assessing them partly in terms of arousal.

The general construct of emotionality was first decomposed into negative and positive emotionality, and negative emotionality was in turn broken down into scales assessing discomfort, fear, frustration, and sadness. Positive emotionality was decomposed into pleasure from intense stimuli, pleasure from low intensity stimuli, and relief. Self–regulation was decomposed into sensory– and response– modulating components, which were in turn broken down into scales assessing attentional focusing, attentional shifting, behavioral inhibition, and behavioral activation. (Derryberry & Rothbart, 1984, p. 156)

Rothbart and Derryberry theorized that regulatory systems of temperament, which in 1984 they redefined as emotional and affective–motivational processes, coordinate attention and response, and ultimately govern virtually all facets of experience and behavior. From this perspective, temperament can exercise an anticipatory or remedial function, enabling the infant to modulate and restructure reactivity. It thus "brings to light the individual's developing capacity for control over self and environment" (Rothbart & Derryberry, 1981, p. 38). (See Table 2.2.)

Goldsmith and Campos

Goldsmith and Campos (1982) attempted to provide an integrative operational definition culled from the definitions and data provided by other researchers. They defined temperament behaviorally as a set of characteristic individual differences in the intensive and temporal parameters of behavioral expressions of affective states. In order to determine the line between temperament and other explanatory constructs, Goldsmith and Campos outlined both inclusive and exclusive criteria for a behavioral definition of temperament. Inclusion criteria were:

1. Temperament is an individual differences construct.
2. Temperament is a dispositional construct. Temperament dimensions are stable, although the degree and nature of stability may vary.
3. In infancy, the dimensions of temperament are affect related (i.e., they are emotional in nature).
4. Variation in temperament refers to individual differences in the intensive and temporal parameters of expression of temperament dimensions. (Goldsmith & Campos, 1982, p. 177)

TABLE 2.2. Dimensions of affect and arousal related to temperament.

Affect/arousal	Dimensions of temperament (Rothbart, 1981)
Mood	
Personal	
Happiness and/or pleasure	Smiling & laughter
Fear	Fear
Persistence of negative affect, given appropriate stimulation by caregiver	Soothability
Interpersonal	
Recovery time of negative affect, given appropriate stimulation by caregiver	Soothability
Arousal/energy level	
Psychomotor	
Psychomotor arousal/activity	Activity level
Attentional	
"Duration of interest"	Undisturbed persistence

Note. Adapted from Campos et al. (1983, p. 835).

Exclusion criteria were:

1. Temperament dimensions are not cognitive or perceptual in nature. Cognition and perception interact with temperament to produce behavior.
2. Temperament dispositions are not affective states. However, individual differences in the parameters of expression of an affective state can be a function of temperament. (Goldsmith & Campos, 1982, p. 177)

Although they defined temperament in terms of behavioral expressions of emotionality and arousal, Goldsmith and Campos were careful to draw a distinction between emotion and temperament.

Temperament refers to stable individual differences in parameters of hedonic tone, arousal, and discrete emotions like anger or fear, whereas emotion concerns the normative affective and expressive processes themselves. (Campos, Barrett, Lamb, Goldsmith, & Stenberg, 1983, p. 830)

Goldsmith and Campos suggest that the influence of temperament can be seen intrapersonally and interpersonally. In the former domain, temperament affects the quality of an infant's approach to the world. For example, an infant's temperamental tendency to cry in response to new stimuli will, to an extent, prevent the child from experiencing the mastery of problem-solving and concomitant self–esteem. Goldsmith and Campos explain that "intrapersonally, the temperament concept helps to account for individual differences in degree of engagement by problem–solving tasks, in attention to significant environmental stimuli, and in the probability that certain affective responses (e.g., distress, smiling) will be elicited and others not" (Campos et al., 1983, p. 830). Temperament's pervasive interpersonal impact is evident in an infant's perception and functioning in the world. By affecting the infant's response to stimuli, temperament influences the way others respond to the infant, and by coloring social interactions, temperament creates a set of expectations in significant others that tends to reinforce the expected behavior in the infant.

Goldsmith and Campos specified that although an infant's overall temperament is stable, behaviors expressing individual traits need not be stable from the neonatal period onward. Organizationally stable functions however, serve as the mechanism by which infant temperament influences the development of later appearing personality traits (Goldsmith & Campos, 1982). (See Table 2.3.)

Thomas and Chess

Thomas and Chess (Chess & Thomas, 1984; Thomas & Chess, 1977, 1980; Thomas, Chess, & Birch, 1968, 1970; Thomas et al., 1963) derived their operational definition of temperament during the initial 22 months of the New York Longitudinal Study (NYLS), an ongoing investigation that began in 1956, with the goal of understanding the dimensions of temperament

TABLE 2.3. Dimensions of affect and arousal related to temperament.

Affect/arousal	Dimensions of temperament (Thomas & Chess, 1977)
Mood	
Personal	
Balance of positive/negative affect	Mood
Balance of positive/negative affect (with associated motor activity) given a novel stimulus	Approach/withdrawal
Degree of modulation of initial reaction to novel stimuli	Adaptability
Measure of affect	Threshold
Measure of affect	Intensity
Interpersonal	
Degree of modulation of initial reaction to novel stimuli	Adaptability
Arousal/energy level	
Psychomotor	
Psychomotor arousal activity	Activity level
(Possible relationship)	Rhythmicity
Attentional	
Latency of response to new stimulus	Distractibility
(Possible relationship)	Threshold
Duration of interest	Attention span/persistence
(Possible relationship)	Intensity

Note. Adapted from Campos et al. (1983, p. 835).

in children and delineating the course of behavioral development. Their 1968 definition of temperament is as follows:

. . . temperament is the behavioral style of the individual child—the how rather than the what (abilities and content) or why (motivations) of behavior. Temperament is a phenomenologic term used to describe the characteristic tempo, rhythmicity, adaptability, energy expenditure, mood, and focus of attention of a child. . . . (Thomas et al., 1968, p. 4)

They described nine dimensions of temperament that had been derived from their operational definition: activity level, rhythmicity (regularity), approach or withdrawal, adaptability, threshold of responsiveness, intensity of reaction, quality of mood, distractibility, and attention span or persistence.

The instruments used in their assessments covered a wide range of information–gathering methods. The operational and theoretical definitions of temperament by Thomas et al. (1963) were inextricably intertwined. From the results of several longitudinal studies assessing the consistency of temperamental characteristics in individual NYLS children, Thomas

and Chess discerned five general patterns revealing the interplay of continuity and change. These were: 1) clear–cut consistency, 2) consistency
in some aspects of temperament at one period and in other aspects at
other times, 3) distortion of the expression of temperament by other factors
such as psychodynamic patterns, 4) consistency in temperament but qualitative change in temperament–environment interaction, and 5) change in
a conspicuous temperamental trait. Statistically, they found that any individual child might show one or a combination of several of these patterns
(Thomas & Chess, 1977). Independent tests have shown that some traits
remain more stable than others. The dimensions of approach/withdrawal,
adaptability, and quality of mood have proven most consistent. Persistence
and intensity, on the other hand, have shown poor reliability. However,
the NYLS investigators, like Goldsmith and Campos (1982), theorized
that traits need not necessarily exhibit considerable stability over time.
According to the NYLS investigators, the interplay of continuity and
change does not prevent certain stable traits or patterns from forming.
But since both continuity and change are forever present, certain temperamental traits will remain stable in age periods during which others
change. All traits, however, will periodically and inevitably transform to
some extent (Chess & Thomas, 1984; Thomas & Chess, 1977, 1980). If
these hypotheses are correct, then the problems of retest reliability that
others have found in the NYLS dimensions would not necessarily reflect
an inadequacy of methodology, but rather, confirm the developmental
nature of temperament.

Although individual dimensions of temperament have shown varying
degrees of continuity, raw data from the NYLS indicate that certain clusters demonstrate stability over time (Thomas et al., 1970). This is similar
to observations made by Carey, Fox, & McDevitt (1977) and Carey and
McDevitt (1978), who found constellations of traits to be temporally stable.
The research of Thomas, Chess, and Birch also indicates that clusters of
traits can also predict behaviors later in childhood and in adult life (Chess
& Thomas, 1984; Chess, Thomas, & Hassibi, 1983; Thomas & Chess,
1977). However, they cautioned that predicting behavior and adjustment
with certainty for individual children is highly unlikely because it is difficult
to determine which of a particular individual's traits will remain stable
(Chess & Thomas, 1984).

Like the authors of the other major operational definitions of temperament, the NYLS investigators postulated that individual and environment
interact in ways that help shape temperament. Again referring to their
interactionist views, they theorized in terms of the interaction between
two opposing forces: the evolving individual and the relatively inflexible
environment. The NYLS investigators pointed out that studies of temperament typically categorize the temperamental characteristics of any
one child based upon a constellation of behaviors that the child exhibits.
They posited that since the exhibited behaviors result from influences

presented by a range of opposing forces, an individual child's temperament cannot be expected to exhibit linear continuity. They theorized that the intra–individual temporal consistencies found in their own research and that of others merely reflected the consistency of one particular behavioral pattern, and therefore the occasional but transient consistency of the interactional forces determining that pattern.

The NYLS studied 133 children over the course of two decades. Because six of them developed depressive symptomatology, Thomas, Chess, and Birch's operational definition, methodologies, and theoretical approach are of special interest to those examining whether infant and adult depressive manifestations are homologous.

Summary

Although there is less than complete agreement among the various researchers regarding the component characteristics of temperament, there is some agreement on what temperament is not. It seems clear that temperament is not entirely inborn nor merely a function of past experience. Rather, it results from some combination of each. Considering these points of agreement, a supposition that parental behavior acts in combination with children's temperament to produce affective and adjustment problems seems justified. Such a hypothesis has been tested in the New York Longitudinal Study.

The four approaches to temperament described above share a number of beliefs. All agree that an individual's temperament profoundly affects development and that temperament is among the foundations for later personality. Common to all of the operational and theoretical approaches to temperament reviewed here is the conclusion that an infant's interaction with caregivers determines in part which temperamental characteristics develop. Goldsmith and Campos (1982), Derryberry and Rothbart (1984), Thomas and Chess (1977), and Buss and Plomin (1975) took that conclusion one step further, specifically suggesting that temperament, in turn, significantly affects the quality of a child's social interactions. Their proposed feedback mechanism of temperament influencing social situations, which then affect the child's self–concept and approach to the world, suggests that temperament may also be instrumental in determining not only the child's affective and cognitive development, but also the development of the self. In fact, many researchers have compiled data indicating that temperament does indeed influence a child's cognitive development. Specifically, dimensions of temperament such as persistence, attention span, goal orientation, and distractibility appear to have a direct relationship to mental scale scores (e.g.,Goldsmith & Gottesman, 1981; Keogh, 1982; Matheny, Wilson, & Nuss, 1984; Seegmiller & King, 1974).

Goldsmith and Campos (1982) theorized that temperament serves organizational functions. Therefore, infants who are temperamentally prone to crying perceive the world as more threatening than less fussy infants.

Irritable infants are probably less likely to eagerly explore the environment. As a result, their intellects may develop at a slower pace.

Derryberry and Rothbart's approach to temperament (1984) might account for the correlation of specific dimensions of temperament and cognition by tying them to the self–regulating functions of attentional processes. According to their theory, infants who are prone to crying might simply tend to focus their attention on negative aspects of their situations. Were they temperamentally able to divert their attention to more positive stimuli, the relationship between themselves and their world might be significantly different. Focusing on the environment and orienting themselves to fascinating aspects of it, they might receive a rush of stimuli that is novel, pleasurable, and cognitively enhancing.

All four of the major approaches to temperament concur that not all behavioral differences are temperamentally related. Rather, only those differences that exhibit some degree of stability over time suggest the influence of temperament. None of the four approaches considers temperament immutable. Some of the investigators have further qualified their belief in temperamental stability. Goldsmith and Campos (1982) stated that temperamental characteristics in infants need not be continuously evident from the neonatal period onward. Moreover, similar temperamental characteristics may be elicited by different stimuli and may be exhibited by a variety of seemingly unrelated behaviors. Chess and Thomas (1984) suggested that rather than remaining static, all temperamental traits transform to some extent. What temporal consistency has been found in individual temperamental differences exhibited by infants and children suggests that an infant's temperament profoundly affects the quality of the individual's entire set of responses to the world (Buss & Plomin, 1975; Goldsmith & Campos, 1982; Rothbart & Derryberry, 1982; Thomas et al., 1963).

In addition to describing temperamental traits as stable and as having social consequences that further influence development, most temperament theorists distinguish between emotion and temperament. For example, Campos et al. (1983) explained that two infants who both smile at a certain stimulus might smile in different ways. One might smile sooner and with more intensity. Smiling in this example indicates the infants' emotional response to the stimulus. The characteristics of the smiles, however, indicate differences in temperament between the two infants.

Relationship Between Depressive Disorders and Temperament

The New York Longitudinal Study

The results of the New York Longitudinal Study (NYLS), reported in 1984 by Chess and Thomas, indicate a direct relationship between certain temperamental and environmental risk factors and the development of adjustment and behavior disorders in young children, including depression and depressive–like phenomena. Because these investigators followed their subjects from the third month of life through their early adulthood, this particular longitudinal study represents to date the best opportunity to investigate the way in which specific temperamental dimensions and/or clusters can contribute to the genesis of affective and behavioral manifestations.

Of the 113 subjects in the the NYLS, six individuals developed depressive symptoms in late childhood or early adolescence. Because the investigators had studied these individuals from age three months to 22 years, they had an excellent opportunity to explore the origins of the depressive symptoms of their subjects, and to perform quantitative analyses of their early temperamental profiles. The investigators hoped that by identifying the antecedents to adult behavior disorders, they could also outline effective therapeutic approaches.

Thomas and Chess (1984), the two principal investigators, postulated that the environment, which is relatively stable, nurtures and shapes the individual, who is relatively labile, and who in turn acts within and influences the environment. This interactionist view of the relationship between individual and environment seemed to the NYLS investigators to work well with Henderson's (1982) theory of goodness and poorness of fit. "Goodness of fit" suggests that the organism's capacities, motivation, and style of behaving and the expectations of the environment are in harmony. In situations where goodness of fit is present, the potential for optimal development is enhanced and the individual is said to be in consonance with his or her environment.

The NYLS investigators believed that consonance between the individual's style, abilities, motivations, etc., and the environment's expectations and demands results in goodness of fit. They were careful to note, however, that goodness of fit does not demand absolute consonance. They speculated that optimal goodness of fit boded well for an individual's ability to develop in his chosen direction. Conversely, they proposed that dissonance between an individual's expectations and abilities and the environment's expectations and demands results in poorness of fit, which they said can lead to distorted development and maladaptive functioning (Thomas & Chess, 1980). A therapeutic strategy based on this model manipulates either the individual or the environment in order to achieve a better fit between the two.

Sources of Data

The NYLS began in March of 1956 with 138 infants from 84 middle– and upper–middle–class families. The families were predominantly Jewish (78%), but some were Protestant (15%) or Catholic (7%). There was one black and one Chinese family. Forty percent of the mothers and 60 percent of the fathers had postgraduate degrees, and only nine percent of the mothers and three percent of the fathers had no college attendance. One hundred and thirty–three of the initial 138 children remained part of the sample group into early adult life. Of these 133 children, 66 were boys and 67 were girls. The children's mean IQ score at six years of age was 127 (Thomas & Chess, 1984).

A comparison group of contrasting socioeconomic background was also studied. This group consisted of 98 children of working–class Puerto Rican parents and was followed longitudinally from early infancy to age six years. In addition, two longitudinal samples of deviant populations were studied. One consisted of 52 children with mildly retarded intellectual levels. The other sample contained 243 children with congenital rubella resulting from the rubella epidemic of 1964. This group, of special interest because many of the children had physical, neurological, and intellectual handicaps, was studied from two to four years of age, again at age eight, and finally at age 13.

Instruments—Core Sample

The NYLS undertook one of the most ambitious data collection efforts of any longitudinal study to date. Researchers employed a number of different techniques and tapped a variety of sources to obtain information about each child's development. They conducted parent interviews every three months for the first 18 months of each child's life, at six–month intervals until the child reached five years, and then yearly until the child was seven or eight years old. When each child was three years old, NYLS staff members interviewed both parents separately to learn more about their attitudes and parenting practices. School observations and teacher interviews supplied additional data. Since approximately 90% of the core sample group began nursery school between the ages of three and four, the investigators could begin collecting school data at a young age. The NYLS staff made ½–hour observations annually of each child enrolled in nursery school, kindergarten, and first grade. If possible, they observed the child during a free–play period. In addition, another of the study's staff members interviewed the child's teacher. Each child's intellectual development was measured at several points during childhood. At ages three and six, the researchers administered the Stanford–Binet Form L to each child. At age nine, 50 subjects were tested again for intelligence quotient using the Wechsler Intelligence Scale for Children (WISC). The investigators assessed each child's behavior before, during, and after the tests.

Because one of the goals of the NYLS was to determine how temperament influences development, especially the development of affective and adjustment disorders, upon reaching adolescence each individual in the sample was evaluated psychologically. Most of the subjects were assessed in semi–structured clinical interviews between the ages of 16 and 17. During the sessions, the subjects were asked questions concerning self–image, relationship with their parents, siblings, and peers, their school functioning, special interests, substance abuse, and interests and plans for the future. All 113 subjects and their parents were interviewed at some point during the subjects' early adulthood. A primary goal of each of the questions was to identify temperamental characteristics that might relate to those measured earlier in the lives of the subjects.

Dimensions of Temperament

Selected data on the reactivity of 22, two to three month old subjects provided the basis from which the NYLS investigators fashioned a methodology that has since been broadly applied. Through inductive analysis of their early assessments, they categorized the temperament of each infant in terms of nine dimensions. These dimensions proved applicable to the NYLS subjects throughout their childhood years.

Thomas and Chess described the nine dimensions as follows:

1. *Activity Level:* the motor component present in a given child's functioning and the diurnal proportion of active and inactive periods. Protocol data on motility during bathing, eating, playing, dressing and handling, as well as information concerning the sleep–wake cycle, reaching, crawling and walking, are used in scoring this category.
2. *Rhythmicity (Regularity):* the predictability and/or unpredictability in time of any function. It can be analyzed in relation to the sleep–wake cycle, hunger, feeding pattern and elimination schedule.
3. *Approach or Withdrawal:* the nature of the initial response to a new stimulus, be it a new food, new toy or new person. Approach responses are positive, whether displayed by mood expression (smiling, verbalizations, etc.) or motor activity (swallowing a new food, reaching for a new toy, active play, etc.). Withdrawal reactions are negative, whether displayed by mood expression (crying, fussing, grimacing, verbalizations, etc.) or motor activity (moving away, spitting new food out, pushing new toy away, etc.).
4. *Adaptability:* responses to new or altered situations. One is not concerned with the nature of the initial responses, but with the ease with which they are modified in desired directions.
5. *Threshold of Responsiveness:* the intensity level of stimulation that is necessary to evoke a discernible response, irrespective of the specific form that the response may take, or the sensory modality affected.
6. *Intensity of Reaction:* the energy level of response, irrespective of its quality or direction.
7. *Quality of Mood:* the amount of pleasant, joyful and friendly behavior, as contrasted with unpleasant, crying and unfriendly behavior.
8. *Distractibility:* the effectiveness of extraneous environmental stimuli in interfering with or in altering the direction of the ongoing behavior.
9. *Attention Span and Persistence:* two related categories. Attention span concerns the length of time a particular activity is pursued by the child.

Persistence refers to the continuation of an activity in the face of obstacles to the maintenance of the activity direction. (Thomas & Chess, 1977, pp. 20–22)

Once they had described the nine dimensions of temperament, the investigators scored infants in each dimension according to conceptually distinct, three–point scales. Item scores in each category were transformed into weighted scores. In this way, temperamental traits were identified. Specific constellations of traits determined the infants' temperamental profiles. The NYLS investigators reported that in both the core group and the comparison groups, a temperamental profile was clearly discernible even in two and three month old infants. Individual traits reflecting specific temperament dimensions exhibited respectable intra–individual stability in the lives of NYLS subjects during the first two years.

Specific Dimensions and Development of Disorder

Thomas, Chess, and Birch pointed out that in and of themselves, temperamental traits are neither good nor bad. However, they believed that certain temperamental traits that are likely to displease significant others in the environment can help create "poorness of fit," which may contribute to the development of secondary depression and other related disorders. Specifically, they noted that traits reflecting aspects of the dimensions of activity level, distractibility, and persistence might be likely to correlate with poorness of fit (Thomas et al., 1968).

For instance, the NYLS investigators observed that children who are temperamentally active often present caregivers with management problems, especially in urban environments. They speculated that parents and teachers who force active children to behave in ways antithetical to their temperamental proclivities can help create poorness of fit for the child (Chess & Thomas, 1984). The investigators also observed that the character and extent of the poorness of fit that a highly active child can experience may depend in part on other temperamental attributes. Highly active children who are also intense are usually far more prone to mishaps. Therefore, they may be doubly likely to experience poorness of fit. Highly active children who are mild in their responses present fewer management problems than do other highly active children. As a result, their behaviors may not contribute to a poor fit (Thomas et al., 1968).

The investigators noted that temperamentally distractible children, like active children, often find themselves at odds with others. These children's attention is easily drawn away from their activities, and thus they are likely to have problems completing tasks (Thomas et al., 1968). Indeed, the NYLS data showed that distractibility was the single temperamental trait most annoying to parents. The investigators, however, viewed distractibility more positively than did most parents. They observed that, in some cases, distractibility "facilitate[s] a child's social functioning by making him quickly responsive to verbal and nonverbal communication from other individuals'' (Thomas et al., 1968, p. 115).

The third temperamental dimension that the NYLS investigators believed might correlate with poorness of fit was persistence. As with activity level, either high or low persistence could be poorly received. The quality of fit experienced by children at either end of the persistence scale might depend largely on the specific activities in which they were persistent. If the objects of a child's persistence were also seen as valuable by the parent, goodness of fit might ensue. Persistent but intense children, however, who become absorbed in a task for hours, may protest loudly at each failure or frustration the task presents and create stress for their caregivers. NYLS researchers felt that parents presenting persistent children with clear guidelines helped prevent maladaptive interactions that could create poorness of fit between themselves and their children. Maladaptive interactions often occurred when parents demanded that their highly persistent children stop activities in which they were deeply engrossed (Thomas et al., 1968).

Specific temperament dimensions were significant in four of the six cases of depressive disorders found in the NYLS sample. However, depression was not consistently linked to any single dimension. In the four cases of depressive neurosis, one was marked by extreme persistence in childhood, another by distractibility, and two were typed as having "difficult" temperament. One of the two cases with a history of major depression showed consistently low quality of mood in childhood, but the other did not.

Typologies

Even though separate traits showed respectable intra–individual stability, the interactionist perspective of Thomas, Chess, & Birch suggested that all temperamental traits would transform repeatedly over the course of a lifetime. Since they felt that clusters of traits could define an individual's temperament more reliably than could individual traits, they investigated whether these relatively stable trait clusters would significantly influence development. Analysis of the behavioral profiles of the two and three month old children revealed that certain temperamental traits often appeared in clusters in individuals. These commonly clustered traits reflected aspects of adaptability, approach/withdrawal, mood, and intensity. Furthermore, trait clusters showed much higher stability than individual temperament traits. Based on these findings, they defined three common temperamental typologies: the easy, the difficult, and the slow–to–warm–up child (Thomas et al., 1970).

Easy children, who represented 40% of the sample, exhibited "positiveness in mood, regularity in bodily functions, a low or moderate intensity of reaction, adaptability and a positive approach to, rather than withdrawal from, new situations" (Thomas et al., 1970, p. 105). Such children were usually easily managed so that they contributed to their caregiver's well-being. Difficult children, on the other hand, are "irregular in bodily functions, are usually intense in their reactions, tend to withdraw in the face of new stimuli, are slow to adapt to changes in the environment and are generally negative in mood" (Thomas et al., 1970, p. 105). Such difficult children displayed irregular sleeping and feeding patterns, responded negatively to novel foods, routines, places, or activities, and were prone to crying and tantrums. The NYLS investigators found that about 14 (10%) of the 141 children met the criteria for difficult temperament (Thomas et al., 1970). The investigators expected that many difficult children would experience poorness of fit with their environments.

The third temperamental type within which the NYLS investigators grouped their subjects was the "slow–to–warm–up" child. These children have a low activity level, react mildly, adapt slowly, often display negative mood, and tend to withdraw from new stimuli. Although both difficult and slow–to–warm–up children generally withdraw from new stimuli, they differ in that the low intensity of the latter's reactions makes them more likely to withdraw quietly rather than loudly. In addition to having less intense reactions, slow–to–warm–up children do not suffer frequent negative moods and the irregularity of bodily functions typical of difficult children (Thomas et al., 1970). The NYLS researchers found 21 slow–to–warm–up children (approximately 15%) in the sample.

Predictive Analyses of NYLS Data

Clusters of Temperament Traits and Childhood Behavior Disorders. Differences in early temperamental profiles appeared to relate significantly to the likelihood of developing behavioral problems that required clinical treatment in childhood. Only four of the individuals classified as temperamentally easy at age three months developed childhood behavior problems requiring such treatment (Chess & Thomas, 1984). By contrast, 10 (71%) of the children typed as temperamentally difficult at age three months developed significant behavior problems in childhood. All 10 children developed their disorders by age seven years. In each case, qualitative analysis of the child's records indicated that the disorder correlated with the child's difficult temperament. However, in many cases, parental inconsistency, impatience, or punitiveness appeared to compound the child's vulnerability to behavior disorders. Of the 12 subjects who developed behavior disorders in adolescence, only two were classified as having difficult temperament. Notably, both were cases of secondary depression. The NYLS data indicated that slow–to–warm–up children are also at greater than average risk for developing behavior problems. Approximately 50% of the sample's slow–to–warm–up children presented clinical disorders during childhood (Chess & Thomas, 1984).

The fact that some easy, some difficult, and some slow–to–warm–up children developed behavior disorders, and that some, but not all, of the behavior disorders seemed to result from poorness of fit suggested to the researchers that no temperamental pattern or specific temperamental trait unfailingly predicts that a child will develop a behavior disorder. Nor does any pattern or trait guarantee that a child will not. The investigators surmised that "similar causes could lead to different symptoms, and the same symptom could derive from different causes" (Chess & Thomas, 1984, p. 228).

Clusters of Temperament Traits, Environmental Factors and Childhood Behavior Disorders. Most of the predominant operational definitions of temperament specify that child and environment affect each other profoundly. Multiple regression and set–correlation analyses conducted by the NYLS investigators revealed that, independent of temperament type, children whose parents were in conflict also were vulnerable to adult adjustment disorders. The NYLS investigators used the results of these analyses to examine how temperamental and environmental risk factors assessed at age three years might predict behavior disorders and adult adjustment problems.

For this longitudinal study, the investigators classified their subjects into the following four groups, with the first group facing the greatest risk for disorder, the second group the least risk, and the third and fourth groups facing intermediate/high risk:

1. The extreme quartiles for both difficult temperament and severity of parental conflict ($n = 5$)
2. The extreme quartiles for both easy temperament and low parental conflict ($n = 8$)
3. The extreme quartiles for easy temperament and for severe parental conflict ($n = 6$)
4. The extreme quartiles for difficult temperament and for low parental conflict ($n = 3$) (Chess & Thomas, 1984, p. 111).

The investigators scored their subjects for adult adjustment on a ten–point scale, with a score of 10 indicating the best adjustment. They found their expectations about adult adjustment problems substantially correct. While subjects in the total NYLS sample scored a mean of 6.01 on the adult adjustment scale, high–risk subjects scored substantially lower, with a mean of 4.92. Low–risk subjects, with an average of 6.78, scored higher than the overall sample mean. The mean adult adjustment scores for both intermediate risk groups were 6.43, higher than the total group mean, but below the low–risk group mean. These results provide important empirical support for the hypothesis that a child's temperament, coupled with environmental stress, does effect the risk for development of adult adjustment disorders (Chess & Thomas, 1984).

With regard to depressive disorders, the evidence is equally strong in suggesting that parental conflict is a contributing factor. In the two cases of recurrent major depression in the NYLS sample, each had a history of parental depression. Among the four cases of secondary depression, one subject's parents were divorced when he was 12, another suffered the death of his father at age 11. The other two cases each had some history of conflict either between the parents or between the parents and child.

In addition to examining the relationship between risk factors at three years and the development of behavior disorders and adult adjustment problems, the investigators examined the relationship between risk factors at three years and the children's adjustment scores at three years. The results indicated that the combination of difficult temperament and parental conflict had a relatively immediate impact on adjustment and behavior.

Furthermore, NYLS data suggested that in addition to determining vulnerability to behavior disorder, the variables of temperament and environment significantly influence the age of the disorder's onset. Whereas the average rate of onset of a behavior disorder in the sample as a whole was seven years, the average age of onset for high–risk and intermediate–risk subjects was four years. Severity of the disorder also reveals the combined influence of difficult temperament and parental discord. However, almost one half (26 of 57) of the behavior disorders in the total sample were diagnosed as mild. Only one of the four high–risk cases with onset prior to adulthood was diagnosed as mild; the other three were diagnosed as moderately severe. In the low–risk group, of the three subjects developing disorder before adulthood, two were mild cases. One was moderately severe (Chess & Thomas, 1984).

Childhood Antecedents of Early Adult Adjustment

A quantitative study identifying subjects with either very high or very low early adult adjustment scores investigated the patterns and significance of their childhood functioning. The NYLS investigators selected the 13 subjects with the highest early adult adjustment scores (above 8.0) and a matching number of subjects with the lowest scores. They then tabulated the subjects' IQ scores at three, six, and nine years; adjustment scores at three and five years; age of onset of any behavior disorder; and outcome of any disorder appearing in childhood. A review of these data revealed significant differences between the low– and high–score groups.

Only one of the subjects with high early adult adjustment scores had developed a behavior disorder at some earlier time. The disorder was described as a mild, brief, adjustment disorder, which had become apparent at age five and from which the child had recovered by age seven. However, all but one of the low score group had developed a behavior disorder at an earlier time. All disorders had persisted into early adult life, and in eight of these cases the disorder had become apparent in childhood. In five cases, the disorder had appeared before age five.

The investigators also examined the highest and lowest scoring adult adjustment groups to determine what temperamental and parental types of conflict characterized the groups. They found that the high–scoring group was fairly heavily populated by individuals who at age three had been typed as having easy temperaments, and that the low–scoring group had many individuals who had been typed difficult and who came from families with severe parental conflict. No individuals from families with severe parental conflict appeared in the low–scoring group. The investigators noted that the numbers in all groups were too small to be statistically significant, but they did observe that their findings suggested that "young adults with the highest level of functioning were more likely to have had easy rather than difficult temperaments at 3 years, and that the young adults with the lowest level of functioning were more likely to have parents in severe conflict with each other at age 3" (Chess & Thomas, 1984, p. 137).

In drawing conclusions about the significance of childhood and adolescent functioning to adult adjustment, the investigators considered the following data most notable. First, with one minor exception, no individual in the high–scoring group had at any time exhibited a behavior disorder. Second, none of the individuals in the NYLS group who had recovered from earlier behavior disorders appeared in the high–scoring group. Third, high scorers were predominantly of easy temperament and characteristically persistent. Fourth, with only one exception they were of superior intelligence. Fifth, although some of the parents of high scorers had been in conflict when the child was three years old, all parents had been consistent in emphasizing specific standards and goals and in supporting the child's attempts to reach those goals. From their quantitative data, the NYLS investigators concluded that individuals scoring in the high adult adjustment groups had benefited from the consistent, positive reinforcement that they had received from their environment.

Case Studies of NYLS Subjects' Depression: A Temperament Perspective

Six of the NYLS subjects developed depressive symptoms of varying degrees. None of the six NYLS individuals developing depression or depressive disorders exhibited florid psychotic symptoms at any time. Two met *DSM–III* criteria for major depression, three met criteria for dysthymic disorder (depressive neurosis), and one met the criteria for adjustment disorder with depressed mood. The NYLS investigators' 22–year data on each individual offer insight into possible temperamental markers and/or contributors to depression.

The NYLS investigators viewed primary depression in their characteristic interactionist fashion. They theorized that biochemical factors alter an individual's mood, making the individual incompetent to deal with environmental stresses. This produces a poorness of fit between individual and environment that in turn intensifies the depressive affect of the biochemical disturbance (Thomas & Chess, 1980). The investigators' strategy for intervention in primary depression sought to minimize the poorness of fit by pharmacologically ameliorating the biochemical disturbance while manipulating certain aspects of the depressed individual's environment in order to reduce various kinds of environmental stress. For secondary depression, their interventionist strategy emphasized identifying which of the individual's temperamental, motivational, and behavioral patterns were contributing to poorness of fit with the environment, and then adjusting those patterns through psychotherapy (Chess & Thomas, 1984).

Case Report. Richard, the second of the NYLS cases of depression, had been assessed during infancy and childhood as temperamentally persistent. He presented symptoms of behavior disorder when he was five years old, at which time he was diagnosed as suffering from a severe adjustment disorder, characterized by temper tantrums.

Richard's behavior improved when he was transferred to another school at which his persistence was encouraged, but in fourth grade he again began to exhibit explosive responses to frustration. By age 10 he had developed a helpless, fatalistic attitude toward his own behavior, accepting the judgment of his teachers and peers that he was a "bad" boy. He also began to show depressive symptoms at this time. Richard's father died when he was 11. Because his family history showed no significant incidence of mental illness, Richard was diagnosed as suffering from a depressive neurosis. Thomas and Chess (1984) surmised that the boy's adjustment disorder had evolved into a dysthymic disorder. In spite of psychotherapy, his dysthymic disorder did not significantly improve, although his condition seemed occasionally and temporarily to take a turn for the better. At age 22, Richard reported success in his work, but dissatisfaction with himself in both professional and social competence. The diagnosis of depressive neurosis was reaffirmed. Richard's temperamental persistence was considered to be a contributing factor to poorness of fit in childhood.

Case Report. Norman, another of Thomas and Chess's (1984) six depressive cases, may have evolved depressive disorder from an earlier adjustment disorder. For Norman, the adjustment disorder became evident at 30 months, and the depressive symptoms at 17 years.

As an infant and child, Norman consistently tested as temperamentally distractible with a short attention span. The investigators reported that Norman's parents typically responded to these characteristics with intolerance. Symptomatology of an adjustment disorder exhibited at 30 months included sleeping difficulties, nocturnal enuresis, poor eating habits, and nail tearing.

In the adolescent interview, Norman seemed dejected and depressed. He had a remarkably low self–image and the investigators diagnosed his condition as depressive neurotic. Evidence precluding a diagnosis of primary depression included the lack of a family proclivity towards depression and the presence of significant intra–family stress. Norman's psychological difficulties continued through the end of his participation in the NYLS. At age 20, he experienced a hypomanic episode. During the early adult interview, the investigators added a diagnosis of severe narcissistic personality disorder to their assessment of his depressive neurosis.

Discussion. The NYLS investigators drew correlations between similar diagnoses and reported that these correlations applied to the cases whether depressive symptoms first appeared in childhood, adolescence, or early adulthood. They noted that both of the subjects for whom recurrent major depression had been diagnosed had strong family histories of depressive illness. Neither subject appeared to succumb to depression as a result of stressful life events or pathogenic interaction with parents. In contrast, the three subjects diagnosed as suffering dysthymic disorder or depressive neurosis presented the opposite picture—negative family histories for depressive illness, and stress–induced episodes of depression and behavior disorder.

The investigators observed that two NYLS subjects met *DSM–III* criteria for major depression, whereas the three subjects with dysthymic disorder and the one subject with adjustment disorder with depressed mood met the criteria for secondary depression. Because subjects at a range of ages were successfully diagnosed using *DSM–III* criteria, and because the NYLS investigators' diagnoses were largely confirmed by independent diagnosticians (Chess et al., 1983), the NYLS investigators concluded that apparently no significant clinical difference exists between depression in childhood and in later life.

They found that only one (Brad, whose case is presented at the beginning of this chapter) of the two subjects with primary depression had been temperamentally predisposed toward negative mood in the first five years of life. On the other hand, two of the five subjects with secondary depression had shown a mild tendency toward negative mood, although two had shown a preponderance of positive mood. Examining other temperamental dimensions for traits exhibited during the first five years of life by the depressed individuals, the investigators found no data indicating that any one temperamental trait played a statistically significant role in the genesis or evolution of primary or secondary depression.

However, when they examined how their four subjects who were diagnosed as suffering depressive neurosis had scored along each of the nine temperamental dimensions as children, they found that each subject showed one extreme or another for a particular temperamental trait or cluster of traits. One subject showed marked persistence; another had shown distractibility and short attention span; and the other two had each been typed as difficult children. Furthermore, the individuals' early temperamental profiles, the data on the ways in which the individuals had, as children, interacted with parents and others, and the subjects' own account of their childhoods all led the investigators to conclude that for each subject manifesting depressive neurosis, temperament had contributed to the development of the disorder.

The investigators concluded that temperament, parent–child interaction, and environmental stress do not appear to contribute to the genesis of primary depression. They further concluded that whereas biological disturbances seem to be at the root of primary depression, temperament plays a significant etiological role in the development of secondary depression, although no single temperamental trait or cluster of traits reliably predicts secondary depression. (See Table 2.4.)

Other Temperament Models and Descriptions of Depression

Buss and Plomin

With regard to infant and childhood depression, Buss and Plomin's (1975) behavioral genetics model provides further foundations on which to build an important body of knowledge concerning the levels of trait transmission and expression. Models of behavioral genetics are supported by the conclusions of Mahmood, Reveley, and Murray, (1983), whose review of the literature on the genetics of affective disorders revealed an increased risk for depression among the relatives of depressed individuals.

Mendlewicz and Rainer's (1977) adoption studies have ascertained a genetic component in the transmission of affective disorders. These authors found that the frequency of affective disorders was higher (31%) in the biological parents of bipolar adoptees than in the biological parents of normal adoptees (2%). Thus, although affective and temperamental deviations manifest differently, the same methodology and approach may be applied to analyze both of these phenomena. That is, the variability of both temperament and affective disorders may be conceived of as occurring on a unitary continuum that is susceptible to the influences of both genetic and environmental factors.

Rothbart and Derryberry

Rothbart and Derryberry's (1981, 1982) temperament model has profound implications for the study of the development of depression and depressive–like phenomena. They saw self–regulation as consisting in part of attentional processes, and observed that some individuals among their sample groups habitually enhanced and attenuated the sensory and semantic information they received, shifting their attention at will away from negative aspects of their situations. These individuals appeared to be less vulnerable than others to negative emotional states, and indeed seemed capable of finding enjoyment even in negative situations. This observation

TABLE 2.4. *DSM-III* criteria for dysthymic disorder and major depression compared to dimensions of temperament.

DSM-III[a]	Thomas et al. (1963)	Buss & Plomin (1975)	Rothbart (1981)
Dysthymic disorder			
Dysphoric mood	Adaptability Approach/withdrawal Mood	Emotionality Impulsivity	Smiling & laughter Fear Distress to limitations Soothability
Sleep disturbances Loss of energy or fatigue	Rhythmicity Activity level Intensity Attention span/ persistence	Activity	Activity level Duration of orienting
Feelings of worthlessness Decreased productivity	Activity level Attention span/ persistence	Activity	Activity level Duration of orienting

Decreased attention
  concentration
	Activity level
	Attention span/
	  persistence
		Activity	Activity level
			Duration of orienting

Social withdrawal	Approach/withdrawal Mood	Sociability	Smiling & laughter Fear

Loss of interest/pleasure
  in usual activities
	Approach/withdrawal
	Mood
	Attention span/
	  persistence
		Emotionality
		Sociability
			Duration of orienting
			Smiling & laughter

Irritable excessive anger (esp. toward caregivers)	Intensity Adaptability Mood	Emotionality Sociability	Smiling & laughter Distress to limitations Soothability

Inability to respond with
  pleasure (to reward/praise)
Psychomotor agitation/
  retardation
	Intensity
	Mood
	Activity level
	Approach/withdrawal
		Emotionality
		Sociability
		Activity
			Smiling & laughter
			Soothability
			Activity level

Pessimistic/brooding	Intensity Attention span/ persistence Mood	Emotionality Emotionality Sociability	Fear Smiling & laughter Distress to limitations
Tearful/excessive crying	Intensity Mood		
Suicidal ideation or behavior			
Major depression Dysphoric mood	Adaptability Approach/withdrawal Mood	Emotionality Impulsivity	Smiling & laughter Fear Distress to limitations Soothability
Eating disturbances	Rhythmicity		
Sleep disturbances	Rhythmicity		
Psychomotor agitation/ retardation	Activity level Approach/withdrawal Intensity Attention span/ persistence	Activity	Activity level
Loss of interest/pleasure in usual activities	Approach/withdrawal Mood Attention span/ persistence	Emotionality Sociability	Duration of orienting Smiling & laughter
Loss of energy or fatigue	Activity level Intensity Attention span/ persistence	Activity	Activity level Duration of orienting
Feelings of worthlessness			
Cognitive disturbances			
Suicidal ideation or behavior			

[a]American Psychiatric Association (1980, pp. 213–214, 222–223).

suggests that individuals who habitually exhibit depressive symptoms may be temperamentally prevented from discovering that "every cloud has a silver lining." Rothbart and Derryberry's system schema is closely related to some recent approaches to depressive phenomena, such as the model of Siever and Davis (1985) that is organized around the concept of "dysregulation." This model posits that "persistent impairment in one or more neurotransmitter homeostatic regulatory mechanisms confers a trait vulnerability to unstable or erratic neurotransmitter output" (p. 1017).

In summary, Rothbart and Derryberry's model helps to explain the role played by affect in self–regulating mechanisms. Delineation of self–regulatory mechanisms and affective components of the infant's experience provide us with a conceptual framework for understanding depressive affect as either a catalytic element that triggers changes in the reactive responses or as a by–product of dysregulation.

Goldsmith and Campos

One of the central tenets of the temperament theory of Goldsmith and Campos is that temperament is affect related (Goldsmith & Campos, 1982). This also implies a close relationship between temperament and affect disorders, such as depression. Goldsmith and Campos also agree with other temperament theorists that temperament plays a role in social interaction. Between these two concepts, there is a clear role for temperament in the genesis of depression as either a difficulty in reactivity or a response to a social maladaptation. Their research has concerned itself with determining how the temperament dimensions outlined by other researchers may be used to describe affective states. In their view, for example, the NYLS addressed affects explicitly in only one dimension, mood. Goldsmith and Campos (1982) took a different position, viewing temperament in terms of affect and arousal, and recast the temperament dimensions of the NYLS in affective terms.

They also noted in the Buss and Plomin (1975) approach a clear but less specific relationship to emotion systems. Rather than correlating to a single affect, Buss and Plomin's dimension of "emotionality" consists of several affects: "fear," "anger," and "distress." "Impulsivity" is neither affect nor arousal related, but rather reflects the parameter, "latency" in response. In Rothbart and Derryberry's (1981) dimensions, they find a relatively strong relationship to specific affects. They note that Rothbart and Derryberry "postulate a connection between temperament and affect in that the emotion systems constitute one of the response systems for reactivity" (p. 170). Facial expressions and other emotional reactions represent examples of responses through which reactivity and self–regulation are expressed. For example, "smiling and laughter" relates directly to the affect of "happiness or pleasure." "Distress to limitations" correlates with "anger." Tables 2.1–2.3 exemplify their approach to mapping the various studies' temperament dimensions onto dimensions of affect and arousal.

Methodological Issues in the Study of Temperament

Regardless of the disparities between various constructs of the dimensions of temperament, most investigators agree that the term *temperament* refers to a general disposition and not to any specific occurrence of an overt expression. Another point of agreement among most investigators is that temperament and the nature of personality change with maturation (Bell et al., 1971; Birns et al., 1969; Buss & Plomin, 1975; Escalona, 1963; Fries, 1944; Goldsmith & Campos, 1982; Kagan, 1971; Korner et al., 1981; Lewis & Starr, 1979; Rothbart & Derryberry, 1982; Shirley, 1933; Sroufe & Waters, 1977; Thomas et al., 1963). Taking these observations into consideration, an accurate determination of temperament requires that the instruments used anticipate that the traits or dimensions measured may differ at subsequent developmental stages. Assessing specific temperament dimensions across too broad an age range with a single instrument may overlook the expression of temperament and introduce error into the data gathered.

Most investigators have acknowledged that differences between individuals are not always related to temperamental characteristics. Rather, other developmental considerations, such as intelligence, may account for the perceived differences. Waters (1978) admonished investigators to develop instruments recognizing the relevance of situational context.

Given the potential for misconstruing of data, an instrument–oriented review integrating the empirical findings of temperament studies seems crucial. Hubert and colleagues (Hubert, Wachs, Peters–Martin, & Gandour, 1982) offered the first such comprehensive review. They noted that what evidence on instrument reliability exists has largely been gleaned by measuring the same temperamental dimension with different instruments at different times, and then checking for uniformity in the measurements. Most instruments have shown only moderate and somewhat inconsistent levels of test/retest reliability. When reliability tests have used interrater comparisons, the results have been more encouraging.

These reliability tests have produced, in some cases, a disappointingly low level of correlation. Furthermore, they reported that instrument validity measurements are scant. Measurements performed reveal inconsistencies both in concurrent and convergent validity. However, considering the opportunities for misinterpretation of data with which the available instruments are fraught, the degree to which the data have proved consistent is both surprising and reassuring. Throughout the studies of temperament, the dimensions of approach/withdrawal and activity level have shown laudable reliability.

Conclusion

This chapter reviews the major studies in the area of infant temperament research. Initially, various definitions of temperament offered by key researchers are discussed. While these definitions are somewhat varied in approach, the basic components of the construct of temperament upon which the researchers agree are emphasized.

Armed with this definition, we explored how several research studies, most notably the NYLS, have further developed temperament dimensions and subsequently, temperament clusters. Furthermore, the method whereby these temperament clusters have been tracked longitudinally in several studies to determine the predictive validity of temperament as a measure for depression is discussed.

As such, it should be clear that temperament represents a vital tool for the researcher and the theoretician. Indeed, in subsequent chapters of this book, the construct of temperament is used as a tool for understanding depressive–like phenomena in infants and children. In addition, the manner in which temperament interacts with the infant's incipient attachment behavior and evolving sense of self is explored.

Temperament is also used as a cornerstone for interpreting theories of depression that are discussed later in the book. For example, such questions as how the infant's temperament facilitates or hinders his or her ability to perceive and respond to contingencies are explored. In addition, the question of discrepancy awareness—essentially, the inchoate ability to distinguish between differing stimuli in the environment and to express preferences and dislikes—is analyzed in terms of the temperamental qualities the infant brings to the environment. Finally, in discussing learned helplessness depression, the temperament construct contributes to an understanding of how an infant may be susceptible to developing this form of depression.

One issue common to virtually all investigations of temperament is its role in the development of personality. The acknowledgment that temperament plays some role in this development is based on the assumption that temperament regulates virtually all intereaction with the environment. Rather than being immutable, both temperament and environment are assumed to change constantly in response to the demands of each other. However, the suspicion that an individual's endogenous characteristics can be affected somewhat by extrinsic factors does not preclude the probability that those characteristics carry their own inertia. Various studies have indicated a significant degree of stability for individual traits. Although no conclusive, indisputable evidence has been presented revealing the mechanism by which temperament affects personality development, enough evidence has accumulated correlating early temperament with later personality to suggest that infant temperament might well be counted among the characteristics holding clues to the etiology of depression and other affective disorders.

A dearth of theoretical approaches, operational definitions, and trustworthy instruments through which theories and definitions may be formulated still hampers the study of temperament. Further temperament—related research, therefore, should aim to develop highly reliable instruments. These instruments may help illuminate valid and reliable correlations between temperament and affective disorders. By assimilating the conclusions of such studies, clinicians familiar with aspects of the temperaments and home situations of individual infants might be alerted to watch for signs of a developing disorder.

CHAPTER 3

Correlates of Attachment to Depressive Phenomena

What is believed to be essential for mental health is that the infant and young child should experience a warm, intimate and continuous relationship with his mother (or permanent mother–substitute) in which both find satisfaction and enjoyment.

John Bowlby (1969, pp. xi–xii)

Depressive disorders are defined exclusively in terms of affect by many researchers. Others consider affect (in particular, negative affect) to be only one of several constituents of depression. But whether or not depression is defined by the role that affect plays, there seems to be nearly universal consensus that affect and depression are strongly related.

Considering the close relationship between affect and depression, it may be hypothesized that clues to the genesis and nature of infant and preschool depression can be found by investigating the hierarchical organization with which the affectional bonds develop from infancy onward. An added benefit of this type of research is the disclosure of individual differences among these bonds and their organization into specific patterns. Recognition of such patterns is a preliminary step for early diagnosis. This chapter reviews such studies in order to derive an understanding of how maladaptive interactions between infants and their primary caregivers might disrupt affectional bonds and how such disruptions may lie at the root of depression.

Bowlby (1958, 1961, 1969) articulated one of the first affect–attachment models. According to Bowlby, by the age of one year almost all children have formed a unique bond with a parent or parent–substitute and the breaking of this bond is painful. Bowlby noted that when children are separated from their mothers during hospitalization, their reactions tend to follow a three–stage pattern similar to the mourning process in adults. He referred to these stages as anger, despair, and detachment. In the first stage, the child protests the separation with tears and actively seeks for the parent. During the despair stage, the child stops searching for the parent. In the final phase, called detachment, the infant reenters a normal round of activities, but if reunited with the caregiver at or after this stage, he or she will be unresponsive. Thus, the attachment has been broken.

Significantly, the experience of loss was found to be unrelated to needs for food, warmth, or even contact, all of which were routinely available to the child from the nursing staff. Taking exception to the prevailing attachment theories, Bowlby postulated that attachment was a primary drive attributable to the process of natural selection, and not a form of learned behavior and/or an expansion of the feeding process. He defined attachment as a set of instinctual responses—such as smiling, crying, and following—which bind mother and child, and he suggested that the original biological purpose served was one of protection from predators. The maintenance of proximity between mother and child is the behavioral means of accomplishing this goal.

Ainsworth and Wittig (1969), through their Strange Situation Procedure, provided a means of exploring individual differences in attachment. They examined the behavioral range of one year olds by inducing stress in a paradigm encompassing episodes of momentary separation from and reunion with the mother. The Strange Situation offers investigators assessing individual differences in the quality of infant–mother attachment a verifiable, reliable and valid instrument (Ainsworth, Bell, & Stayton, 1971; Blanchard & Main, 1979; Connell, 1976; Main & Weston, 1981; Rosenberg, 1975; Waters, 1978). Especially when used in conjunction with other laboratory instruments and with home observations, the Strange Situation highlights the underlying affective component beneath attachment behaviors and defensive strategies (avoidance of the caregiver).

Waters (1978), Matas, Arend, and Sroufe (1978), and others examined predictive validity of individual differences in attachment at one year for normal and abnormal child development. Positive affect was shown to correlate with secure attachment from infancy through three and one half years (Waters, Wippman, & Sroufe, 1979). Findings such as these suggest that specific patterns of attachment in infancy could mediate the development of affective disorders.

An infant's earliest attachment relationships may provide a model for later relationships, as some researchers have theorized. Sroufe (1983) postulates that there is developmental coherence across transformations in behavior. Main, Kaplan, and, Cassidy (1985) describe the "inner working model" of attachment as "a set of conscious and/or unconscious rules for the organization of information relevant to attachment" (pp. 66–67). For example, an infant who expects rejection from a primary caregiver usually exhibits avoidant behavior toward that particular caregiver (Gaensbauer, Harmon, & Mrazek, 1980; George & Main, 1979; Lewis & Schaeffer, 1979; Main & Stadtman, 1981; Main, Tomasini, & Tolan, 1979; Main & Weston, 1981).

Assuming that depression and depressive–like phenomena are affect related, Sroufe's contention that attachment behaviors will transform in coherent ways leads to the question of whether maladaptive behaviors will also transform in similar ways. If so, affect–related problems of attachment that can be demonstrated by the Strange Situation may be precursors of depressive–like phenomena at a later age.

Correlations between attachment behavior and affective development can be addressed by discussing the nature and function of both attachment and avoidant behavior, and the interactivity of attachment behavior systems with other behavior systems. This chapter reviews studies that have distinguished individual differences among human infants in their attachment behaviors. It explores how caregivers' behaviors shape the quality of infants' affectional ties. Finally, the chapter probes possible developmental consequences of insecure infant–caregiver attachments and their relationship to the process of detachment.

Case Report

Johnny was a healthy, full–term baby admitted to an institution at three weeks of age. A nurse on Johnny's unit, Elizabeth, was immediately attracted to the infant. Although Elizabeth was responsible for all the babies on the unit, she placed Johnny's crib in a position where she could give him extra attention. She enjoyed playing with Johnny and frequently spoke or sang to him. Despite this increased attention, however, Elizabeth's time was limited. Johnny was often fed in his bed with the bottle propped; his contact with Elizabeth spanned only brief periods of each day.

Upon evaluation at three months of age, Johnny appeared healthy and alert. He smiled readily. His visual perception was advanced and, significantly, he was able to distinguish between Elizabeth and the examiner. Sophisticated gazing behavior was observed and he was able to differentiate a human face from a mask face. Johnny's language acquisition at this age was better developed than that of other institution children. He cooed, chuckled, squealed, and exhibited a distinct vocal–social response. These behaviors were most prevalent when Johnny had contact with another person. However, despite his mature level of social interaction, in some respects Johnny also showed behaviors typical of institution children. Most notably, he became stiff and unrelaxed when held by anyone other than Elizabeth.

When Johnny was five months old, Elizabeth began to withdraw the level of special attention that had characterized their relationship. She explained that Johnny would soon be leaving her nursery and that parting with him was extremely painful. Thus, she slowly began to disengage herself from Johnny's care and eventually, curtailed special contact with the infant.

Johnny was next seen for evaluation at six months of age. Although he still responded to the examiners in a friendly manner, marked disturbances in his developmental course had begun to surface. He had become silent and a notable change in his relationship with people was observed. Johnny no longer showed displeasure at the loss of social contact. He was also less discriminating than before in reactions to both people and his physical environment. For example, he no longer distinguished between Elizabeth and the examiner. He was still visually preoccupied by people, however, and responded to tactile stimulation by smiling. Nevertheless, there had been an overall decline in development. Sitting behavior was poor, with much slumping and some head lag. In addition, Johnny rocked a great deal when alone.

At age six and one half months, Johnny was moved to a second nursery where none of the caregivers developed a special relationship with him. At nine months, he was transferred yet again. One of the nurses on this ward, Thelma, took a special interest in him. Johnny was evaluated shortly thereafter, when he was 41 weeks old. He was basically amiable and friendly, but there was less smiling than before. Essentially he had become a silent baby whose use of vocalization was minimal. He cried rarely and, when heard, the cry was woeful with little recognizable affect. Although he seemed to enjoy social contact, he showed no displeasure at loss of contact, and emotional interaction was described as shallow, bland, and non-specific.

At approximately nine and one half months, Johnny began to cry at night when Thelma was away. At such times, he could not be comforted. When seen again several weeks later, however, the examiners were impressed with both an increase in the degree of playful social interchange and with Johnny's strong displeasure at the loss of social contact; a re sponse not observed since Johnny was five months old. This improved developmental trend coincided with an increased intensity in the relationship between Thelma and Johnny.

When Johnny was 14 1/2 months of age, Thelma became ill and was away for two weeks. During this time, Johnny lost his appetite and vomited on several occasions. Upon evaluation, he was found to be lethargic, apathetic, and depressed. He had lost some weight and displayed a somber expression. He did not respond to the attentions of the examiners (Provence, 1983).

Johnny's case is notable in that the ebb and flow of his developmental progress corresponds to the presence of a significant "other" in his environment.

Description of Attachment Behavior

Environment and Adaptation

The recognition that behavioral equipment, like anatomical and physiological equipment, can contribute to survival and propagation only when it develops and operates within an environment that falls within prescribed limits is crucial to an understanding of both instinctive behavior and psychopathology. (Bowlby, 1982, p.46–47)

In his discussion of the characteristics of instinctive behavior, Bowlby (1982) suggests that the dichotomy between "innate versus acquired" characteristics can more profitably be seen as a continuum with environmentally stable characteristics at one end and environmentally labile at the other. Morphological characteristics such as eye color and shape of limbs, as well as behaviors traditionally described as "instinctive" fall at the stable end; body weight, immunity reactions and learned skills lie at the labile end. The behavioral systems that appear to be environmentally stable may still be influenced by changes in the environment. Adaptation, in the biological sense, is always for the purpose of greater survival. The attachment system is only one of many adaptive systems created by the evolutionary process.

. . . the genetic biases in a species . . . provide for a balance between [behaviors] which lead the infant away from the mother and promote exploration and acquisition of knowledge . . . and those which draw mother and infant together and promote the protection and nurturance that the mother can provide. (Ainsworth & Bell, 1979, p. 51)

Function of Attachment Behavior

Bowlby views attachment as a flexible, adaptive, functionally related, organizational system—a network of responses that an infant employs to ensure survival of the species. Bowlby suggests that the main function of attachment behavior (e.g., maintaining proximity between mother and infant), in biological terms, is protection from predators. A fortuitous side effect of such proximity is the increased ability to learn from the mother. Ainsworth held that, since a secure attachment serves as the child's base for exploration, caregiver moderation in regard to the affectional tie in effect nurtures both the affectional tie and the infant's cognitive and social development (Ainsworth, 1973; Ainsworth et al., 1971).

Bowlby (1969) contends that attachment behavior is instinctive and independent of secondary drives such as feeding. He cites the attraction of human infants to purely social stimuli, without any component of feeding. Also, attachment behaviors are frequently directed at young children or others whom the infant would have no reason to associate with caregiving. Woolf's (1969) studies on the development of smiling clearly indicate an inborn bias toward the human figure.

Organization of Attachment Behavior

Bowlby (1958) postulates a number of instinctual responses that, during the first year of life, become integrated into attachment behavior. These include, but are not limited to, sucking, clinging, following, crying, and smiling. He states that attachment behavior tends to become organized into more sophisticated, often goal–corrected systems, of which there are two main classes: signaling behavior, which brings mother to child, and approach behavior, which brings child to mother. Attachment behavior, like much of early human behavior, may be organized from instinctive behaviors into genetically programmed goal–corrected systems (Bowlby, 1958, 1961, 1969). These behaviors need not be defined in terms of motivation, but instead are set in motion by environmental effectors that trigger the genetic program. Specific behaviors may be modified by experience or change in environmental factors.

Bowlby (1982) introduced the concepts of *set–goals* and *feedback* to govern both starting and stopping of actions. He suggests that certain behaviors, such as those involved in attachment, can be conceived of as part of a continuously monitored system. The purpose of the behavior is to bring the system into an equilibrium, that is, to achieve a set–goal. In attachment, mother and child continually re–evaluate the goal in light of internal changes and changes in the environment. Bowlby conceives of this evaluation process as a feedback system that measures the degree to which the entire mechanism conforms to the set–goal.

Bowlby prefers the term *goal–corrected* to *goal–directed*. *Goal–directed* behavior implies behavior that is simply designed to ensure proximity between mother and child. If this were the only mechanism governing attachment behavior, there would be no reason for the child to ever leave the mother's side. *Goal–corrected* behavior suggests a more complex system governed by variable set–goals. In the normal pattern of day–to–day activity, mother and child would maintain a degree of proximity consistent with their mutual perceptions of the environment. If the environment presents no immediate danger, mother and child tolerate degrees of exploratory distance. If, however, either mother or child become alarmed for any reason, forms of signaling or approach behavior are initiated. This implies that attachment behavior organizes itself into a dynamic relationship that involves both mother and infant.

Definition and Measurement of Attachment Behavior

Definitions

Researchers interested in attachment have had difficulty arriving at a precise definition of the concept. They view it alternately as either a set of behaviors or as a relationship. Bowlby's earliest descriptions of attachment focused on a set of instinctive behaviors that had the biological function of maintaining proximity between mother and child for the child's protection. Thus in his book *Attachment* (1969), he commonly refers to "attachment behavior." However, he points out that one cannot study the infant and mother separately since there is what he describes as a "dynamic equilibrium" between the mother and infant (Bowlby, 1969, p. 236).

In contrast, Ainsworth speaks of attachment as a relationship. She defines attachment as an "affectional tie that one person forms to another specific person" (Ainsworth, 1973, p.1). Nevertheless, her Strange Situation Procedure is only designed to measure child behaviors. Ainsworth defines an attachment figure "as providing a secure base from which a child may venture forth to explore the world" (Ainsworth & Wittig, 1969), thus linking the attachment system to an exploratory behavior system.

Hinde (1982) contends that since even the earliest signs of attachment behavior from the child are mediated by contact with another person, any attempt to measure attachment behavior must take both the infant and mother into account. He objects to quantitative measures focused exclusively on either baby or mother, arguing that:

. . . measures of behavior within an ongoing relationship are likely to reflect the characteristics of both partners: Frequency of crying depends on the mother as well as the baby, and latency to pick up depends on the baby's past behavior as well as on the mother. (1982, p. 65)

Strange Situation Procedure

Ainsworth and Wittig's Strange Situation Paradigm (1969) has given researchers their first major tool for measurement of attachment behavior. The Strange Situation Procedure was described as:

. . . [a] setting to systematically observe the effect of the presence and absence of a mother–figure on the response of infants or young children to strangeness or other fear–arousing stimuli . . . We were interested especially in the extent to which an infant could use his mother as a secure base from which to explore, in his reaction to a stranger, and in his response to brief separation from his mother. (Ainsworth et al., 1971, p.17)

Ainsworth expected that under normal conditions, infants' propensity for exploration would find a mutable balance with their propensity for attachment. In fact, Ainsworth noted that field and laboratory studies of animals conducted by other investigators reveal that the balance between attachment and exploration behaviors in infants follows a developmental trend with exploration becoming more evident with maturation. However, throughout infancy, separation or perceived danger activates attachment behaviors to reunite mother and infant (Ainsworth & Bell, 1979). Therefore, although they are both genetically programmed, exploration (which by definition includes confronting the unknown) and attachment (which by definition precludes exploring the unknown) might reasonably be viewed as conflicting motivations in threatening situations. To discern the characteristics of specific attachment relationships, the Strange Situation progressively taxes the infant's capacity for coordinating and maintaining adaptive responses in a situation inviting exploration while simultaneously presenting mild threats. The Strange Situation's scoring system has proven adequately reliable when used in laboratory observations (Ainsworth,

Blehar, Waters, & Wall, 1978; Connell, 1976; Main & Weston, 1981; Waters, 1978).

Procedure. The procedure consists of a series of eight episodes involving mother, baby, and a stranger (and experimenter in the introductory episode). Subjects in the experiment are introduced into a room containing a 9x9–foot clear space and three chairs arranged in a triangle. One of the chairs, a child's chair, has toys on it. When the procedure begins, the baby is placed between the two adult chairs, facing the toys. The eight episodes are observed through one–way glass from an adjacent room. Episodes proceed as shown in Table 3.1.

Subjects. The original data were drawn from 23 white, middle–class mother–infant pairs. The infants were 51 weeks old. In a second sample (Bell, 1970) of 33 pairs, the infants were 49 weeks old.

Classification of Behavior. Bowlby's (1969) control theory provides the theoretical foundation for the attachment classification system used in the Strange Situation. His theory states that specific instinctive behaviors such as smiling, following, babbling, etc. are organized into more complex systems that are governed by a single set–goal. These systems, in turn, interact with other systems of behavior with possibly contradictory goals, i.e., a system of proximity maintaining behaviors interacting with a system of exploratory behaviors. These complex systems are also mediated by feedback from the environment and other organisms. Still further, all the be-

TABLE 3.1. Strange Situation Procedure.[a]

Episodes	Participants	Duration	Behavior highlighted by episode
1	Mother, baby, experimenter	30 sec (approx.)	(Introductory)
2	Mother, baby	3 min	Exploration of strange environment with mother present
3	Stranger, mother, baby	3 min	Response to stranger with mother present
4	Stranger, baby	3 min	Response to separation with stranger present
5	Mother, baby	Variable	Response to reunion with mother
6	Baby	3 min	Response to separation when left alone
7	Stranger, baby	3 min	Response to continuing separation, and to stranger after being left alone
8	Mother, baby	Variable	Response to second reunion with mother

[a]From Ainsworth, M. D. S., Bell, S. M., & Stayton, D. J. (1971). Individual differences in strange-situation behavior in 1-year-olds. In H. R. Schaffer (Ed.), *The origins of human social relations* (p. 20). London/New York: Academic Press. Reprinted by permission of ©The Developmental Sciences Trusts.

haviors of the child interact with complementary and independent systems
of behavior in the mother. The mother–child relationship is viewed by
Bowlby as a dynamic system with its own set–goals and interactive feedback. Bowlby suggested that attachment figures are capable of both comforting and alarming infants. As seen in the Strange Situation Procedure,
the child may initiate seeking behavior if he or she becomes distressed
by the mother's absence. When the mother returns, the child may be sat-
isfied by the simple sight of the mother or the child may seek physical
contact. If an infant perceives attachment figures as both threatening and
also as the only source of protection, the resulting conflict is virtually
irresolvable. When this occurs, anger and resistant behavior toward the
caregiver gradually ensue.

One major system balanced against the attachment system is the system
of behaviors promoting exploration on the part of the child. Although the
attachment system promotes learning by giving the child an opportunity
to model the mother's behavior, it is equally important that the child explores his or her environment independently, to gain experiential knowledge.

Attachment behavior has the dual purpose of creating and cementing
a secure relationship with the mother figure and of escaping or avoiding
an alarming stimulus (by retreating to the mother, or bringing the mother
into the situation). From observations of the Strange Situation Procedure,
Bretherton and Ainsworth (1974) identified four behaviors at work in the
interactions between the child and the stranger.

1. *Attachment*—Exhibited by retreating to mother and making contact or
   hiding behind mother, etc.
2. *Fear/Wariness*—Includes crying (at stranger), withdrawal, leaning
   away, gaze aversion, retreat to mother, rejection or snubbing of a toy
   offered by the stranger.
3. *Exploratory*—Interest in the stranger (like interest in the toys in the
   Strange Situation Procedure) is indicative of the exploratory system.
   It is assumed that unfamiliar objects and situations offer the greatest
   possibilities for producing fear, therefore the exploratory and fear/alarm
   systems are closely related, and may be activated by the same stimulus.
   It was observed that the stranger was almost always of greater interest
   than the toys.
4. *Affiliative*—Attempts on the part of the infant to engage the stranger
   in an affiliative response were exhibited by smiling (at stranger), vocalizing, approaching, touching, or accepting an offered toy.

A fifth class of behaviors was defined as representing a combination of
wary and affiliative elements, i.e., a "coy response" simultaneously combining gaze aversion and smiling. This coy response may also take the
form of a partial approach (Bretherton & Ainsworth, 1974, p. 153).

Several systems can be simultaneously active, as Sroufe, Waters, and

Matas (1974) found in examining affective response to novel stimuli in infants (i.e., laughter versus crying). They observed that infants have a disposition toward both responses and that both approach and avoidance systems can be active at once, depending on context. The internal state of the baby will affect the threshold of fear response. If the baby is tired or hungry, the threshold of fear response may be lowered, and stimuli that would evoke laughter at other times would cause the infant to cry.

Originally, Ainsworth and Wittig (1969) hypothesized that an infant's behavior during a separation episode might provide the best indication of the quality of attachment. The children in the first Strange Situation study were originally classified with regard to demonstrated separation anxiety. The investigators initially divided the observed infants into three distinct groups. Those in Group A were described as "avoidant." These infants showed minimal disturbance on separation. Infants who showed definite separation anxiety were classified as "securely attached" and assigned to Group B. The third group, Group C, contained infants displaying resistant or ambivalent attachment behavior. They showed separation anxiety combined with some maladaptive behavior. Later it was observed that reunion behavior served as a better gauge of quality of attachment. The three groups were therefore further divided into eight subgroupings designed to reflect separation, reunion, and exploratory behaviors.

The eight subgroups are divided as follows (see Ainsworth et al., 1971, pp.22–25):

Group A: Avoidant. Infants showed little or no tendency to seek proximity or contact with mother and treated the stranger very much the same as the mother. They evinced little distress during separations or distress at being left alone. Subgroups within Group A were distinguished by their reunion behavior.
A1—Avoidant reunion behavior. These babies tended not to approach mother at reunion, to resist being picked up, or wanted to be put down after a short time.
A2—Ambivalent reunion behavior. These babies approached and then turned away from the mother, or first approached and then ignored the mother. When picked up, they may cling momentarily and then show signs of wanting to be put down.
Group B: Securely Attached. Actively seeks proximity and contact with mother. Infants cried or smiled at reunion and clearly preferred mother to stranger. Not all Group B infants showed distress at separation, but those who did were not placated by the presence of the stranger.
B1—Smiled at reunion, seemed interested in establishing interaction, but did not especially seek proximity. Little or no distress during separation.
B2—Approached on reunion, desired contact. Little or no distress during separation.

TABLE 3.2. Atypical attachment classifications compared.

Classification	Attachment behaviors	Affect	Other behaviors	Comments	Sample
Radke-Yarrow et al. (1985), A/C classification	Moderate to high avoidance. Moderate to high resistance. Moderate to high proximity seeking	Affectless Sad, with signs of depression	Odd or atypical body posture or movement		99 children assessed at 24 & 36 months 0% infants had this classification with normal mothers (N = 31) 20% infants with mothers with major depressions (N = 55) 29% infants with mothers with bipolar depression (N = 14)
Main et al. (1985), insecure-disorganized/ disoriented	Disordered temporal sequences of attachment behaviors (e.g., strong avoidance following strong proximity seeking)	"Dazed behavior": odd or atypical body posture or movement suggestive of depression, confusion, or apprehension	Contradictory behaviors, e.g., approach with head/gaze averted Incomplete movements	"Characterized behavior as attempt to control parent, either through directly punitive behavior or through anxious, overly bright	17.9% or 34 of 189-infant sample

		Undirected affective expressions			
Main & Weston (1981), unclassifiable infants	Seeks proximity but affectless	Affectless	Low relatedness and strong conflict in play session	'caregiving'' behavior, (inappropriate role reversal),'' p. 85 Proximity seeking present in high-stress situations and in repeated separations in otherwise avoidant infant. This group may be erroneously classified as securely attached	12.5% of 152-infant sample
Crittenden (1983), A/C classification	Moderate to high avoidance Moderate to high resistance Moderate to high proximity seeking		Disturbed behaviors such as head cocking, huddling, rocking, etc.	Suggested ambivalence/ avoidance was manifestation of anxiety, and these A/C infants were the most anxious	12.3% or 9 of 73-infant sample

Note. See also Londerville and Main (1981; p. 293), who found 4 of 36 (11%) subjects were classifiable as A/C babies.

B3—Strong response to reunion, may cry. The babies in this group may
or may not show distress at separation, but at reunion they definitely
seek physical contact more than those in Subgroups B1 or B2.

B4—Sought proximity throughout all episodes. Babies in this subgroup
showed some insecurity even before separation episodes and showed
little exploratory behavior. They tended to cling to the mother. Clearly
distressed during separation.

Group C: Ambivalently Attached. This group had fewer common characteristics, except for a general quality termed *maladaptive behavior.*
They shared an inability to use the mother as a secure base for exploration. Some Group C babies showed no inclination to explore. Some
explored actively but did not seem to enjoy it.

C1—Ambivalent contact with mother, perhaps marked by clinging,
pushing, hitting, etc. Distressed throughout separations. Exploration
mixed with anger or anxiety.

C2—Very passive, both in lack of exploration and in reunion behavior.
May or may not show distress at separation.

Although the Strange Situation has generally been considered reliable
only through the second year in normal non–handicapped populations,
Main and colleagues (1985) have recently developed a test for attachment
classification in six year olds. They observed that insecure attachment
was characterized by restricted or rule–bound behavior, attention and
emotional expression. These attachments appear to require greater out-
ward organization than secure attachments to balance the disorganization
of the underlying relationship. (See Table 3.2 for atypical attachment classifications, and Table 3.3 for chronology of attachment development.)

Stability and Correlations of Behavioral Patterns

The attempt to predict stable behavior patterns from early measures of
attachment does not imply that specific behaviors occur consistently over
the years. Rather, it is assumed that new behaviors will supersede old
ones as the infant matures, while maintaining degrees of predictive value
throughout different organizations. Attachment patterns have demonstrated considerable temporal stability. Waters (1978), for example, demonstrated stability from 12 to 18 months. More significantly, however,
attachment patterns demonstrated at an early age can reliably predict many
aspects of functioning later in life. These relationships have important
implications for the development or prevention of depression. Matas et
al. (1978) showed autonomous functioning to be better developed in more
securely attached toddlers (24 months). Arend, Gove, & Sroufe (1978)
and Waters et al. (1979) were able to make predictions from attachment
at 15–18 months to functioning in preschool and kindergarten. Sroufe's

TABLE 3.3. Comparative chronology of attachment development.

Age	Schaffer & Emerson	Bowlby	Ainsworth & Wittig
0 Weeks	Asocial stage,	Orientation and	Undiscriminated
8 Weeks	undifferentiated	signals without	attachment
	seeking of arousal	discrimination of	Differential
16 Weeks	Undifferentiated	figure (0 to 8–12	responsiveness at
24 Weeks	attachment behavior	weeks)	close range,
32 Weeks	Attachment begins to	Orientation and	discrimination of
	focus on specific	signals directed	mother
40 Weeks	people	towards	Differential
48 Weeks		discriminated	responsiveness at
1 Year		figures (12 weeks to	a distance, crying
		6 months)	when mother
2 Years		Maintenance of	leaves room
3 Years		proximity to a	Active initiation and
		discriminated figure	maintenance of
		(6 months–1 year to	contact
		3rd year)	
		Formation of a goal-	
		corrected	
		partnership (2–3	
		years to adulthood)	

report on individual differences in pre–school children (1983) found correlations between Strange Situation tests done at 12 months and several aspects of behavior in four and five year olds. Sroufe found that children who were securely attached were predictably better able to manage their impulses and feelings. Securely attached children were also found to have greater self–esteem. This finding is noteworthy since high self–esteem measures are generally absent in depressed children. Significantly, securely attached children were found to be less dependent on teachers than anxiously attached children. Anxiously attached children were rated higher in seeking help in areas relating to "self–management, social–management, and seeking attention in negative ways" (Sroufe, 1983, p.60).

Waters et al. (1979) compared positive affect and attachment in 36 infants at 18 months and 45 infants at 24 months. The infants were observed during free play sessions with their mothers, and observers looked for positive affective sharing as evidenced by smiling, showing toys, or combinations of smiling, showing, and vocalizing. In the observations at 18 months, 95% of the securely attached infants spontaneously smiled at their mothers, versus 42% of the avoidant and 40% of the resistant infants. Forty–seven percent of the securely attached, 25% of the avoidant, and none of the resistant infants showed toys. Of the securely attached infants, 21% showed combinations of smiling, showing, and/or vocalizing. None of the anxiously attached infants did. Observers who rated the infants on a three-point-scale for affective sharing gave 58% of the securely attached and none of the anxiously attached infants the highest score. Forty–two percent of the avoidant infants, 40% of the resistant infants, and only 5% of the securely attached infants were given the lowest score.

Sroufe (1983) also found a strong relationship between secure attachment and positive expressions of affect. Securely attached children were rated higher on ability to enjoy themselves and other children in a positive manner. They were also rated lower on anger, aggression, and negative affect. Secure attachment was also found to be correlated with social competence in ratings both by the teachers and other preschoolers. In sociometric studies, the securely attached children were rated as more popular by their peers as well as by their teachers.

Factors Affecting the Development and Display of Attachment Behaviors

The Infant's Temperament

The development of an attachment between mother and infant, although genetically predisposed, occurs differently in every mother–infant pair. Individual or temperamental differences among infants may be the least important factor affecting quality of attachment, since the infant is assumed to be more malleable than either the more developed mother or the established environment. However, it should not be assumed that the infant has no reciprocal effect on his or her environment, or on his or her parents.

In the infant's first months, the tendency toward monotropy combines with learned responses to favor an attachment with the person with whom the infant has the most contact. Not only the quantity, but also the quality of social interaction affects attachment behavior. The mother may have the most contact with the child by default, and yet harbor ambivalent feelings toward the child. Interactions with the infant may differ depending on who initiates the interactions, the mother or the infant. In discussing correlations between Strange Situation tests and observed behavior at home, Ainsworth (1979) notes that some studies (Connell, 1976; Waters, Vaughn, & Egeland, 1980), suggested that Group C babies may as newborns be constitutionally difficult, which would contribute to differences in maternal care. The more temperamentally demanding infant may also get a greater share of attention, as Bowlby (1969) points out. He suggests that apathetic infants, who initiate fewer interactions and are less responsive to initiatives from others, are less likely to reap the benefits of greater learning and socialization that more demanding infants receive. Infants who smile (or cry) more, for whatever reason, are rewarding the people who deal with them with greater response. This tends to increase the likelihood of further interactions. The bulk of evidence, however, suggests that more differences in the quality of attachment are attributable to the mother than to the child.

Maternal Factors

Ainsworth (1979) found that, at home, mothers of infants rated "securely attached" in the Strange Situation test were more "sensitively responsive" to their children than the mothers of children rated "avoidant" or "ambivalently attached." She found that mothers of avoidant infants showed an aversion to physical contact with their children, and tended to express anger more often.

Bowlby (1982) says that the bias of the mother exerts a strong influence—stronger than any innate biases on the part of the infant. Bowlby concludes,

. . . mothers play a much larger [role] than do infants in determining how much interaction takes place. . . . there are clear indications that the pattern of attachment a child [shows] toward his mother–figure is to a high degree the consequence of the pattern of mothering he is receiving. (1982, pp.345–346)

Ainsworth et al. (1971) felt that four types of maternal qualities—sensitivity, acceptance, cooperation, accessibility—contributed significantly to the differences in attachment development among children. They rated maternal behaviors in the Strange Situation Procedure on four scales:

1. *Sensitivity–Insensitivity*—Measured the degree to which the mother was able "to see things from the infant's point of view." Sensitive mothers were respectful of their children's demands. They responded appropriately to the infant's signals and interpreted them correctly. Insensitive mothers, in contrast, tended to initiate contacts and interactions according to their own desires and frequently misinterpreted the infant's signals.
2. *Acceptance–Rejection*—Rated the degree of mother's positive and negative feelings toward the child. Highly rejecting mothers tended to express hostility and anger toward their children. Not surprisingly, Group A (avoidant) infants had the most rejecting mothers. These infants showed little distress at separation.
3. *Cooperation–Interference*—Highly interfering mothers showed a lack of respect for their infant's autonomy. They imposed their will on the infant, without regard for his affective state. Cooperative mothers, on the other hand, took the infant's own scale of values into account. Group A1 infants had mothers who scored high on interference. Non–rejecting, highly interfering mothers had highly insecure Group C1 infants.
4. *Accessibility–Ignoring*—Measured how much attention the mother focused on the infant. Highly accessible mothers were focused on their children much of the time. Highly ignoring mothers tended to focus attention on other things. Non–rejecting, highly ignoring mothers had passive infants in Group C2. Like Subgroup C1 infants, C2 infants were unable to learn to control their environment. They lacked the opportunity for protest because of the mother's distancing.

Attachment Deprivation

Most researchers agree that for secure attachment to evolve, quality matters more than quantity of contact. Nevertheless, prolonged separation from, or deprivation of, an attachment figure has been found to cause severe problems. The infant who is not provided with a model for relationships is likely to experience difficulty developing them in later life. Ainsworth (1973) says, "[t]he most striking long–term effect of prolonged and severe deprivation in infancy and early childhood was found to be inability to establish and to maintain deep and significant interpersonal relations—that is, an inability to become attached" (p. 53).

Robertson and Bowlby (1952) discuss three identifiable phases in an infant's response to separation: protest, despair, and detachment. While these states may theoretically be described as separate entities, the child merges one state with the next and may spend days or weeks in transition among phases or may alternate between two phases (Bowlby, 1969).

Protest can begin immediately after separation or after some delay. This phase may last for a few hours or extend to a week or more. Often the infant manifests protest by loud crying, shaking in bed, or tossing about. He or she may also exhibit an eager response to any sight or sound indicating the return of an absent parent.

During the succeeding phase, despair, the infant continues to exhibit a preoccupation with the missing parent, but behavior also suggests an increasing hopelessness. Physical movement diminishes or ceases. The infant or child becomes withdrawn and inactive, and ceases to make demands.

When the infant enters the detachment phase, the observer may be misled into believing that he or she is recovering from the loss, since the infant may begin to show more interest in the environment. For a child whose stay in a hospital or residential nursery is prolonged, the entire experience of loss is likely to be repeated several times as he or she becomes transiently attached to a series of nurses or caregivers who eventually leave. This series of disturbances may gradually result in the child's withdrawal of commitment and eventually lead to cessation of attachment behavior. A child who reaches this state may become increasingly self–centered and show enthusiasm only for material goods. Although some researchers have suggested the term *withdrawal* for this phase, Bowlby proposes *detachment*—a natural counterpart of attachment—as a more accurate term, and describes it as "a rejection of mother as love object, which may be temporary or permanent," (p. xiii) following a period of absence.

Yarrow (1964), in his critique of Spitz and Wolf's study (1946) of infants separated from their mothers in an institutional setting at age 6–8 months, reported that 19 of the infants displayed reactions of acute anxiety, active rejection of adults, symptoms of severe depression, decreased activity level, loss of appetite, and withdrawal from people and environment. Some of the infants continued to deteriorate until they died. The investigators also noted a progression in severity of disturbance over time and concluded that infants could not endure separation for more than five months without risking irreparable damage, such as behavior indicative of depression and depressive–like phenomena.

Bowlby (1980), in a discussion of infants in their second year of life who were temporarily separated from their parents, concluded that the ability to remember a "model" of the missing parent during a temporary separation may be observed in many children at age 16 months or older, who are in the care of substitute mother–figures. Observation of this memory ability was linked to the child's response at separation; maladaptive behavior appeared to be associated with the child's awareness of the missing parent.

The Function of Avoidant Behavior

Avoidant Behavior in Adult Animals

Researchers interested in attachment and avoidance in humans have derived some of their theories from observations of comparable behavior in animals. Ethologists have observed that visual avoidance is common among adult animals. Tinbergen and Chance both advanced theories emphasizing that avoidance in animals functions in the service of proximity. They agreed that animals exhibit avoidant behavior when their survival instincts conflict with their tendencies toward flight or aggression. However, the two ethologists held differing opinions of the specific mechanisms by which avoidance achieves proximity and survival of the species. Tinbergen (Tinbergen & Moynihan, 1952) posited that an animal practices avoidant behavior for its presumed effect on the social partner. According to Tinbergen, avoidant behavior serves a signal function. Unlike certain approach signals such as calling and clinging, which make direct appeals to the attachment figure for increased proximity or for contact, avoidant behavior convinces the attachment figure that its "fight or flight" responses are unnecessary. Therefore, the signal function proposed by Tinbergen is one of deception. An animal's avoidant behavior signals nothing directly. Rather, it conceals signals that might defeat the animal's attempt to gain proximity or contact.

Chance (1962) put forth two interpretations of visual avoidance in animals. In one interpretation, he posited that avoidance specifically serves proximity. However, unlike Tinbergen, Chance suggested that the intent of avoidant behavior is its presumed effect on the performer, not on the social partner. He proposed that visual avoidance serves a "cutoff" function, ensuring that stimuli from the environment that might otherwise trigger flight and aggression are obscured and rendered ineffective.

Chance's interpretation suggests a further advantage of avoidant behavior. According to his model, visual cutoff allows an animal to regain control of its own behavior when overpowering stimuli from a social partner threaten to compel the animal toward behavior that is not self–serving. Based on this interpretation, avoidance does not specifically serve proximity. Rather, it allows the animal maximum flexibility in choosing whether or not to remain proximate.

Avoidant Behavior in Human Infants

Many researchers (Ainsworth, 1972; Ainsworth et al., 1971; Gaensbauer et al. 1980; George & Main, 1979; Lewis & Schaeffer, 1979; Main, 1977; Main et al., 1979; Main & Stadtman, 1981; Main & Weston, 1981) have found that infants expecting rejection from a primary caregiver exhibit avoidant behavior toward the caregiver. Investigators have described various types of avoidant behaviors in human infants. Moving, looking away from, and failure to respond to the caregiver have all been interpreted as related to avoidance. Such behavior can be accommodated by Bowlby's and Ainsworth's theories. If approaching a caregiver elicits rejection or provokes caregiver behavior that the infant interprets as threatening, avoiding the caregiver may afford the infant an opportunity to obtain at least an acceptable degree of proximity to the caregiver. Even overt anger toward a caregiver (typed by most of the above–cited investigators as an example of avoidant behavior) may be considered to function in the service of attachment if, as Bowlby suggested, it can prod the caregiver to approach the infant.

If the avoidant behavior exhibited by human infants toward their primary caregivers is considered in light of Tinbergen's and Chance's ethological theories, three mechanisms emerge by which avoidance might serve to ensure proximity. First, avoidance may convince attachment figures that both fight and flight are unnecessary. In this way, avoidance might appease historically rejecting caregivers sufficiently so that they tolerate some proximity with their infants. Second, avoidance may allow infants to remain proximate to caregivers whose behavior infants perceive as threatening. Finally, avoidance may simply "buy time" for infants, letting them quell any frightened responses to troubling caregiver behavior and to choose responses most likely to ensure their own survival.

Many investigators studying avoidant behavior in infants concur with the ethologists (Bowlby, 1969; Chance, 1962; Tinbergen & Moynihan, 1952) that avoidant behavior betrays an underlying conflict between affiliative– and fear–related behavioral systems. These investigators accept Bowlby's perspective, which postulates that in the face of threats from the environment, infants experience a painful conflict that only contact with the attachment figure can resolve. Taking Bowlby's lead, authorities of avoidant behavior in infants presuppose an adaptive function for attachment that allows an infant to acclimate to environmental stress. For example, Sroufe, Waters, and Matas (1974; Waters, Matas & Sroufe, 1975) reported observing a clear temporal relationship between gaze aversion and heart rate acceleration. They proposed that gaze aversion is a mechanism by which very young infants, who are relatively powerless, cope with stress. Gaze aversion serves a cutoff function, modulating infants' arousal level as expressed by heart rate. This position is reminiscent of Chance's theory concerning organization. Brazelton, Koslowski, and Main (1974) expressed a similar interpretation of the function of visual avoidance. They proposed that visual avoidance in infants is one of the few ways infants have of protecting themselves from unpleasant stimuli. Furthermore, in analyzing the behavior of the members of five mother–infant dyads, they observed that mothers who impose constant affection on their infants provoke their infants to visually avoid them. On the other hand, mothers who take cues from their infants for giving and withholding affection seem to create a secure base from which the infants can learn to satisfy their own needs.

Main (1977, 1981) has suggested that in stress situations, historically rejected infants avoid their caregivers as an alternative to expressing angry behavior toward them. She and other researchers found that anger can be safely expressed in situations out of context, when contact with the caregiver is not crucial (Blanchard & Main, 1979; George & Main, 1979; Main, 1977; Main, Tomasini, & Tolan, 1979; Main & Townsend, 1982; Main & Weston, 1981). Thus avoidance may indeed fulfill a cutoff function.

Precursors of Avoidance Behaviors

Main's Investigations: Normal and Abused Children

Close parallels between the reunion behavior exhibited by many of Ainsworth's infants during the Strange Situation (Tracy, Lamb, & Ainsworth, 1976) and avoidant behavior often observed in infants during reunion with a parent after a separation intrigued one researcher sufficiently enough for her to investigate how avoidant and resistant behaviors may stem from the perception of parental rejection arising from separation. Main set out to investigate how parental rejection might affect security attachments, and how security attachments might in turn influence social, affective, and even cognitive development. Much of Main's work correlates observations made in the Strange Situation with observations of children and their attachment figures made in less taxing laboratory situations as well as in their homes. Bowlby's (1969) theory stated that when a mother physically rejects her infant the child's resulting conflict gives rise to aggression, conflict behavior, and avoidance. Based on this theory, Main expected that experiments would prove infant avoidance to be directly related to parental anger and aversion to contact.

Main's (1973) studies first attempted to examine the effect of attachment quality on exploration and cognitive development. A subsequent study (1977) correlated her observations of reunion behavior at a daycare center with security classifications derived in the Strange Situation. A later study on this same theme (Blanchard & Main, 1979) demonstrated that avoidance exhibited in the daycare setting is significantly related to avoidance exhibited in the Strange Situation.

In addition, Main and Weston (1981) conducted an investigation testing for pervasiveness in an infant's avoidant behavior. The infants in this study were tested in the Strange Situation at 12 months of age with one parent, and at 18 months with the other parent. The investigators found that some infants enjoy entirely different attachment relationships with each parent. The actual comparisons for each parent are shown in Table 3.4. From these findings, the investigators inferred that avoidant behavior may not reflect an endogenous trait. Rather, enduring relationships seem to influence an infant's patterns of attachments.

Infants found to be unclassifiable at this time were described as follows:

Behaves to parent in reunion as secure infant but behaves identically to the stranger . . . extreme avoidance is combined with extreme distress throughout the situation . . . behaves in one reunion as a secure infant but in the other reunion as an insecure infant . . . physical behavior is that of a secure infant—approach, clinging—but infant is affectless with signs of depression. (Main & Weston, 1981, pp. 934–935)

Recently, Main, Kaplan, and Cassidy(1985) declared yet a further type of insecure attachment classification, "insecure–disorganized/disoriented" to describe the majority of the infants who were formerly designated "unclassifiable" in the Strange Situation. These children's behavior in the Strange Situation was characterized by " '[d]azed' behavior on reunion with the parent, stoppage of movement in postures suggestive of depres-

TABLE 3.4. Classifications of infants seen at 12 months and at 18 months with different parents.

Seen with mother	Seen with father			
	Avoidant	Secure	Ambivalent	Unclassified
Avoidant	9	9		1
Secure	11	15	2	1
Ambivalent		2	1	2
Unclassified	2	4		2

Note. From Main and Weston (1981, p. 936). Sixty-one infants were seen in this study, 46 first with mother and 15 first with father.

sion, confusion, or apprehension. . . ." (p. 79). The authors state that the majority of these children had parents who had histories of trauma in their own attachment relationships. (See Table 3.2.)

Summary of Main's Conclusions

From her data, Main reported clusters of avoidant behaviors observed in infants and in mothers of avoidant infants.

Clusters of Behavior Observed in Infants Classified as Insecurely Attached. A variety of subtly avoidant behaviors exhibited by infants in relation to the mother were observed. Some infants classified as insecurely attached showed little attachment behavior either at separation or reunion. What attachment behavior they did show was often abortive. Many did not cry upon separation. For those who did cry, often the tears seemed to relate more to distress at being alone than to distress at separation from the mother. The general absence of tears appeared to be part of an overall absence of strong affect. Many infants treated the stranger with the same neutral affect as they treated the mother. Upon reunion with the mother, a variety of avoidant behaviors served to shift the infants' attention away from the mother. Infants averted their gazes, moved away from the mother, or seized nearby inanimate objects upon which they focused their attention. Some responded to reunion with alternating movements of approach and avoidance. Others simply made clear that they wanted to be put down when they were picked up.

Based on statistical analysis of her observations of clusters of avoidant behaviors evident in infants, Main posited seven characteristics associated with avoidance of the mother by the infant:

1. Avoidance of the mother in the Strange Situation is negatively related to angry behavior toward her (angry crying, hitting, batting away toys) observed in the Strange Situation itself.
2. However, avoidance of the mother in the Strange Situation is positively related to angry behavior toward her seen in other (stress–free) settings. Often it appears out of context.
3. Avoidance of the mother is related to difficulties in other social relationships, that is, with persons other than the mother. Often other persons making friendly overtures are actively avoided.
4. Despite the fact that avoidance of the parent is related to avoidance of (or difficulties with) other adults making friendly overtures, there is no relationship between a given infant's avoidance of his or her mother and father.
5. Avoidance is related to restrictions in affective responsiveness.
6. Avoidance is related to indices of conflict or disturbance—to odd behaviors and to stereotypes.

7. There is no evidence that avoidance is associated either with advances or with deficits in cognitive or other functioning. (Main, 1981, pp. 662–664)

From the above, it may be suggested that avoidant behaviors that are strategically designed to function as a defense allow the infant to modulate an otherwise negative affective experience (e.g., caregiver rejection). As a result of "avoiding," the infant simultaneously maintains and seeks a different experience that will tax him or her with positive affect. Besides the genetically programmed aspect of this behavior, avoidant behavior indicates the perception of discrepancies or non–contingencies with an already internalized representation of either previous experience or of what the infant considers to be a more reciprocal dyadic relationship. As is pointed out in the following chapters, disruption of both contingencies and expectations generally evokes degrees of negative affect in infants as early as three months of age (DeCasper & Carstens, 1981). The experience of disrupted contingency can, in some instances, result in the cognitive, motivational, and self–esteem deficits indicative of learned helplessness depression. Manifestations of avoidance behavior, therefore, hint that such infants are not only vulnerable to, but may already be experiencing, depression or depressive–like behavior.

Behaviors Exhibited by Mothers of Children Classified as Insecurely Attached. Mothers of avoidant infants seemed angry but appeared to mask their anger and showed little facial expression. Whereas mothers of infants classified as securely attached usually responded to infant crying with support and gentleness, mothers of insecure infants exhibited a lack of affect. Often these mothers stated a felt aversion to physical contact.

Drawing on Bowlby's (1969) theory, Main had originally hypothesized that angry resistant and avoidant behavior exhibited by infants in relation to their mothers resulted from their perception of having been rejected. Experimentally, she arrived at the following list of maternal characteristics associated with avoidance of the mother by the infant:

1. Avoidance of the mother is associated with the mother's apparent aversion to physical contact with the infant.
2. Avoidance of the mother is associated with angry and threatening behavior by the mother.
3. Avoidance of the mother is associated with restriction of the mother's affect expression. (Main, 1981, pp. 665–666).

Main found the results of her studies to be concordant with Bowlby's views, and observed that infants for whom a parent has been historically rejecting typically have less positive social interactions, in general, in infancy and later childhood (Main, 1981).

Based on Bowlby's and Chance's theories, Main and Stadtman devised a definition of avoidance that accommodates the experimental observations. Main viewed attachment as an adaptive means to an end and defined avoidance as:

. . . an organized yet incomplete shift in attention which is defensive in character, and which serves as an alternative to behavioral and emotional disorganization. Thus in the stressful separation situation avoidance may function to modulate the painful and vacillating emotions aroused by the historically rejecting mother. (Main & Stadtman, 1981, p.293)

In so concluding, Main also speculated that Tinbergen's and Chance's ethological theories of attachment have at least partial applicability to human infants. Her interpretation of Tinbergen's signal function theory suggested to her that for human infants and children, avoidant behavior may serve proximity in one of two ways. It may function either to elicit care from the attachment figure or to signal the attachment figure deceptively, concealing strongly aroused tendencies toward distress and anger that are in conflict with the need for proximity and that, if exhibited, might drive away the attachment figure. She noted, however, that the concept of avoidance as a care–eliciting signal has yet to be tested experimentally in humans. Furthermore, she observed that interpreting avoidant behavior of infants as a special, deceptive signal, serving proximity and appropriate for use with certain types of parents, does not accommodate the observed similarities between behaviors of infants avoiding parents after major and minor separations.

Chance's "cutoff" theory suggested to Main that infants exhibit visual avoidance when sight of the attachment figure might cause the infants to flee or display anger. Furthermore, cutting off the attachment figure from sight could permit tendencies conflicting with the need for proximity to wane, allowing infants to regain control of their behavior and determine more calmly the preferred course of action. However, Main noted that infants separated from their parents for a period of from one week to several months would probably not have developed a fear of the parent as a result of the absence. As a result, fear resulting in avoidant behavior restraining flight seemed unlikely. Main deemed anger a more appropriate response than fear to a major separation, and left open the question of whether avoidant behavior in infants could be equated with cutoff in the service of proximity. She noted that experiments confirming this hypothesis have not been conducted.

Main's research has far reaching implications in terms of development of the self. Main et al. (1985) defined individual differences in attachment organization as differences in the mental representation of the self. The attachment relationship, as Main and her colleagues (1985) view it, consists of an "internal working model" of the events occurring within that relationship—the infant's experience of actions and results related to the attachment figure. If attachment is an internal organization of a model of another's behavior, then when that behavior is unpredictable or inconsistent, the internal model is likely to be disorganized. The developing model of the self must in turn reflect disorganization and lack of consistency, and may be a precursor to affective disorder.

In this view of attachment, both maternal and infant characteristics will significantly affect the evolution of attachment. Londerville and Main (1981) found that children judged to be securely attached were more compliant and cooperative relative to nonsecure children. They also found that mothers of securely attached children used gentle physical interventions and warmer tones. Considering the results of the Main et al. (1979) study, which identified mothers of securely attached infants as significantly more sensitive and accepting, the Londerville and Main data suggest that sensitive mothers not only allow their children more satisfactory security attachments, but encourage their children to behave in ways that reinforce the mothers' warmth and sensitivity. In other words, a cycle is created, with the mother's behavior being reinforced and even mimicked by the child, and with the child's behavior encouraging the mother's warmth.

Reviewing recent studies of abused infants prompted Main (Main & Goldwyn, 1984) to postulate another form that the cycle of behavior between mother and child can take. The investigators noted that a general difficulty with the control of aggression, an aversive response to others' distress, and self-isolating tendencies are typical of child–battering parents. Interestingly, abused infants show similar behavioral tendencies as early as one to three years of age. Furthermore, these three behavioral characteristics develop not only in children who are actually abused physically, but in children who have been maternally rejected in more subtle ways. For example, Main's own studies showed that rejection by the mother can lead the infant to avoidance, hostility, and affectless response to her, as well as to others. In essence, the investigators were positing that the experience of nonviolent rejection can create a continuum of psychological processes in which "normal" rejection proved as damaging as "abnormal" rejection.

In addition, the processes of avoidance in mother and infant appear to be similar. In light of Main and Weston's (1982) interpretation of avoidance as a shift in attention to maintain self–organization under threat, Main and Goldwyn (1984) sought to identify whether adult women whose children were avoidant in the Strange Situation had a similar cognitive shift in relation to their own mothers. They also sought to determine whether that cognitive shift had led mothers to adopt any impersonal, hostile, and self–isolating tendencies that might have typified their own mothers. To investigate these hypotheses, the researchers drew on preliminary findings taken from an ongoing study of social development in normal families. Main and Goldwyn relied on the Berkeley Adult Attachment Interviews to discern information concerning descriptions of relationships, memories, how mothers (as children) had assessed their relationships with their own mothers, and how they currently assessed the same relationship. A significant positive relationship between apparent rejection by the mother in childhood and inability to recall childhood memories became apparent, as did a relationship between rejection by the mother and idealization of the mother. Furthermore, the data showed that mothers' rejection by their own mothers strongly related to their own infants' avoidance. Main and Goldwyn concluded:

A mother's apparent experience of her own mother as rejecting is systematically related to her rejection of her infant and at the same time to systematic distortions in her own cognitive processes. These distortions (idealization of the rejecting parent, difficulty in remembering childhood, incoherency in discussing attachment) are each significantly related to the mother's rejection of her own infant. (Main & Goldwyn, 1984, p. 203)

Other Studies Involving Infants at Risk for Affective Disorders

Main's findings that parental rejection profoundly affects a child's social interaction beyond infancy suggest that parental rejection and the resulting avoidant behaviors might also predict the development of affective disorders. Longitudinal studies conducted by Gaensbauer, Harmon, Cytryn, and McKnew (1984); Zahn–Waxler, Cummings, McKnew, Davenport, and Radke–Yarrow (1984); and Radke–Yarrow, Cummings, Kuczynski, and Chapman (1985) of children at risk for affective disorder by virtue of a parent's manic–depressive disorder indicate that such children do exhibit behaviors that are considered symptoms of affective disorder.

The study conducted by Zahn–Waxler and associates followed seven boys, each of whom had a manic–depressive parent. Beginning when the boys were 12 months of age, their cognitive, neurological, physical, social, and emotional functioning were assessed, and these measures were compared to assessments made of 20 control group children. The sample group exhibited excessive shyness and dependency, hyperactivity, temper tantrums, poor impulse control, and inappropriate affect to a significantly greater degree than did children in the control group.

When the children were age two and one–half, their peer interactions were observed in a laboratory setting. The sample group showed more inappropriate and displaced aggression, as well as less altruism toward peers. When their aggression was aroused, it remained internalized. When it was expressed, it was still displaced.

Some of the symptoms of affective disorder noted among the sample group at age 12 months are reminiscent of the severely avoidant behavior exhibited by children typed insecurely attached by Main. Specifically, Main's observations of angry crying, hitting, batting away toys, and open petulance (George & Main, 1979; Main, 1977) seem similar to Zahn–Waxler's observations of tantrum behaviors and poor impulse control. Zahn–Waxler and associates noted that the emotional dysregulation, with concomitant poor social relationships, illustrates one process whereby depression may develop. Taking this conclusion one step further, one might infer that insecure attachments also indicate a process by which depression may develop.

Gaensbauer (1982), using the Structured Playroom Paradigm, had found that insecure attachment was more often associated with a less stable caregiving environment than was secure attachment, and that change from secure to insecure attachment was associated with higher stress event scores than was stable secure attachment. Gaensbauer et al. (1984) studied a variety of specific environmental influences to determine their effect on social and affective development in infants at risk for affective disorders. Seven male infants having one parent diagnosed as manic–depressive were studied from 12 to 15 months of age and again at 18 months, and then compared with a control group for sex, age, race, and socioeconomic status. The investigators found the sample group developed a higher frequency of avoidant attachment patterns. Six were classified as avoidant by age 18 months. The control group, on the other hand, demonstrated secure attachments throughout the study.

Furthermore, the sample group in this study manifested maladaptive affective patterns at various intervals. They seemed angrier with their mothers during both low–stress, free–play situations and testing situations than did controls. Incidence of distress in the sample group roughly matched those for anger. The sample group also seemed to experience significantly less pleasure during maternal reunions and during Bayley testing situations. The investigators' measurements of affiliative and attachment behaviors and affect expression all indicated an increasing severity of disturbance with age for the sample group, with many members of the group seeming to be quite disturbed by age 18 months. Gaensbauer and associates concluded that disturbance in the quality of attachment between mothers and infants is more noticeable the older an infant is, and that disturbed caregiving environments, when compounded by a genetic predisposition toward affective disorder, increase the likelihood of the child developing affective disorders. The investigators predicted that diagnosis of depression in infancy would be augmented by analyzing and incorporating the psychosocial environment in particular infants at risk of affective disorder.

Drawing from the hypothesis (Bowlby, 1969, 1973) that insecure attachment creates in the infant an image of himself as unlovable, and that depressed parents may transmit a picture of low esteem to the child, Radke–Yarrow et al. (1985) attempted to examine the behaviors in depressed families that may create or transmit such a message. Ninety–nine children, ages two to three years, of mixed race, sex, and socioeconomic status were examined over a course of several weeks. The large majority had mothers with some history of depression (14 bipolar depressive, 42 major unipolar depressive, 12 with minor depression, and 31 with no history of affective disturbance). In the control group, both parents were free of history of affective disturbance. In the other families, fathers varied in their history. Some were diagnosed as depressive, but alcoholic, schizophrenic, and antisocial personalities were excluded. Mothers were rated on their level of functioning during the child's lifetime, with zero meaning the mother was in need of continuous care and 100 denoting superior functioning. The mean score for bipolar mothers was 47.6; for unipolar, 54.2; and for mothers with minor depression, 76.3. Mothers with no history of depression were not rated.

Each mother–child pair was observed in several episodes of the Strange Situation over several weeks. Children's behavior was observed and rated on reunion with mothers. The moods of the mothers were observed by the same observers and also reported by the mothers.

In addition to the standard classes of attachment behavior noted by Ainsworth (1969, 1972), Radke–Yarrow et al. (1985) observed a fourth classification of infants who showed mixed avoidant and resistant characteristics. This group showed similarities to Crittenden's (1983) A/C classification, Main and Weston's (1981) unclassified group, and the "insecure–disorganized/ disoriented" children identified by Main et al. (1985). (See Table 3.2.) These children displayed both strongly avoidant and strongly resistant behaviors on reunion. They also exhibited one or more of the following: affectlessness or sadness with signs of depression; odd or atypical body posture or movement; moderate to high proximity seeking.

Nearly three quarters of the children of normal mothers and mothers with minor depression were rated securely attached while less than half (45%) of the children of mothers with major affective disorder were rated securely attached (53% of the offspring of unipolar depressive parents, and only 21% of the offspring of bipolar depressive parents). Of the insecurely attached children of normal parents, all were in the avoidant category. Of all the children of mothers with major affective disturbance, 31% were avoidant, 4% were resistant, and 20% fell into the A/C category. The absence of a father appeared to increase the rate of insecure attachment in children whose mothers had major affective disorders. A disproportionate number of the children in the A/C category fit this family picture.

Relevance of Avoidant Behavior

Avoidance as a disorder was empirically shown to be a reliable diagnosis for children using *DSM–III* criteria (Earls, 1982). Investigation of avoidance from a psychoanalytic perspective suggests it acts as a pathological defense exhibited by children whose mothers are depressed or schizophrenic (Fraiberg, 1982). In her own sample, Fraiberg (1982) reported unfluctuating avoidant behaviors exhibited consistently by infants whose mother's avoidance of them had reached a pathological extreme. Total avoidance of the mother may occur as early as three months of age.

Fraiberg noted that even though infants in her sample avoided their mothers totally and consistently, the particular avoidance behavior they employed was selective and discriminating. They did not necessarily avoid their fathers or even strangers. This observation may conflict with Main's observation that children insecurely attached to one parent tend to exhibit conflict behavior with strangers (George & Main, 1979; Main & Stadtman, 1981; Main & Weston, 1981).

Noting that Kaufman (1977) had theorized that the biological responses of fight–flight and conservation–withdrawal are precursors of the psy-chobiological states of anxiety and depression, Fraiberg equated "screaming into the wilderness" with conservation–withdrawal, and the calm, consistent avoidance of the mother as fight–flight. Therefore, she termed pathological avoidance an early psychobiological defense mech-anism, predictive of affective disorders.

Conclusion

Avoidant behavior expressed with one parent often predicts that the infant will exhibit avoidant behavior and its related affective disturbances with peers and other adults. Evidence also exists suggesting that adults who, as infants, had behaved avoidantly with a caregiver eventually behave avoidantly with their own children as well. Avoidant behavior assumes both subtle and overt forms. It is expressed as mildly as simple gaze aver-sion and as fiercely as angry resistance and tantrums. In its more aggressive forms, avoidance is generally expressed out of context, so that the behavior seems displaced, disordered, and unpredictable. Avoidant behavior is commonly observed in infants whose parents appear angry, inexpressive, and disliking of physical contact. Interestingly, avoidant behavior is also commonly observed among infants in daycare, presumably because the infants interpret being placed in daycare as rejection by the parent.

Although both attachment theory and recent functional interpretations of infant behavior suggest that conflict situations (such as major separations or parental rejection) should trigger attachment behaviors, Bowlby's bi-ological theory—which posits that the attachment system in humans is flexible, adaptive, and goal oriented—offers a reasonable, ontogenic ex-planation for avoidant behavior. Seen in this light, avoidant behavior is a form of strategically disguised attachment behavior. Furthermore, Chance's theory of avoidant behavior as an attempt to achieve flexibility and organization in behavioral responses to conflict situations offers an explanation of the proximate cause of avoidance in infants. Together, these theories afford a somewhat workable understanding of the process by which an infant may avoid a parent. Nevertheless, repeated instances of avoidance may suggest that the infant is experiencing recurrent internal conflicts. From the seeds of this recurring conflict, affective disorders may emerge.

CHAPTER 4

Correlates of Object Permanence and Constancy to Depressive Phenomena

Many theories trace depression and depressive–like phenomena to some deviation, whether cognitive or affective, during the emergence of the self. Since the self is created by interactions with the environment, it is imperative to understand how infants and children develop in their relations with animate and inanimate objects. Through the impact of objects on a growing child's representational abilities, an interactional style will evolve, shaping cognitive and affective development. Moreover, the interactional style that the infant brings to the world of objects may ultimately determine his or her vulnerability to depression.

Two milestone concepts have dominated the literature on the development of representational thought. Object permanence, a cognitive construct, and object constancy, a psychoanalytic construct, have similar origins. Object permanence originates in the child's physical interactions with the world, and object constancy, in his or her psychic and emotional interactions with the environment. These processes share a common developmental course, subject to many of the same constructive and destructive influences. Often these two facets of development have a common developmental outcome. Thus, when impairments occur in the course of development, they tend to originate at the same maturational point, disable the same mental processes, and result in the same fate—loss of the ability to represent both the cognitive and affective aspects of early relationships. Since these relationships provide the substance from which the self is ultimately formed, derailment of developmental processes with respect to interactions with animate and inanimate objects can culminate in loss of the ability to represent the self positively. This phenomenon may lie at the root of depression in early life.

The development of object constancy and object permanence depends, to a large extent, on the caregiver's empathic responses to the infant. Through such responses, the infant feels encouraged to explore the world and to overcome the helplessness and loneliness that accompany new mental and physical independence. Empathic responses permit the infant to identify with the mother emotionally, fostering self–control and the ability to view others independently. As the infant's memory develops, the mother's empathic responses provide comfort and nurturance when the mother is absent.

If the mother is unable to provide these empathic responses, cognitive deficits will appear once the infant can cognitively and affectively represent himself or herself. But there may be precursors earlier in life: the infant will not construct a sense of self, and the spheres developed up to that point will also show deficits, i.e., the common manifestations of depression, as defined by deficits in object constancy and object permanence. By the same token, as the infant develops new competencies in object permanence and object constancy, he or she faces greater risks in terms of his or her awareness. The more fully developed the sense of self, the greater the impact and the potential symptomatology of full–blown depression when development is arrested or impaired. This chapter traces the development of representational thought as it is manifested through object permanence and object constancy.

Case Report

In 1980, Solnit reported on the case of Cindy, a child of 20 months involved in a custody dispute between two adoptive homes. Until this age, Cindy, the child of a black mother and white father, had been living in the foster home of Mrs. T, a black widow in her mid–40s.

When Cindy's biological mother relinquished parental rights and the child became available for adoption, the welfare department informed Mrs. T of their decision to place Cindy in a white middle–class family. Among reasons given for this decision were the fact that Mrs. T had been granted foster custody only, the potential that Mrs. T's worsening health might interfere with Cindy's care, and the opportunity for Cindy to live in a two–parent home that offered greater financial advantages.

To support her effort to retain custody of Cindy, the attorney Mrs. T consulted brought in professionals from a mental health clinic for young children. The clinicians found Cindy at age 22 months to be progressing well in Mrs. T's care, and to be receiving the necessary attention and stimuli for healthy physical, emotional, and intellectual development. She was assessed as being alert, well nourished, and well nurtured. Her interest in toys and other test objects was assessed as normal. She especially enjoyed cubes, pegboards, and picture books, and her attention span was good for a child of her age. Her social development was progressing appropriately, and although she approached the examiner tentatively at first, she adjusted with normal rapidity. Her relationship with Mrs. T appeared warm, and the foster mother supplied reassurance and congenial, supportive responses, appropriate to the degree of success in the situation.

Although the examiner recommended against the decision to remove

Cindy from Mrs. T's home, a judge ruled in favor of the welfare department
when Cindy was 26 months old. After a period of one month in a temporary
home—during which time Cindy suffered sleeplessness, loss of appetite,
and temper tantrums—the child was placed in her prospective adoptive
home.

Mrs. T's attorney, in a continuing effort to re–establish custody with
Mrs. T, arranged for a second psychiatric evaluation of the child at 27–
plus months, a few weeks after moving into her adoptive home. The panel,
two psychiatrists and a social worker, were asked to make recommen-
dations on the advisability of returning Cindy to Mrs. T's care. The investigators found Cindy to be "depressed" and stated that she "had lost
ground in social, verbal, and neuromuscular development" (Solnit, 1980,
p. 5). The evaluators did not perceive a close relationship between Cindy
and her adoptive mother; however, the mother praised the child's placid
temperament and easy adjustment to other family members. With respect
to her emotional behavior, the investigators found Cindy to be too receptive to strange adults (suggestive of insecure attachment) and to have
an inattentive, restless, and disorderly way of playing. One evaluator also
pointed out Cindy's tendency to give more attention to objects than to
people.

Although the panel recommended that Cindy be returned to Mrs. T,
the ruling again went in favor of the adoptive parents. Mrs. T's attorney
was dissuaded from appealing the decision, because by this time Cindy
(now age 39 months) had been away from Mrs. T for 12 months. During
that period she appeared to have begun successful adjustment to her new
home and her adoptive parents were pleased with her progress. Another
change of home, albeit to one where she had previously fared well, was
viewed as being too disruptive.

Object Permanence

Object permanence is a form of perceptual constancy signifying the infant's
awareness that objects exist independently of those who view them, and
continue to exist when not in view. Cohen, DeLoache, and Strauss (1979)
defined perceptual constancy as ". . . the perceived stability of an object
in the face of marked changes in sensory stimulation that it provides the
perceiver" (p. 419). The general term *constancy* derives from academic
and experimental psychology, and refers to the ability to organize external
stimuli (usually visual) into categories irrespective of spatial changes, variations in color, etc. Object permanence refers to a belief in the continued
existence of an object even though it is partially or completely hidden.
Corman and Escalona (1969) defined the concept of object permanence
as meaning ". . . that the child has learned to conceive of things as external, relatively permanent, and existing independent of . . . his percep-

tions and actions in relation to the object" (pp. 351–352). Permanence, according to Piaget (1954), refers to an attribute of constancy whereby objects retain their essential character. A third type of perceptual constancy distinguished among infants, egocentric constancy, refers to the perceived constancy of an object despite changes in the observer's location.

Development and Significance of Object Permanence

Prior to the acquisition of representational thought, children cannot conceive of external images as distinct, functioning entities independent of the actions that the child may perform on them, or independent of the child's perception. Piaget refers to this period of cognitive development as the *sensorimotor period,* lasting roughly through the second year of life. During the sensorimotor phase, the infant successfully accomplishes acts that he or she is incapable of representing mentally. The infant views the world egocentrically, through actions rather than representations. As this period progresses, sensory and motor activities separate and the infant begins to convert temporary mental representations into stable mental constructs referred to in Piagetian terminology as *schema.*

According to Piaget (1970), these schema, which allow for cognitive development, result from the dynamic equilibrium between subject and object, with logical thinking developing primarily through reciprocal responses during social interaction (Decarie, 1978). Continuous interaction of the infant with the external world gives rise to progressively more sophisticated cognitive structures. Kagan (1979) defines a schema as ". . . an abstract representation of an event that retains the relations [to] physical dimensions of an original experience—be it object, sound, smell or dynamic sequence" (p. 164).

Schemata that develop during the first two years of life (sensorimotor schemata) were defined by Escalona (1963) in the following manner:

. . . formal aspects of early experience (sensorimotor schemata) lead to adaptations [accounting for] properties . . . of the real physical world that, once they find mental representation, constitute the basic elements of thought . . . such functions . . . as anticipation, intentionality . . . the constancy of the object world, spatial and temporal coordinates . . . are 'learned' on a sensorimotor level, at first without a counterpart in terms of corresponding ideas or structures. . . . development of intelligence . . . in terms of . . . an expanding cognitive apparatus, is predicated on such early body learning. (p. 198)

Thus the "learning" that takes place during the first two years of life forms the basis by which future information is understood, and children's earliest social interactions give them a sense of the "logic" by which one event leads to or causes a specific result or reaction. From these first responses, infants develop a sense of self and a sense of the external milieu around them. Since the person with whom the infant interacts most is the mother, it is she and the quality of her responses that will determine in large part what knowledge of himself or herself and the world the infant will acquire. (See Table 4.1 for a comparison of attachment formation and the development of object permanence.)

Development of the ability to represent objects mentally commences approximately during the sixth month and evolves gradually through 18 months of age and onward. In Piaget's chronology, representational thought is not firmly established until the third year, during what he refers to as the representational phase. During this phase, the young child recapitulates knowledge gained through sensorimotor development, and restructures it in terms of thought rather than action. Objects initially integrated into the actions of the child begin to assume independent existences containing their own forces and phenomena. As the child's subjective involvement decreases and recedes, his or her understanding of external phenomena increases dramatically. All of these developments enhance evocative memory; the ability to evoke a mental representation without visual clues of its existence (Piaget, 1954). According to Piaget, when a child can evoke such a memory, he or she has reached the first level of object permanence. Longitudinal and cross–sectional studies have generally confirmed Piaget's sequence of cognitive development, although the chronology of development has varied to some extent. Object concept scales have enabled researchers to measure when infants develop various cognitive capacities and have been widely used to measure object permanence and related developmental milestones (Corman & Escalona, 1969; Decarie, 1965; Kopp, Sigman, & Parmalee, 1974; Uzgiris & Hunt, 1966).

These developmental gradations in cognitive functioning, during which a child gains an understanding of the independence of surrounding objects, have profound implications for a child's affective development. With growth in the ability to represent objects mentally comes the ability to represent the self and others. The child relies on these memories of others, particularly the mother, for comfort in times of stress. Bemesderfer and Cohler (1983) note that the capacity to maintain mental representations facilitates establishment of satisfying relationships with others. Since the concept of permanence does not develop abstractly in a vacuum, but through interactions with others, inadequate or inappropriate responses from the environment—primarily from the mother—may hinder the definition of self. The loss or arresting of self–definition may herald the onset of depression or depressive–like phenomena. Indeed, Garber (1984) argues that the cognitive symptoms of depression—low self–esteem, guilt, and hopelessness—cannot emerge before representational thought allows for self–definition.

Garber's observation exemplifies a tendency to emphasize the links between depression and the development of the self, the latter occurring simultaneously with the establishment of representational capacity. While the acquisition of representational capacity, as measured through attainment of object permanence, allows for the expression of specific types of self–oriented depressive symptomatology, it is by no means a prerequisite for the cognitive symptoms of depression to emerge. An infant's cognitive response to objects, and the expectancies associated with objects with which it interacts, may assume significance before an infant or toddler has achieved full representational capability. Indeed, McCall and Mc-Ghee's (1977) discrepancy theory suggests that specific types of environmental stimuli can alter an infant's affects even at a very young age. They theorize that moderate discrepancies in stimuli presented to infants will result in optimal attention and positive affect, while extreme discrepancies in stimuli presented to infants will produce the opposite, a low level of attention and negative affect. Thus, the disappearance of familiar objects, or highly discrepant presentation of such objects, may elicit a depressive response akin to that evoked by object loss. The use of smiling as a gauge of infant and toddler reactions to their ability to retrieve "lost" objects in experimental settings betrays the strength of the relationship between the quality of affect and an infant's interactions with objects—animate and inanimate—in the environment. This relationship has been demonstrated empirically with infants as young as seven months old by Nachman and Stern (1984) and by McDevitt (1975) with nine month old infants. According to this argument, the ability to represent objects mentally, which infants refine over the second year of life, can promote positive affect by giving infants new tools to retrieve "lost" objects. Ramsay and Campos (1978) have noted that the smiling indicative of representational capacity in the infants they studied (between 10 and 16 months of age) might reflect the infants' sense of mastery at deploying new cognitive tools to alleviate uncertainty. (Discrepancy theory and its relationship to depressive phenomena are discussed in greater depth in Chapter 8.)

Although cognitive development culminating in object permanence establishes many of the conditions for healthy affective growth, both with respect to the self and with respect to objects, the relationship cannot be viewed unidirectionally. It has been shown, for example, that security of attachment, an aspect of affective development, will influence environmental exploration that contributes to cognitive growth. The impact of a strain on affects also reveals the bidirectional nature of the relationships; that is, stressful affect states can impair cognitions and ultimately lead to, or intensify, depressive reactions. Recently acquired representational capacity may be especially vulnerable, as Greenspan (1981) argues. With the deterioration of representational capacity, a youngster loses the ability to represent both important attachment relationships and the self. Withdrawal, self–abasement, insecurity, and worthlessness may result. Separations, under such circumstances, may prompt depressive responses according to Greenspan.

TABLE 4.1. Comparison of attachment formation and development of object permanence.

Phases of development of attachment[a]	Stages of object permanence
I. Phase of undiscriminating social responsiveness (0–3 months)	I. 0–1 month
Capacity to orient to salient features of environment; orienting behaviors of visual fixation, visual tracking, listening, rooting, and postural adjustment when held; primitive behaviors—sucking and grasping; special signaling behaviors—smiling, crying, vocalizing; these behaviors easily disrupted by competing stimuli	Reflexive interaction with the environment; no active search behaviors; no discernible concept of object permanence (Bower, 1972; Corman & Escalona, 1969)
	II. 1–4 months
	"Primary circular reactions"; reflex-based habits; active search behaviors (looking and hearing); no representation of object (Bower & Paterson, 1973; Gratch et al., 1974)
	III. 4–10 months
II. Phase of discriminating social responsiveness (3+ months)	"Secondary circular reactions"; habit schemes; adjustments to displacement of object; qualified search for disappeared object; developing sense of object permanence (Goldberg, 1977; Meicler & Gratch, 1980; Moore et al., 1978)
Discriminates between and differentially responsive to familiar and strange figures; emergence of differential smiling, vocalization, crying; more active and varied proximity-seeking and contact-maintaining behaviors	

III. Phase of active initiative in seeking proximity and contact (7–36 months)

More initiative in promoting proximity and contact; locomotion and voluntary movements evident in attachment behavior; more active and effective greeting responses; following, approaching, clinging, and other active contact behaviors; later: "goal-corrected" behaviors and attachment by age 12 months

IV. Phase of goal-corrected partnership (36+ months)

Inference about attachment figure's "set-goals"; attempts to alter these caregiver actions and goals; reciprocity of increasing sophistication

IV. 10–12 months

Increased ability to manipulate environment; active search for completely disappeared objects; enhanced eye and hand coordination; attributes of permanence (Bremner, 1978a,b; Butterworth, 1977; Gratch et al., 1974)

V. 12–18 months

"Tertiary circular reactions"; ability to follow disappearing moving object; person permanence; libidinal object constancy (Harris, 1975; Ramsay & Campos, 1978; Saal, 1975)

VI. 18–24 months

New cognitive strategies for object representation; maintains a model in the physical absence of model; reconstructing complex movements; object permanence, complete and active search (Bell, 1970; Decarie & Simineau, 1979; Wachs, 1975)

[a] Ainsworth (1973, pp. 10–13).

Object Constancy

The psychoanalytic theory of object constancy entered psychiatric theory as a developmental concept, correlating with both a level of attainment in object relations and an aspect in the process of emerging object relations. Several authors define "libidinal object constancy" as the achievement of a specific libidinal attachment to the love object, coupled with a mental representation that develops after the phase of need satisfaction in object relations (Cobliner, 1965; Decarie, 1965; Fraiberg, 1969; Freud, 1965; Hoffer, 1952, 1955; Nagera, 1966; Spitz, 1965, 1966). Indeed, the concept of object constancy has been redefined many times since it was introduced by Hartmann in 1952 when he stated that:

. . . the ego needs, in order properly to develop, a secure relation not only to the drives but also to the object. . . . But ego development and object relations are correlated in . . . complex ways . . . it is a long way from the object that exists only as long as it is need–satisfying to that form of satisfactory object relations that includes object constancy . . . .(p. 163)

Anna Freud describes object constancy as an example of libido development in which "the image of a cathected person can be maintained internally for longer periods of time, irrespective of the real object's presence in the external world" (Freud, 1965, p. 61). Solnit (1982) refers to object constancy in a similar fashion, as the capacity to retain a tie to primary love objects emotionally and in memory, and to evoke their nurturing presence in their absence. However, Freud added an important nuance omitted from many psychological definitions of object constancy that she viewed as being limited to the cognitive aspects of the attachment—namely, the child's capacity to keep an inner image of the object in the absence of the object. This definition more closely resembles Piaget's (1954) cognitive concept of person permanence—a concept derived from object permanence but applied to people rather than objects—since Piaget felt that the representational abilities reflected in attainment of object permanence might be detected earlier in relation to people due to their greater intrinsic appeal to young infants. But Anna Freud's definition of object constancy incorporates a greater affective component. She wrote:

What we mean by object constancy is the child's capacity to keep up object cathexis irrespective of frustration or satisfaction. . . . Before constancy, the child withdraws cathexis from an unsatisfactory or unsatisfying object. Also in times when no need or libidinal wish is present, the object is considered as non–existent, unnecessary. The turning toward the object takes place again [only] when the wish or need arises. (1965, p. 506)

This additional component in the definition of object constancy was noted by Kaplan (1972), who emphasized the ability to maintain cathexis despite angry feelings, as well as the need to consolidate ambivalent feelings into a unified representation. Rinsley (1986) makes a similar distinction between the cognitive and affective elements of object constancy. According to Rinsley, the former encompasses the transition from reliance on recognition memory to generate a mental image of the mother to the use of the evocative memory for calling upon a mental representation of the mother in her absence. The latter refers to an evolving libidinal tie to the mother.

Significance of Object Constancy

Despite disagreements about precisely what object constancy represents, there is broad consensus about the importance of the concept's role in object relations, and hence about its impact on the climate in which the early self is formed. Most of what is known about the implications of achieving object constancy still lies in the realm of theory derived from clinical observation, and has not been empirically demonstrated in the same manner as object permanence. Measures of the relationship between attachment and object constancy, as evaluated by procedures such as the Strange Situation, might provide some empirical basis for inference. However, no such parallels have been drawn in the literature, which is still largely theoretical. Heard (1978) has made a theoretical attempt to integrate theories of object relations and attachment, observing a common concern with how the internal representation of the self derives from the internal representation of significant early attachment relationships. For example, Heard suggests that feelings of worthlessness and inadequacy may emanate from an internal representation of an inability to exert control over attachment figures. (See Table 4.2 for a comparison of the phases of object constancy with the development of attachment.)

Inasmuch as object constancy itself develops progressively, its impact must also be viewed within a developmental framework. The contribution of object constancy to development will vary with the nature of the specific developmental tasks confronting infants through early life and beyond. In the earliest stages of life, object constancy enables an infant to retain ties to primary love objects emotionally and in memory, and to evoke their nurturing presence even in their absence (Solnit, 1982). Many researchers have noted the significance of object constancy for the development of mature object relations (Bemesderfer & Cohler, 1983; Hartmann, 1952; Solnit, 1982). The changes brought about by object constancy allow the senior toddler to replace self–centered and demanding object–relations with more ego–determined object relations. Esteem and consideration for the object are now possible. Object constancy also allows for greater trust and affection as well as confidence in the object (McDevitt & Mahler, 1986).

More importantly, however, object constancy, as an expression of certain achievements in early object relations, creates the preconditions nec-

TABLE 4.2. Comparison of object constancy and development of attachment.

Phases of object constancy[a]	Phases of development of attachment[b]
I. Autistic phase (0–2 months)	I. Phase of undiscriminating social responsiveness (0–3 months)
Consciousness dominated by internal bodily sensations; stimulus barrier (which shields against overstimulation) replicates prenatal state; primary goal is tension-reduction	Capacity to orient to salient features of environment; orienting behaviors of visual fixation, visual tracking, listening, rooting, and postural adjustment when held; primitive behaviors—sucking and grasping; special signaling behaviors—smiling, crying, vocalizing; these behaviors easily disrupted by competing stimuli
II. Symbiotic phase (2–5 months)	II. Phase of discriminating social responsiveness (3–6+ months)
Association of mother features with her actions; stimulus barrier replaced by child/mother symbiosis; rudimentary affective exchanges with mother that are the basis for later social relationships	Discriminates between and differentially responsive to familiar and strange figures; emergence of differential smiling, vocalization, crying; more active and varied proximity-seeking and contact-maintaining behaviors
III. Separation-Individuation phase (5 to 25–36 months)	III. Phase of active initiative in seeking proximity and contact (7–36 months)
A. Differentiation (5–9 months)	More initiative in promoting proximity and contact; locomotion and voluntary movements evident in attachment behavior; more active and effective greeting responses; following, approaching, clinging, and other active contact behaviors; later: "goal-corrected" behaviors and attachment by age 12 months
Discrimination of, and then preference for, mother; first active distancing from mother; quality of attachment relates to degree of stranger and separation distress	
B. Practicing (10–15 months)	IV. Phase of goal-corrected partnership (36+ months)
Awareness of bodily separateness; advent of self-produced locomotion; increased affective bond, internal image of mother; low stranger distress; low-keyed in mother's absence	Inference about attachment figure's "set-goals"; attempts to alter these caregiver actions and goals; reciprocity of increasing sophistication
C. Rapprochement (16–24 months)	
Evocative memory and representational thought; increased sensitivity to approval/disapproval; increased separation and stranger distress; ambivalent desires for attachment/separateness	
D. Object constancy (25–36 months)	
Libidinal object constancy: mother-concept that can be recalled in her absence, is invested with strong feelings, and portrays her as separate person with both positive and negative attributes	

[a] Mahler (1958); Mahler et al. (1975); Mahler and McDevitt, 1968.
[b] Ainsworth (1973, pp. 10–12).

essary for successful separation from the caregiver (first object) (Freud, 1965; Whiteside, Busch, & Horner, 1976) and for developing a definition of the self. In the course of a normal pattern of separation/individuation, a toddler will have to confront the potentially depressive realization of his or her own physical and psychological separateness from his or her mother, a realization that is initially greeted with elation, but which eventually may provoke feelings of loneliness and helplessness (Mahler, 1972; McDevitt, 1979). As the toddler increasingly appreciates his or her inability to exercise an omnipotent influence on his or her mother, feelings of frustration and anger often arise (McDevitt, 1979), forcing a reevaluation of the relationship. Mahler (1972) describes the period as the "rapprochement crisis." During this time the internal representation of the mother is fragile and transitional. According to McDevitt and Mahler (1986), aggressive and hostile feelings may, for the first time, dominate the young child's intrapsychic world as he attempts to adjust to his independence and to accept limitations imposed by his mother. In fact, anxiety and ambivalence may be so intense that the child may feel impelled to employ regressive behaviors, such as clinging, simply to preserve the object representation. With object constancy, the young child can begin to resolve the ambivalence and stabilize the representation.

Since the self is initially defined in the context of relations with others, achieving stable object representation, whether measured by the more limited or the more comprehensive definitions of object constancy, is an essential prerequisite for protecting the fragile, emerging self. Rinsley (1986) suggests that the potentially negative impact of troubled object relations on the developing self may be traced to points as early as the first months of life. He posits that a negative self–perception, whether it appears in childhood or later in life, may stem in part from a negative self object formed through negative feeding–bonding experiences during the month after birth. Object constancy implies that the love object will continue to be desired and not replaced with another object if the love object is absent or fails to fulfill the infant's desires (Mahler, Pine, & Bergman, 1975). In a sense the phenomenon of object constancy may be viewed as guaranteeing the continuity of the self, and as such, as insulating the infant from vulnerability to depression. Greenspan (1981) notes that when representational abilities first develop, they are highly susceptible to regression through alterations in affective states. With the consolidation of representational abilities that develops through object constancy, however, the young child can tolerate greater disruptions in affective states that threaten either loss of the object or loss of the self as defined in respect to the object. When the climate for development of early object relations is suboptimal (in attachment theory, when insecure attachments form) progress toward stable self representation may falter or regressions may occur. Both outcomes expose the self to uncertainty and to the possibility of cognitive and affective loss. Without a stable and independent representation of the object, loss of the object may ultimately mean loss of the self. In the absence of appropriate outlets for a child's developing sense of object constancy, the child may suffer from object loss that threatens not only the object but loss of the self contained in the object (Joffe & Sandler, 1965).

The unfolding development of object constancy transpires in two basic stages related to parent–infant bonding, according to Solnit (1982). During the first stage, the need satisfying attachment of the infant to the mother provides an opportunity for reciprocal relationships based on the mother's empathic responses to the child. During the second stage, the infant values the object for attributes other than the ability to satisfy, such as for imitation, identification, and fantasy projection. Solnit's summary of the role of object constancy captures its far–reaching implications for development. According to Solnit, the achievement of object constancy:

. . . enables the child to move from need–satisfying limitations to the capabilities that can be characterized as ego functions. These are . . . expressed in memory, speech, thought as trial action, and in the elaboration of personal relationships which serve social–psychological needs. Object constancy is a developmental capacity that provides the child with a sense of himself and his parents and enables him to become increasingly independent in forming new personal relationships. . . . (p. 216)

Factors Affecting Object Constancy

Object constancy depends, to a large extent, on the development of particular cognitive capacities. Object permanence, as manifested by evocative memory, makes object constancy possible. As Fraiberg (1969, p. 28) noted, "[t]here is no 'object concept' without 'mental representation,' no 'mental representation' without 'object concept.' " For Piaget, the development of an object concept is inextricably linked to the evocation of a mental representation of the object itself. That object constancy presupposes certain cognitive capacities does not, however, suggest that although these capacities must be fully developed before object constancy can be established, they are not sufficient for libidinal object constancy to be attained. The developmental processes culminating in object permanence and object constancy are more accurately depicted as parallel, with the products of cognitive development integrated into a child's overall emotional development, and the products of rewarding emotional growth fostering exploration, communication, and intellectual achievement.

Moreover, while cognitive developments help propel the evolution of a mature form of object constancy, other factors, such as the development of empathy, may also underlie the development of object constancy. Hoffman (1984) has suggested that the attainment of person permanence, which contains many of the same components as object constancy, corresponds chronologically to the development of empathy. This hypothesis appears plausible given the importance of the caregiver's empathy in fostering the infant's empathy, which, in turn, contributes to the infant's realization of the caregiver's separate autonomous existence and the "reflected" independence of the infant. The overall quality of the interactional environment in which a young child's early object relations mature will have a profound effect on his success in attaining object constancy. The mother's emotional availability, in particular, will influence a child's progress toward object constancy by affecting the child's ability to resolve ambivalence typical of the period (McDevitt and Mahler, 1986). Maternal anxiety or depression may interfere with an infant's earliest interactions with his or her mother and lay memory traces that ultimately take shape in a negative identity (Rinsley, 1986).

Development of Object Constancy

Object constancy emerges in a phase–specific developmental progression in which each transitional phase is characterized by a readjustment in self–object relations (McDevitt, 1975). Each level in this progression must be achieved in order for the next to occur. At each new level of object constancy, the sense of self and the way in which it relates to others matures. Although there is general agreement on the evolutionary nature of the attainment of object constancy—and thus on its evolving significance in development—the specific chronology is still not clearly understood. Part of the difficulty lies in the variety of definitions associated with the concept, since the definition of the milestone will, to a large extent, dictate the types of capacities needed to achieve the milestone. For example, attaining object constancy defined as maintenance of cathexis without splitting the object representation into good and bad identities requires a more sophisticated level of mental representation than attainment of constancy defined as maintenance of cathexis irrespective of presence or needs satisfaction. Outlining a clear chronology is further complicated by the complexity of the interactions between cognitive development—attainment of object permanence—and object constancy. Some degree of consensus has, nonetheless, formed around the progression delineated by Mahler in her theory on the development of object relations (Mahler, 1963, 1965, 1966; Mahler & McDevitt, 1968; Mahler et al., 1975). This theory provides a useful foundation for identifying points of increased vulnerability to depression in the growing child.

Mahler's developmental sequence commences with what she terms "the autism phase," during which the neonate is insulated and protected from incoming stimuli. Autism is a time of inwardness. The infant is protected by a stimulus barrier against extremes of stimulation, and can only distinguish between such states as tension and relief. As the mother cares for the child, the infant learns to associate qualities of the maternal succor (voice tone, oral sensations during suckling) with the maternal figure and with her activities. Failure to achieve this association can lead to childhood autism, a failure to distinguish self and world, and in a psychopathological sense, may result in maladaptive behavior such as self–mutilation, head banging, and self–biting, which have been interpreted as attempts to establish a boundary between self and world (Campos et al., 1983). (See Table 4.3 for a comparison of the progression in obtaining object permanence and object constancy.)

As the infant continues through Piaget's sensorimotor stage, at two months of age he or she enters a new phase of object relations which Mahler termed the "symbiotic phase." The transition from autism to symbiosis corresponds roughly with the Piagetian shift from reflective interaction with the environment in Stage 1 (0–1 months) to primary circular reactions in Stage 2 (1–4 months).

The symbiotic phase persists until about the fifth month of life, during which the "stimulus barrier" is replaced by a belief that there is a symbiotic union between child and mother, and the infant develops a specific libidinal attachment to the mother, or at least to a specific part of her body, such as her breast. During this time the infant does not intrapsychically separate his or her own wishes from the satisfaction of these wishes.

Sensitive, attuned mothers respond to cues from the child, such as cooing and smiling, with caregiving behavior that reduces the child's tension, just as cues from the mother (voice tone, facial expression) accompany ministrations to the child's needs. Such primitive affective exchanges lay the groundwork for empathy, as they mutually mediate cues between the child and the mother.

Mahler theorizes that the symbiotic phase is crucial for subsequent social relationships, not just the specific mother–infant relationship. Building up a cumulative memory trace of the mother and investing that primitive representation with positive emotions via the mother's empathic responses to the child's needs, facilitates organization of the infant's memory. These memory traces help the infant to differentiate between the mother and the external world, and between the self and the outer environment of objects. In addition, these memories lay the groundwork for the splitting of the mother into a "good" mother and a "bad" mother.

Development arrested in the symbiotic phase can lead the child to manifest a maladaptive relationship to reality—what Mahler calls symbiotic psychosis (Mahler, 1958; Mahler & McDevitt, 1968). Continuing to desire symbiosis, the infant shows lack of self–other boundaries and exhibits undifferentiated fusion with the external world, exhibited by feelings of contentment or confusion resulting in panic or rage. Symbiotic psychosis results in the establishment of a parasitic relationship with whomever can fulfill the infant's needs (Campos, Hiatt, Ramsay, Henderson, & Svejda, 1978).

TABLE 4.3. Comparison of object constancy and object permanence.

Phases of object constancy[a]	Stages of object permanence
I. Autistic phase (0–2 months) Consciousness dominated by internal bodily sensations; stimulus barrier (which shields against overstimulation) replicates prenatal state; primary goal is tension reduction	I. 0–1 month Reflexive interaction with the environment; no active search behaviors; no discernible concept of object permanence (Bower, 1972; Corman & Escalona, 1969)
II. Symbiotic phase (2–5 months) Association of mother features with her actions; stimulus barrier replaced by child/mother symbiosis; rudimentary affective exchanges with mother that are the basis for later social relationships	II. 1–4 months "Primary circular reactions"; reflex-based habits; active search behaviors (looking and hearing); no representation of object (Bower & Patterson, 1973; Gratch et al., 1974)
III. Separation-Individuation phase (5 to 25–36 months)	III. 4–10 months "Secondary circular reactions"; habit schemes; adjustments to the displacement of object; qualified search for disappeared object; developing sense of object permanence (Goldberg, 1977; Meicler & Gratch, 1980; Moore et al., 1978)
A. Differentiation (5–9 months) Discrimination of, and then preference for mother; first active distancing from mother; quality of attachment relates to degree of stranger and separation distress	IV. 10–12 months Increased ability to manipulate environment; active search for completely disappeared objects; enhanced eye and hand coordination; attributes of permanence (Bremner, 1978a,b; Butterworth, 1977; Gratch et al., 1974)
B. Practicing (10–15 months) Awareness of bodily separateness; advent of self-produced locomotion; increased affective bond, internal image of mother; low stranger distress; low-keyed in mother's absence	V. –18 months "Tertiary circular reactions"; ability to follow a disappearing moving object; person permanence; libidinal object constancy (Harris, 1975; Ramsay & Campos, 1978; Saal, 1975)
C. Rapprochement (16–24 months) Evocative memory and representational thought; increased sensitivity to approval/disapproval; increased separation and stranger distress; ambivalent desires for attachment/separateness	VI. 18–24 months New cognitive strategies for object representation; maintained in a model in the physical absence of model; reconstructing complex movements; object permanence, complete, and active search (Bell, 1970; Decarie & Simineau, 1979; Wachs, 1975)
D. Object constancy (25–36 months) Libidinal object constancy; mother-concept that can be recalled in her absence, is invested with strong feelings, and portrays her as separate person with both positive and negative attributes	

[a]Mahler (1958); Mahler et al. (1975); Mahler and McDevitt (1968).

Mahler notes that by about 20 weeks the infant's cognitive capacities allow for primitive representations that will direct the course of object relations. For example, infants begin to understand that objects can disappear and continue to exist. They can also anticipate the reappearance of objects temporarily moved behind a screen (Bower, Broughton & Moore, 1971). These newly acquired skills will prove indispensable as the infant enters the separation–individuation phase of object relations, a phase which begins at five months and lasts until 25 to 36 months of age. This phase consists of two interrelated facets: the developing sense of object relations and the developing sense of self. A consolidation of individuation by the end of the third year occurs when the two aspects have gained stability and have been integrated. Mahler emphasizes the importance of viewing these two aspects as being interrelated, since one aspect may diverge because of a developmental lag in the other. With each subphase of separation–individuation, the child establishes a new definition of self and self–object relations, as well as more complex cognitive and emotional structures, and integrates such ego functions as emotion, memory, and cognition. (According to Mahler's theory, separation–individuation consists of four subphases, differentiation, practicing, rapprochement and "the child on the way to object constancy" [Mahler, 1972, p. 488].)

Differentiation actually begins at the peak of the symbiotic phase (five to six months of age), prior to separation–individuation proper, and continues until the ninth or tenth month. As the infant's bodily dependence decreases, he or she ventures away from the mother, though remaining in close proximity to her. Establishment of the libidinal attachment helps the infant begin to recognize that the mother is not just an undifferentiated aspect in a symbiotic relationship, but is also a partner in the infant–mother dyad. Infants demonstrate the attachment by preferential gazing in the mother's direction, by smiling at her, and by quiet behavior in her presence. During her absence, infants display a longing for the mother, since the memory is still not sufficiently developed to cognitively and affectively sustain the caregiver when she is out of visual range (McDevitt, 1975). They often manifest low–keyed behavior, withdrawing inwardly and becoming insensitive to affect or external stimuli when the caregiver is removed (Mahler & McDevitt, 1968). A marked absence of stranger distress, which Mahler theorizes is inversely related to the degree of trust in the mother (Campos et al., 1983), reflects satisfaction of the symbiotic phase and recognition of the mother as a satisfier of desires.

The second subphase, "practicing," overlaps with subphase I, beginning at between seven and 10 months and lasting until 15 to 16 months of age. The "practicing" that the infant engages in during this period is related to his or her increasing bodily independence and realization of the separatedness of both animate and inanimate objects. Practicing relating to the love objects, particularly the mother, goes on during both the early and later periods of the subphase, as the infant imitates the mother's actions, affects, and behaviors. The infant's progressive, more sophisticated bodily independence allows for exploration of the environment, as motor skills are rehearsed and developed. As the ability to ambulate around the world increases, so too does the infant's understanding of the world, generating confidence to explore further as physical independence increases. During explorations, the child displays less need for physical proximity to the mother; this reflects the increased awareness of the separateness of other people. However, the infant will return periodically to "home base" for physical contact.

While nothing so demonstrates the child's separateness from the mother as the advent of self–produced locomotion, an increasingly stable mental representation of the mother enables the infant to tolerate brief separations from her by the end of the subphase. A notable relationship develops between the mother's absence and the child's distress. The separation distress that first appears in pronounced form during this time will persist until the child attains full object constancy. With the gradual acquisition of object constancy, behavioral expression of the distress may change. It may diminish from a global sense of distress in the early stages of differentiation to a more specific distress focused more purely on the mother. When the child perceives that the mother is absent, the infant evinces a more low–keyed pattern of gesturing, is less interested in the surroundings, and is less daring in motility. In the mother's absence, the child begins to use evocative memory to recall the love object. Often a child at this time appears preoccupied and inward, a state Mahler et al. (1975) describe as "reminiscent of a miniature anaclitic depression" (p. 75).

Indeed, the child's affective response to the mother's absence reflects the dynamics of the caregiver–infant interaction. The more positive the relationship, the more positive the evocative image in her absence, since the infant can now recapitulate enjoyable activities in games and symbolic play. Children who have a symbiotic relationship with their mothers appear to express little variability in mood when she is not present, while children who are developing a reciprocal social relationship express greater variations, crying for prolonged periods upon reunion with the mother (Bemesderfer & Cohler, 1983). Mahler speculates that the typical elation displayed by children during this period relates in part to the escape from the "re–engulfment" of the symbiosis characteristic of an earlier phase (Mahler et al., 1975).

Corresponding to the acquisition of object permanence and later to the cognitive shift from sensorimotor thinking to preoperational thinking (which requires the child to restructure previous cognitive achievements in light of new mental development) is the infant's entrance into a new phase of object relations, rapprochement, which lasts from 15 to 22–24 months of age, and sometimes far beyond.

This stage is critical for determining a toddler's susceptibility to depressive symptomatology, as many observers note (Anthony, 1983; Mahler, 1972; McDevitt, 1979). The sharper delineation of self and the intra-psychic representation of the other has by now become integrated into the toddler's psyche (Mahler et al., 1975). Even under the most favorable circumstances, psychoanalytic theory postulates that the diminution in illusory omnipotence that accompanies separation can stimulate a sense of helplessness and loneliness. A natural tendency toward depressive re-action is typical at this period and may be evident in a variety of behaviors including exaggerated separation reactions reminiscent of responses to object loss (Mahler et al., 1975). Whether these symptoms subside as nat-urally as they arose, or whether they endure may have a lasting impact on the child's depressive predisposition.

Mahler cites the example of a child who hurts himself, and who reacts with perplexity if the mother is not automatically there to minister to him (Mahler et al., 1975). The return to the "stranger anxiety" that originated in the differentiation subphase contributes to the "rapprochement crisis" during which the child learns that the parents are separate figures with their own interests. During these crises, the image of the mother is unst-able, cathected by both aggressive and libidinal forces, and hence the corresponding definition of the self is unstable.

Limitations that the mother imposes arouse anger, frustration, and dis-appointment, and the child alternately clings to or fights with the mother, who is gradually seen as a separate autonomous individual, not merely as an appendage of the child's needs. As a result, the primary love object becomes an ambivalent figure, both a source of love and protection, as well as a disciplining, limiting figure. The primary love object is "split" into a "good mother" and a "bad mother," and the child copes with this dichotomy by corresponding mechanisms of defensive "splitting" of the object representation. Repeated contact and empathic responses from the mother eventually help stabilize the mother's image, and the child begins to resolve these ambivalent feelings, thus achieving the beginnings of object constancy in the fourth subphase of the separation–individuation process.

Failure to resolve the ambivalence of the rapprochement crisis can cause the naturally occurring depressive symptoms to persist beyond the de-velopmentally expected period. Introjection of the "bad" maternal rep-resentation or a representation that continues to be "split" may create pathological helplessness, passivity, and separation anxiety from non-pathological symptoms that appear at the peak of separation–individuation (McDevitt, 1979). When ambivalence lingers and the young child fails to develop an integrated representation of the mother, the child may form a depreciated self–concept, viewing himself or herself as ineffective at reconciling conflicting emotions produced by encounters with the envi-ronment. This self–concept may rest at the core of subsequent depression (Bemesderfer & Cohler, 1983).

Most researchers assign a critical role to maternal empathy and re-sponsiveness in helping the young child navigate this crisis period (Anthony, 1983; Bemesderfer & Cohler, 1983; Mahler, 1972; McDevitt, 1979). A mother who is both available to the child and accepting of his or her ambivalence will help temper the child's conflict, neutralizing the hostility with which the object, and, in turn, the self, is cathected during this period (McDevitt & Mahler, 1986). Factors such as maternal depression, which diminish maternal responsiveness, may thus be responsible for the degeneration of nonpathological, age–expected depressive symptoms into pathologic helplessness and solitude (Anthony, 1983; Bemesderfer & Cohler, 1983; McDevitt, 1979). By delaying the formation of an integrated intrapsychic image of the mother, maternal depression and other environmental stressors can cause the child at risk to develop "ambivalent dependency, pathological defense mechanisms, the turning of aggression to self, feelings of helplessness, and the establishment of a specific vulnerability . . . [to] a depressive tendency, to . . . depressive moodiness, and to future clinical depressions" (Anthony, 1983, p. 12).

The final stage of separation–individuation, culminating in object constancy, occurs when a unified representation of the object becomes intrapsychically available. This substage lasts from 24 to 36 months, and sometimes extends far beyond. As the ambivalent characteristics of the rapprochement subphase resolve, the mental representation of the mother becomes stabilized; she is invested with libidinally cathected energy rather than aggressive energy, she "exists" whether need satisfying or not, or whether she is present or temporarily absent, and the representation is not subject to regression or splitting into part objects, e.g., good mother/bad mother.

Libidinal object constancy and individuation can now be seen as formalized, integrated structures. As Mahler et al., noted, "the constancy of the object implies more than the maintenance of the representation of the absent love object. . . . It also implies the unifying of the 'good' and 'bad' object into one . . . representation" (1975, p. 110). McDevitt and Mahler (1986) contend that this attainment implies more than an ability to maintain a libidinally cathected representation of the object. It also entails the full internalization of the object image into the psychic structures themselves. The mother's empathic responses continue to be extremely important in order to provide a sense of nurturing comfort and security, which in turn allow the child to concentrate on accomplishing other achievements. The rapid development of verbal skills now takes precedence over communication through gesturing. Make–believe games, role playing, and the development of a fantasy world are in evidence, and playtime takes on a more constructive quality. The child is able to tolerate the absence of the mother within familiar surroundings, and even appears to be more contented in her absence than presence, given the constraints established by Mahler (1965). Mahler notes that this subphase is the period in which object constancy, as outlined by Hartmann (1952), is attained (Mahler, 1965).

Conclusion

A child who progresses in a healthy way to attainment of object constancy can reap the psychic rewards of replacing helplessness with mastery, and has the psychic apparatus to tolerate a wide range of affects that, until now, might have threatened a precarious representational capacity and the self which it helped craft (Greenspan, 1981). As Bemesderfer and Cohler (1983) pointed out:

Separation–individuation and the process of achieving psychic autonomy involve not only children's ability to practice individuation, but the internalization of the mother's more or less empathic response to this process, which leads to . . . [achieving] an intimate relationship, characterized by appropriate closeness and distance . . . [and] the ability to deal with affects engendered through experiences with others. . . . (p. 188)

CHAPTER 5

Correlates of the Self to Depressive Phenomena

The infant's emerging acquisition of a sense of self represents a crucial developmental milestone. *Self,* as discussed in this chapter, is a concept embracing both cognitive and affective correlates.

There are several reasons why the emerging sense of self signifies a pivotal point in development. The evolution of a sense of self allows the infant to experience an enriched understanding of his or her environment and also gradually permits the infant to comprehend his or her functioning as a separate, independent, and autonomous entity. In addition, with an incipient self that enables the infant to differentiate between his or her physical–psychological being and the external world, the potential for self-attribution is achieved. Self–attribution may be negative or positive, and much data indicate that the accumulated effects of self–attribution manifestations are reflected in the construct of self–esteem. Pertinent to this discussion is the fact that self–esteem abnormalities have been directly correlated with depressive phenomena. Indeed, many have argued that although the infant may frequently evince fleeting and transient displays of negative affect, such manifestations do not represent bona fide depressive phenomena *until* the advent of a sense of self, and the concomitant capacity for negative self–attribution.

If this premise is accepted, it becomes essential to pinpoint the precise chronological stage at which the incipient sense of self emerges, because implicitly the achievement of this developmental milestone precedes the onset of depression. By achieving this milestone, the infant acquires, for the first time, the potential for moving down the debilitating path toward depression. This chapter, in reviewing the literature on the infant's evolving sense of self–recognition, delineates that crucial juncture when the self may be empirically ascertained.

The self, in coordination with affective and cognitive capacities, is involved in the regulation and development of both normative and maladaptive behavior. Self–esteem, whether referenced positively or negatively, is a significant component of the sense of self. Positive self–referencing runs parallel with normative developmental adaptation, while negative self–referencing, in contrast, appears to be an important catalytic element in the development of depression (Abramson, Seligman & Teasdale, 1978; Beck, 1967) and is related to the severity of depression (Kuiper, Derry, & MacDonald, 1982). Furthermore, the depressive phenomena are characterized by a defective perception of self–boundaries which, in turn, results from a failure to establish adequate patterns of self– and object–representations (Fast, 1976).

Self-concept has been the subject of numerous studies, some tracing the construct to social interactions (Lewis, Brooks–Gunn, & Jaskir, 1985; Schneider–Rosen & Cicchetti, 1984) and some to cognitive development (Bertenthal & Fischer, 1978). McDevitt and Mahler (1986) urge that the process of self–definition be viewed as multiply determined, shaped by interactions and identifications with parents, as well as by memory organization and mental representation. Wylie (1979) presents a volume of studies on predictors and correlates of self–esteem, but notes that the results of such studies are diverse and that they "sustain no integrated, substantive summary" (p. 39). In view of this diversity, it is necessary to seek and systematically test the predictors and correlates of self–concept within a developmental framework. New research procedures and designs must strive to capture the complexity of the developmental process. In addition, they must account for individual differences in evaluating the way in which the self–concept recapitulates the developmental processes leading to formation of the sense of self. Damon and Hart (1982) noted that the developmental model outlines the way in which sense of self clearly reflects the contours of self–esteem. Other researchers, such as Reich (1960), have suggested the existence of an intermediate step by which self–esteem results only after the self is measured against an "inner image."

Some investigators suggest that the sequential developmental process of self–understanding follows a trajectory that is directed toward progressively differentiated levels of abstraction. In their review of the literature, however, Damon and Hart (1982) stressed that tools for measuring children's self–concept must tap the changes that occur in self–understanding throughout childhood. Ultimately, self–awareness evolves into self–recognition (Kagan, 1984). The development of self–recognition— one aspect of the evolving self–concept—does not emerge fully at a particular epoch, but gradually progresses through various stages of formation of the self–recognition concept (Amsterdam & Levitt, 1980; Bertenthal & Fischer, 1978).

Werner (1957) and Phillips and Zigler (1961) have stated that "there is a continuum of growth underlying psychological processes . . ." and that "whenever development occurs, it proceeds from a state of relative globality and lack of differentiation to a state of increasing differentiation, articulation, and hierarchic integration" (Werner, 1957, p. 126). This characterization applies to the emergence of a child's self–concept. Initially, globality is manifested by the strong fusion between the self and objects. This fusion is ever–present, but its strength diminishes over time. Along similar lines, Ornstein (1981) has stressed that the notion of progressive differentiation between the self and objects implies a further and sharper demarcation of these two constructs as the child develops.

Whether one can mark distinct stages in the evolution of the relationship between self and object, it is clear that these concepts emerge in the course of development. As is discussed in Chapter 3, depression and depressive–like phenomena in early life have significant correlates in both normal and disordered development to object relations. This discussion examines the other side of the equation, focusing on the incipient self as a source of vulnerability to depression. Of the many factors influencing the growth of a self–concept, it is the relationship between attachment behaviors, as they facilitate the ability of infants to represent themselves, and the self that proves to be critical for an understanding of depression.

One subset of depression (discussed in Chapter 8) is learned helplessness. According to the re–formulated Learned Helplessness Paradigm (Abramson et al., 1978), a self–esteem deficit is one of the mandatory prerequisites for developing this form of depression. Indeed, the Learned Helplessness Paradigm stipulates that only when the capacity for self–attribution is present is the individual vulnerable to experiencing both the affective and cognitive correlates of depression. In assessing the data collected in this chapter, documentation is made of the way in which the self (as manifested through negative self–esteem) may contribute to the experience of depression and also to how negative self–attribution may, in and of itself, serve as a catalytic element in the onset of depression.

Case Report

When Diane was 19 months old, her mother jumped from a cliff to her death. Although the facts of the suicide were repeatedly explained to the child for several weeks after the event, Diane would inquire about her mother's whereabouts incessantly. Over the next several months, Diane developed symptomatology of overeating and dependency. She also became prone to long crying spells. Eventually she began expressing the fear that the people close to her would be hurt or die, and she developed a habit of falling down and hurting herself.

By the age of four, when Diane entered therapy, her accident proneness had mushroomed beyond the usual childhood scrapes and bruises to the point where the child was displaying dangerous self–destructive behavior. Diane also had spells of diarrhea and she related to her therapist terrifying nightmares of being kidnapped by a witch.

During play sessions with dolls, Diane frequently dropped the toys under the table—seemingly in an accidental fashion. She also fell a number of times for no apparent reason. On numerous occasions she fantasized with the dolls, creating a fairy story about a child who frequently became dizzy and fell off high places. In addition, most of her story telling centered on children who were beaten, burned, or otherwise physically abused.

According to Diane's father and others, the child's mother had been an excessively withdrawn and depressed woman, especially in the period just prior to the suicide. Diane's father, although not psychologically disordered, was assessed as being generally non–communicative and withholding of emotion. Prior to therapy, there had been no parental figure with whom Diane had forged a meaningful bond.

During the second year of analysis, Diane's progress became apparent. She declared that at the time of her mother's suicide she had been "unable to love herself." She engaged in a fantasy story about a doll, whom she named "Diane," and played a game called "being with Mommy." She commented that "Diane loves Diane," and said that the therapist should have his own namesake doll to love when he was lonely. Diane also speculated whether her mother would have committed suicide if she had had a "Mommy" doll.

By the end of Diane's therapy, when she was six years old, the self–destructive behavior had long since ceased. Diane was able to express her love of the therapist, as well as feelings of sadness, openly and without fear. During the last session, Diane said goodbye to the therapist, as well as "goodbye" to her mother. The therapist interpreted the comment as a recognition that feelings for her mother had been revived during the analytic relationship and that Diane had finally worked through the process of separation of self that she had not achieved with her own mother (Lopez & Kliman, 1979).

Defining Self–Concept

Harter (1982) emphasized that clear, operational definitions of "self–concept" and "self–esteem" are rare, and that vaguely defined terms often confound the application of results summarized in the literature. She also noted that concepts related to "self" are manifold, and tend more toward a "prefix usage" than unequivocal constructs. Among the "prefix usages" that one encounters in the literature are: ". . . self–recognition, self–concept, self–image, self–theory, self–esteem, self–control, self–regulation, self–monitoring, self–evaluation, self–criticism, self–reward, self–perception, self–schematas . . . .to name the most prevalent exemplars" (Harter, 1983, p. 276).

The methods used to ascertain which of these many aspects of self–concept are present at various stages of life depend on, and are often limited by, the age of the subject. When the subjects are infants not yet capable of verbalizing, the empirical data are derived primarily from studies using the visual self–recognition approach involving mirrors, pictures, and other visual cues. Since this approach is of necessity a narrow one, it may not represent or tap into the full spectrum of self–awareness possessed by young infants. Nevertheless, whatever conceptual limitations are imposed by the use of visual cues to determine the initial boundaries of the self–concept, it is also true that the visual self–recognition procedure has been the most successful technique to date for inferring supportive evidence of a developmentally determined self–concept (Damon & Hart, 1982).

By adopting a developmental view of the self, most researchers agree that "reflection" or "self–awareness" is a prerequisite for self–experience, and that this capacity emerges during the second year of life, along with what Piagetian researchers term the initial phases of "representational intelligence," the development of representational thought and recall memory. Kagan (1982) defines self–awareness as the "capacity to hold cognitive representations on the stage of active memory" (p. 376). The self–awareness initially formulated during the second year of life is progressively reformulated to achieve greater levels of complexity as developmental changes occur (Emde, 1983). Of particular importance, "the most fundamental biological principle of [the] self" (Emde, 1983, p. 170) is "self–regulation."

Amsterdam and Levitt (1980) defined various aspects of the self from the perspective of "self–consciousness," including: "1) an awareness of oneself; 2) an awareness of oneself as distinct from others; 3) an awareness of being the focus of attention of others; and 4) the explicit . . . awareness of being the focus of one's own attention" (p. 68). The foregoing definitions refer to aspects of "self–awareness," and the terms apply to affective states such as shyness, embarrassment, or coy behavior. These states denote self–conscious behavior usually resulting from the subject being the focus of attention. In defining the etiology of self–consciousness, Amsterdam and Levitt examined developmental stages during the first year of life. They noted that as early as three to four months of age, infants exhibit some sense of self as differentiated from others, as evidenced by the stranger anxiety reactions on the part of eight month olds. By 14 months, the researchers note evidence of affective self–consciousness that includes a spectrum of feelings including shame, embarrassment, vanity, pride, and coyness. Self–recognition is marked by the infant's ability to recognize himself or herself in a mirror, an achievement occurring between 18 and 24 months of age. The visual ability to identify the mirror image precedes both the verbal ability to identify the "self" and the capacity to use a name or the pronoun "me" for self–reference (Amsterdam & Levitt, 1980).

Examining emotional development and self–knowledge, Lewis and Brooks (1978) observed that self–awareness involves an evaluation of internal stimuli or bodily changes that are conceptualized in a perceptual–

cognitive dynamic similar to information processing of other stimuli, the difference being that the former information is within the body. They suggested that the ability of the organism to cause events and to evaluate changes within the perceptible environment requires some level of self–concept, as well as cognitive ability. They stated that:

Evaluation of . . . changes assumes consciousness of self–awareness as well as [cognition] . . . the evaluation process itself requires an agent of evaluation. It is . . . difficult to construct a sentence of evaluation of internal stimuli that does not use a self–referent. The source of the stimuli and the agent evaluating the stimuli are the same; this interface we call *self.* (Lewis & Brooks, 1978, p. 210)

The Development of Self–Concept During Infancy

The use of mirrors to test for self–recognition dates back as far as Charles Darwin (1877), who wrote in his diary that his nine month old son would look at a mirror and say "Ah" when his name was mentioned. Darwin suggested that this was an indication of his son's first conscious realization of self–recognition. Almost a century later, researchers still relied on mirror tests to measure self–recognition.

Dixon (1957) used mirrors to evaluate the development of self awareness in a longitudinal study of five infants (twins and three unrelated infants) from the age of four months to 12 months. A four–phased developmental sequence of self–discovery, beginning early in the first year, emerged when Dixon measured the infants' responses (smiling at the image, reaching out to the image, talking to it, etc.) to mirrors placed in their cribs.

Stage 1 (4th–6th month) This stage is defined by the infant's episodic unsustained interest in his or her image, but sustained attention and greater activity and recognition (smiling, looking, or cooing) of the mother's image in the mirror.

Stage 2 (lasting until approximately six months) The infant takes an interest in his or her own reflection (smiling at and talking to the image), but his or her reaction is not different from the reaction to the image of another infant. Nevertheless, the mother's image is still more interesting than the infant's own image.

Stage 3 (beginning at approximately seven months) The infant takes a specific interest in his or her reflection. During this stage, the infant exhibits "reality testing," by observing the image carefully while rising up and down slowly, or opening and closing the mouth with deliberation. The infant can also distinguish between his or her image and that of another infant, preferring to interact with the other infant's image.

Stage 4 (between 12 and 18 months) The infant turns away when confronted with his or her own image, rather than "basking in reflected vanity." During this stage, the infant avoids his or her own image, crying at the image or smiling coyly while averting his or her gaze. The infant is now capable of differentiating between his or her own image and that of the "other."

The sequential development of the self and the self–constancy outlined by McDevitt and Mahler (1986) also dates a consolidated self–concept to the middle of the second year when, among other things, the infant can recognize himself or herself in the mirror, differentiate between the pronouns "me" and "you," and claim possession of different objects. The process actually begins around the third month and follows a course roughly parallel with the development of object constancy. Although McDevitt and Mahler acknowledge that the earliest feelings of self are not observable, they suggest that such feelings probably coalesce around feelings associated with body parts. The differentiation subphase brings partial awareness of the self's body parts as distinct from the body parts of the object. Improved locomotion, one of the major advances of the practicing subphase, helps the infant delineate more precisely between his or her own body and the object world. At the same time, and continuing throughout the rapprochement subphase, the young toddler, aided by the advent of representational thinking, begins to gain an awareness of his or her mental self. By the fourth and final subphase of separation–individuation, the toddler has not only integrated the various body parts into a single body self, but has acquired a broader sense of his or her own feeling states, perceptions, and capabilities.

Dixon pointed out that the developmental sequence in the infants was similar, and that by as early as one year of age, the infants' behavior suggested true self–recognition. However, it is possible to fault this study on methodological grounds, since the sample was small, and it is unclear precisely what features of self–recognition were being examined.

Amsterdam's study of self–recognition (1972) did not fully support the conclusions of Dixon for early infancy self–recognition (Damon & Hart, 1982). Instead, Amsterdam concluded that "full self–recognition" does not exist until 20 to 24 months of age, much later than indicated by other researchers.

The study, which is valuable because of its clearly defined technique, tested 88 infants longitudinally from three through 24 months of age. Unbeknownst to the infants, their noses were rouged and their reactions to their altered images were recorded and examined at various ages. Amsterdam assumed that in order to note a difference in a facial feature, the infant must first possess a distinct set of features by which to compare the difference between his or her nose and the reddened version. Touching the reddened nose signified that the image in the mirror violated a stable set of features that the infant expected to see. Locating the red spot would first require the infant to make an association between his or her face and the mirror face, thus exhibiting the earliest evidence of the self as an object.

Results of Amsterdam's study indicated three phases of reaction to the mirror image:

Stage 1   The infant initially reacts to the image as a "sociable playmate," as evidenced by prolonged and repeated vocalizations and smiling coupled with delight and enthusiasm. During this stage, the child playfully approaches the "other mirror child." Most of the subjects (85%) from six through 12 months of age showed such behavior.

Stage 2   Through the second year, children do not display "naive joy" at the mirror image. Instead, they display a wariness toward the image, often withdrawing from it. However, they intermittently smile or vocalize toward the image.

Stage 3   At 20 to 24 months of age, 65% of the children showed that they recognized their images.

Amsterdam found evidence for the first two stages outlined by Dixon, but did not agree that the infants relate the mirror image to the self during this period. She criticized Dixon for placing too little emphasis on elements surrounding the experience with the mirror, stating that reactions were related to these changes in environment, not to self–recognition. The data reveal that 54% of the group of subjects ages 18 to 24 months showed recognition of their mirror images, including only one 18– and one 19–month–old child. A noticeable increase occurred after 20 months, by which point two thirds of all the subjects evidenced well–established recognition behavior. Thus, Amsterdam would not date true self–recognition until the end of the second year.

Amsterdam's study has significant implications for understanding the etiology of depression and depressive–like phenomena in infancy. Through the motor activity of touching their noses, the infants in the study were viewed as having achieved a sense of self–recognition. That is, by immediately locating their reddened noses, they were signaling an awareness that the mirror image was different or discrepant from their internal self schema. Thus, the researcher concluded that the infant had indeed demonstrated a sense of self. In addition, however, the study is reminiscent of the notion posited by DeCasper and Carstens (1981) and Ramey and Finkelstein (1984) that infants are capable of perceiving and responding to discrepancies or non–contingencies from the first hours of birth. The implicit contribution of Amsterdam's work, then, is that by approximately 20 months of age infants not only perceive discrepancy in the external environment, but have acquired the capacity to recognize discrepancy within the internal representation of their sense of self. Once the potential for internal discrepancy awareness is achieved, inferentially the infant becomes capable of formulating both positive and negative self–attributions. It is with the advent of negative self–attribution that depression becomes a viable possibility. Amsterdam's study implies that at a particular chronological stage in development, infants possess a sufficient sense of self to engage in a process of internal discrepancy awareness. When this process is not intact, negative self–attribution, with its accompanying negative affect, becomes possible.

Lewis and Brooks–Gunn (1979) obtained results similar to those of Amsterdam, except that their examinations of responses to the rouged noses of 15 month old infants indicated an earlier acquisition of recognition of featural factors than reported by Amsterdam, who noted this behavior at 20 to 24 months. Lewis and Brooks–Gunn used the rouged face technique to determine when self–reference occurred, but in their studies the infants' responses to the rouge were compared with a control condition (no rouge), and self–recognition was determined not based on mirror–directed behavior, but inferred from self–directed behaviors of two types: mark–directed and body–directed. In their first study of 96 infants aged nine to 24 months, mark–directed behavior was evident in one third of the sample, and was highly age related: no nine to 12 month olds noticed the mark; one quarter of the 15 to 18 month olds did notice it; three quarters of the 21 to 24 month olds noticed the mark. In terms of body–directed behaviors, 40% of the sample exhibited such behavior, and these behaviors were evidenced in all age groups, even the nine to 12 month olds.

In another study, Lewis and Brooks–Gunn (1979) examined behaviors before a mirror and in videotaped situations of infants beginning at five to eight months, through 21 to 24 months. At five to eight months the infants gave no evidence of self–recognition, self–and–other differentiation, or evidence that they had developed a set of features permitting them to recognize their own image. However, researchers found a variety of self–directed behaviors. Infants smiled at their images, touched their bodies, examined their images intently, and engaged in rhythmic behaviors such as clapping. Between nine and 12 months of age, the infants showed some elements of self, other, and object–recognition, and of differentiating the self from others and objects. This was evidenced by the observation that the infants now used mirrors to reach out for objects, and turned toward objects and persons reflected in the mirror. At 15 to 18 months, the first indications of feature recognition occurred when some infants were able to point to a picture of themselves when their name was said, or when they ignored or frowned at peer pictures. By 21 to 24 months, the children distinguished between themselves and others in both contingent and non–contingent situations, and used their names and an appropriate personal pronoun.

Lewis and Brooks (1978) postulated that a common developmental sequence underlies emotional experiences, cognitive growth, and self–knowledge, and that to understand any one of these three, it is necessary to examine what elements unite them in the infant's development. They presented a schema that outlined four major periods in a child's first two years. (See Table 5.1.)

Period One (birth to three months) This period ". . . is characterized by biological determinism and is primarily reflexive. The distinction

TABLE 5.1. Self-representation versus object permanence.

Stages of self-representation[a]	Stages of object permanence
I. 0–3 months Responses biologically determined and reflexive; developing distinction between self and other in perceptual clues; no emotional experience	I. 0–1 month Reflexive interaction with environment; no active search behaviors; no discernible concept of object permanence (Bower, 1972; Corman & Escalona, 1969)
	II. 1–4 months "Primary circular reactions"; reflex-based habits; active search behaviors (looking and hearing); no representation of object (Bower & Patterson, 1973; Gratch et al., 1974)
II. 4–8 months Emergence of social activity and behavior; consolidation of self-other, self-permanence merges; differentiation of self-action from others; cognitive growth/primary and secondary circular reactions; learns effect on object and social world	III. 4–10 months "Secondary circular reactions"; habit schemes; adjustments to the displacement of object; qualified search for disappeared object; developing sense of object permanence (Goldberg, 1977; Meicler & Gratch, 1980; Moore et al., 1978)
III. 9–12 months Truly social organism; established and differentiated emotional experience; reflexive imitation; means–ends; emergence of object permanence	IV. 10–12 months Increased ability to manipulate environment; active search for completely disappeared objects; enhanced eye and hand coordination; attributes of permanence (Bremner, 1978a,b; Butterworth, 1977; Gratch et al., 1974)
	V. 12–18 months "Tertiary circular reactions"; ability to follow a disappearing moving object; person permanence; libidinal object constancy (Harris, 1975; Ramsay & Campos, 1978; Saal, 1975)
IV. 12–24 months Self-recognition and categorical self clearly established, including fixed categories of self-representation (e.g., gender); beginning of representational behavior; empathy and emergence of complex emotional expression, language, complex means-ends, symbolic representation	VI. 18–24 months New cognitive strategies for object representation; maintains a model in the physical absence of model; reconstructing complex movements; object permanence, complete and active search (Bell, 1970; Decarie & Simineau; Wachs, 1975)

[a]Lewis and Brooks (1978).

between self and other, possibly on the basis of perceptual rather than cognitive cues, is being made. Emotional experience does not exist, as emotional expressions and states are usually produced by strong stimuli changes, characterized as unconditional responses. Cognitive growth is characterized by reflexive responses to stimuli changes" (p. 218).

Period Two (four to eight months) Characterized by " . . . the emergence of social activity and the establishment of social as well as biological control of behavior. The self/other distinction is consolidated and self–permanence emerges . . . secondary circular reactions are developed, and the infant learns its effect on the object and social world" (p. 219).

Period Three (9 to 12 months) Characterized by ". . . the emergence of a truly social organism, one that knows about itself [and] others. . . . Emotional experiences are firmly established. . . . Within the cognitive sphere, this period [witnesses] . . . the appearance of object permanence, reflexive imitation, and means–ends. . . ." (pp. 219–220).

Period Four (12 to 24 months) Characterized as ". . . the beginning of representational behavior, including social representation and self–representation. Several features of the categorical self become more or less fixed (e.g., gender). More complex emotional expression, dependent on complex cognitive skills, emerges (e.g., empathy)" (p. 220). Cognitively, language development, complex means–ends, and symbolic representations emerge.

Piaget's theory (1952, 1954) divides cognitive development into four major periods: sensorimotor, preoperational, concrete operational, and formal operational. The sensorimotor period begins at birth and extends to approximately the end of the second year. Piaget further segmented this first period of cognitive development into six stages. The conclusion of this period can be objectively followed by tracing specific achievements, (e.g., sensorimotor schemes, object permanence, etc.). Stage 1 ranges from birth to the end of the first month; Stage 2 ranges from the first month to the fourth month; Stage 3 ranges from the fourth to the tenth month; Stage 4 lasts until the 12th month; Stage 5 lasts until the 18th month; and Stage 6 lasts until the end of the second year. The final stage of the sensorimotor period is characterized by the infant's ability to internally represent. Representation may be viewed as Harris (1983) defined it, namely: "[as the] internalized execution of a sensorimotor scheme rather than its overt execution" (p. 695). Sensorimotor schemes have also been referred to as circular reactions, defined as "organized act[s] that tend to produce stimuli that lead to . . . subsequent re–elicitation" (p. 692).

The notion of a common developmental sequence in cognitive development and self–representation was studied by Bertenthal and Fischer (1978), who compared self–recognition behaviors to the sequence of behaviors that relate to the development of object permanence. Their research sought to demonstrate that self–recognition develops sequentially and gradually through a succession of types of behaviors. Forty–eight infants between the ages of six and 24 months were tested, and equally divided into six age groups (6, 8, 10, 12, 18, and 24 months). They assessed object permanence using the Uzgiris–Hunt Scale (Uzgiris & Hunt, 1975), and apportioned object permanence items to stages that paralleled the five stages of self–recognition. (As observed by Harris (1983), object permanence is ultimately premised on the infant's grasp of the object, based on the precise trajectory and displacement of the object, and on the infant's ability to comprehend how his or her own action can transform an invisible object into a visible object.)

The following are the five self–recognition tasks that Bertenthal and Fischer paired with cognitive–developmental stages of object permanence:

Tactual Exploration Task   For this task each infant was situated facing the mirror. An infant had three minutes to look at and simultaneously touch some part of his or her mirrored image.

Hat Task   For this task each infant was placed before the mirror and dressed in a vest designed to hold a hat above the infant's head by means of a rod and wire. To demonstrate attainment of Stage 4 in cognitive development (during which the infant begins to conceive of objects as being autonomous and independent of his or her own subjective state [Ginsburg & Opper, 1978]), within two minutes the infant had to look to the mirror image of the hat and then immediately focus on the real hat, or attempt to grab it. Such behavior would demonstrate a behavioral connection between the mirror image and focus on the real hat.

Toy Task   This task involved placing the infant in front of the mirror, and lowering a toy to a point behind the infant until its image in the mirror was just above the infant's eye level. Within 30 seconds, an infant who had reached Stage 5 in cognitive development (during which the infant can comprehend a complex series of displacements and search for the object in the proper place [Ginsburg & Opper, 1978]), would look in the mirror, see the toy, and turn toward it.

The Rouge Task   The Rouge Task involved touching the tip of the infant's nose with a dot of rouge. After a period of free–play, a mirror was brought into the room and the infant was placed in front of it. Demonstration of Stage 6 in cognitive development (during which the infant can reconstruct a series of invisible displacements of an object [Ginsburg & Opper, 1978]), required that within three minutes the infant would touch the rouged nose or verbally indicate that something was different.

The Name Task   This procedure called for the infant to be placed at the mirror, for the mother to stand outside the mirror's reflective field, and for her to point to the mirror image of the infant and ask three times successively, "Who's that?" Immediately upon completion of the questions an infant who had reached Stage 7 (as proposed by Bertenthal

& Fischer, 1978) had to reply with his or her name or an appropriate pronoun.

This study revealed moderately high correlations between the stages of self–recognition and object permanence, although there were some differences between the two measurements. Self–recognition lagged behind object permanence to a significant degree at 12 and 18 months, but no significant differences at the other stages were demonstrated. The differences noted were attributed to infants at Stages 5 to 7 in object permanence. The researchers found no consistent relationships between self–recognition and object permanence across age groups. Sometimes the two skills were highly advanced, and sometimes object permanence was more advanced than self–recognition. The authors suspected that the child may not integrate these diverse skills into a self concept until he or she is older than two years.

Emde (1984) summarized many of the qualities of the infant's concept of self that emerges by 15 to 20 months of age. He noted that recognition studies (Amsterdam, 1972; Lewis & Brooks–Gunn, 1979) have addressed a self–concept, including a sense of "continuity over time and space" (p. 39). The development of self–recognition relates to the capacity for unique, differential identification of the self–image. Verbal self–description, personal noun/pronoun reference, and the child's emotional reactions to success and failure all indicate growing self–awareness. In psychoanalytic thought, this crucial period between 15 and 20 months marks the beginning of the representational self and object world (Sandler & Rosenblatt, 1962) in which the toddler has established an acute awareness of his separateness. This inaugurates the rapprochement crisis described by Mahler et al. (1975).

Furthermore, Emde (1984) has suggested that as the child moves from early infancy to early childhood during the second to the third year, the sense of continuity and stability are reflected in many realms, including: 1) self–awareness; 2) self–consciousness; 3) symbolic play; 4) advanced cognitive abilities (i.e., causality, awareness of social rules); 5) "socialization" of affect expressions; 6) organization of inner states. The last two acquisitions relate to the affective state of the child and signify important attainments. Development of empathic abilities additionally influence the transformation of the self–concept.

Self–Concept Among Preschoolers and Older Children

Among preschoolers, self–concept may be more of an action concept than a body–image concept according to Keller, Ford and Meacham (1978), who examined dimensions of the self–concept in three to five year olds.

They found that children in these age groups significantly prefer to make action–referent over body–referent statements. Notably, they detected stability in self–concept during this age period, and suggested that major changes in the self–concept might not occur until the child enters school, a period in which new task demands and a well–defined change from the home to the school come into play.

Ability to distinguish clearly between mind and body brings a new level of self–awareness, as several researchers have observed. Broughton (1978) wrote that in early childhood, the self is initially conceived of as a body part, and that the mind, self, and body are not separately distinguished. At about eight years of age, a second level of self–concept emerges, when children come to understand that mental and physical aspects are distinct from identification with a particular body part.

Another developmental sequence, outlined by Selman (1980), begins with an initial level, the physicalistic conceptions of self, similar to Broughton's first level in which children make virtually no distinction between inner states and outer experience. At about age six, children understand that inner psychological "reality" is different from physical "reality." Not until age eight do children understand that these two "realities" are not necessarily compatible, and that differences occur between outer reality and the inward psychological state. That is, the child understands that he or she can have an inner state that is not expressed in external behavior: for example, the denial of a desire. As the distinctions between inner and outer reality become clear, the child begins to appreciate that the self can be the object of its own reflection, independent of behavior.

This model includes two final levels in the development of self–awareness. The next level is exemplified by the concept that the self can be aware of itself and that one can consciously observe the various experiences that the self undergoes. At the final level, the adolescent is able to conceive of conscious and unconscious experiences, and comprehends that some aspects of mind influence behavior without being accessible to consciousness. For the adolescent, according to Selman, self–reflection begins with the notion that one can control one's experience, but that there are still some undefined limits to such behavior.

During the entire period of development outlined by Emde and Broughton, in order for a normative self–concept to develop, i.e., one that is "cohesive," "stable," and "vigorous," the environment for the self must provide "phase–appropriate responses" and be ". . . actively responsive to the infant's . . . mirroring and idealizing needs" (Ornstein, 1981, p. 444). The role of the parents is particularly important for regulating the "empathic capacities of the child's psychological environment" (Ornstein, 1981, p. 452) and encouraging the growth of the child's empathic attitudes, which safeguard the child against pathology by strengthening the self–concept. In addition, however, the child's accomplishments during each subphase of separation–individuation will shape the child's self–concept. McDevitt and Mahler (1986) note that the autonomous accomplishments— including learning, mastery, exploration, and competence—of the practicing subphase provide a critical supply of narcissistic reserves.

The interplay between empathic response from the environment (generally provided by the caregiver) and the infant's evolving capacity to draw causal inferences from affective cues, emerges clearly in the work of Kagan (1981, 1982, 1984). Kagan suggests that the overt signs of this interplay of external and internal factors are embodied in the child's exhibition of goal–directed or mastery–oriented behavior. Such behavior is, according to Kagan, vital evidence of the development of the self.

Concentrating on the maturation of the self during the second and third years of life, Kagan (1981) determined that at 24 months of age children become aware of the self's ability to direct action, and that self–descriptive statements of pronoun and verb (e.g., "I play") become more frequent accompaniments to activity. Among Kagan's sample, self–descriptive utterances did not appear until the period of 17 to 19 months, with a major increase between 19 and 24 months of age; by 27 months of age, the level of sophisticated expression was marked. Kagan postulated that self– awareness is reflected in such self–descriptive statements, since it is virtually impossible to frame statements about the self without using personal pronoun references. In his 1984 study, Kagan outlined other precursors to self–consciousness. During the period of change between 17 and 24 months, a sense of right and wrong develops and can be applied flexibly. Children also acquire the ability to infer another's psychological state and to empathize. Together, these developments promote the notion that violence is wrong. Children can, by this point, experience anxiety at the prospect of task failure and can reflect, to some extent, on their own abilities.

Kagan's 1982 study drew more explicit connections between mastery or goal–oriented behavior and self–awareness during the last half of the second year of life. The combination of causality inference and empathy, and the ability to match disapproval with certain actions, prepares the infant for evaluating his or her actions more keenly. Along these lines, the infant shows what Kagan refers to as "smiles of mastery," positive affective responses to attainment of a goal, which appear to be "private" rather than "public" smiles, and represent communications between the child and himself or herself. Kagan notes that such smiles are rare at 17 months, increase after 19 months, and peak at 25 months. He interprets these smiles as a signal that the infant has "generated a goal for an external action sequence, persisted in gaining that goal, and smiled upon attainment" (Kagan, 1982, p. 390). That is, smiles of mastery may represent displays of the ability to attribute causal outcome to the "self."

The finding of "smiles of mastery" by Kagan at approximately two years of age has significant ramifications not only for charting the development of a self–concept, but also for identifying when infants and children may first become susceptible to depression and depressive–like phenomena.

Although Kagan was investigating infants and focusing on self–concept development, his findings implicitly correlate with the studies of Dweck and Reppucci (1973), who investigated attributional style and self–concept among eight year olds. These latter investigators identified two groups of children who displayed almost diametrically opposite modes of self–attribution: mastery–oriented children and the learned helpless, who exhibited symptomatology of depression. For those categorized as mastery oriented, Dweck and Reppucci wrote that such children attribute success to their own abilities, and do not "give up" when confronted with repeated failure on tasks. Borrowing Kagan's terminology, such mastery–oriented children seem programmed toward achieving "smiles of mastery" feelings, even in the face of failure. In sharp contrast, the learned helpless children deteriorated when confronted with failure tasks. These children, according to Dweck and Reppucci, do not take responsibility for either their success or failure. Rather, outcomes are perceived as being non–contingent and adverse circumstances are viewed as insurmountable. That is, such children seem to lack the requisite psychological equipment for a belief that they can "master" a difficult situation. Thus, by eight years old, mastery–oriented children appear to possess an internal coping mechanism for striving to overcome failure and achieve the positive affect associated with accomplishment, while learned helpless children seem to lack this mechanism and respond in a debilitated fashion.

Kagan's data pinpointing "smiles of mastery" capacity at approximately two years of age suggest, that at that chronological point in the development of the self, children begin the process of self–attribution. Once this capacity is evident, the child may either move in the direction of mastery orientation or learned helpless behavior. Thus, it may be argued that by two years of age the requisite internal mechanism, including most notably a self–concept, is sufficiently developed for the child to become vulnerable to depression and depressive–like phenomena.

Development of Self–Concept During School Years

Changes in linguistic abilities present clues to how children view themselves, as observed in Secord and Peevers's (1974) comparisons of self–descriptions by third graders and preschool children. For preschoolers, descriptions of active statements about the self are phrased in absolute terms ("I ride a bike"), whereas third graders use comparative terms ("I can ride a bike better than my brother"). This shift indicates that the older children have widened competencies permitting them to express comparisons.

Self–identity becomes sharply focused, particularly in certain aspects, during school years. A study by Guardo and Bohan (1971) examining aspects of self–identity among children six to nine years old, demonstrated that children felt they could not change gender, change into animal form, or become a different child; suggesting that in this age range (concrete operational in Piagetian terms) children possess "constancy" in the irreversible nature of their gender identity and individuality.

Thus, it appears that self–awareness, especially the ability to reflect upon the "me" as an object of observation by the "I," does not develop until the middle years of childhood, although some researchers would assert that the true ability for introspection does not fully develop until the period of formal operations in Piagetian terms (11½ years onward). Nevertheless, some elements of self–recognition are present at 18 months of age, and subsequent development further refines the infants' self–awareness with regard to gender, age and other facets of identity (Harter, 1983).

Development of Self–Regulation

Self–regulation refers to the ability to monitor one's behavior. The development of self–regulation allows the infant and child to move from external to internal control. It is a multi–faceted concept for which there is no direct measure. However, measures of attachment, temperament, and self–recognition, which measure the child's highest level of competence in the face of a developmental challenge, do provide an indirect index of how well the child manages to establish a homeostatic relationship between his internal and external worlds. The development of self–regulation emerges in phases related to self–initiated behaviors. Kopp (1982) has outlined a developmental taxonomy plotting the transformations of self–regulation through five phases: neurophysiological modulation (birth to 2–3+ months); sensorimotor modulation (3–9+ months); control (12–18+ months); self–control (24+ months); self–regulation (36+ months). (See Table 5.2.)

Neurophysiological modulation involves neurophysiological and reflexive adaptations to the environment. These include some control of arousal states and organized patterns of functional behavior, and the activation of processes protecting the neonate from strong stimuli. During this phase the infant's neuroendocrinological mechanism exerts a strong effect on his or her development. The second phase, sensorimotor modulation, refers to sensorimotor adaptations (intentional motor responses to changes in events) in accord with perceptual or motivational contingencies. Individual differences in biological predispositions (e.g., temperament), as well as external factors (e.g., attachment behaviors of the caregiver), figure prominently in sensorimotor modulation.

TABLE 5.2. Self-regulation versus object permanence.

Stages of self-regulation[a]	Stages of object permanence
I. Neurophysical modulation (0 to 2–3 months) Neurophysical and reflexive adaptations to environment; some control of arousal states; some organized patterns of functional behavior; protective processes to defend against strong stimuli	I. 0–1 month Reflexive interaction with the environment; no active search behaviors; no discernible concept of object permanence (Bower, 1972; Corman & Escalona, 1969) II. 1–4 months "Primary circular reactions"; reflex-based habits; active search behaviors (looking and hearing); no representation of object (Bower & Patterson, 1973; Gratch et al., 1974)
II. Sensorimotor modulation (3–9+ months) Intentional motor responses to stimuli; these sensorimotor adaptations guided by both temperament and attachment relationships; differentiation of self-action from others	III. 4–10 months "Secondary circular reactions"; habit schemes; adjustments to the displacement of an object; qualified search for disappeared object; developing sense of object permanence (Goldberg, 1977; Meicler & Gratch, 1980; Moore et al., 1978) IV. 10–12 months Increased ability to manipulate environment; active search for completely disappeared objects; enhanced eye and hand coordination; attributes of permanence (Bremner, 1978a,b; Butterworth. 1977; Gratch et al., 1974)

V. 12–18 months
"Tertiary circular reactions"; ability to follow disappearing moving object; person permanence; libidinal object constancy (Harris, 1975; Ramsay & Campos, 1978; Saal, 1975)

VI. 18–24 months
New cognitive strategies for object representation; maintains a model in the physical absence of model; reconstructing complex movements; object permanence, complete and active search (Bell, 1970; Decarie & Simineau, 1979; Wachs, 1975)

III. Control (12–18+ months)
Ability to initiate, maintain, modulate, or cease physical acts, communications, and social signals; some compliance; intention; appraisal of different features of environment; self-initiated inhibition of prohibited behavior; awareness of social or task demands defined by caregivers

IV. Self-Control (24+ months)
Capacity for representational thinking and evocative memory; symbolic representation of objects in their absence; sense of personal continuity and independence; increased awareness of what is acceptable to caregivers

V. Self-Regulation (36+ months)
Ability to delay/inhibit action at the request of others; compliance; modulates behavior according to established precepts, based on stored memory of conventions that govern behavior, in the absence of external monitors; elaboration of sense of self; self-conscious behavior; affective memory; increased adaptation to environment

[a]Kopp, (1982).

The third phase is control, characterized by ". . . the emerging ability of children to show awareness of social or task demands . . . defined by caregivers, and to initiate, maintain, modulate, or cease physical acts, communication and emotional signals accordingly" (Kopp, 1982, p. 204). Features of this phase include ". . . compliance and self–initiated inhibition of a previously prohibited behavior . . . intent, appraisal of differential features of the environment . . . awareness of what is [and is] not acceptable to caregivers" (p. 205).

Self–control emerges as the infant develops the capacity for representational thinking and evocative memory. These cognitive expansions allow for symbolic representations of objects even in their absence, and permit children to form an understanding of their own continuity and independence, and to make associations between the caregiver's expectations. Characterizations of the fourth phase are compliance, the ability to act, to delay action upon request, and to modulate behavior according to established precepts based on "stored memory" governing behavior in the absence of external monitors. In addition, there is a further elaboration of a sense of self and the origination of self–conscious behavior.

The difference between self–control (Phase 4) and self–regulation (Phase 5) is one of degree rather than kind. Both self–control and self–regulation depend on the capacity for representational thought and recall. The chief differences are in the limited flexibility of children in Phase 4 to adapt themselves to situational changes, and their diminished capacity for delay, in contrast to the enhanced adaptive abilities of Phase 5 behavior.

Relation of Self to Attachment

Developmental psychopathology holds that adaptation at one stage of an individual's life will have profound consequences for adaptation at subsequent levels. Not surprisingly, attainment of one of the earliest and most significant developmental milestones, attachment, has proven to relate strongly to another crucial milestone, development of many facets of the self. Several studies demonstrate the relationship of the developing self to early social interactions as measured in attachment formation. Ainsworth, Blehar, Waters, and Wall (1978) have suggested that as security in attachment increases, so does the sense of self. Sandler (1986) argues for a concept of development of the self that closely mirrors development of object relations. He relates, for example, development of self–esteem to development of esteem for the object. Others, such as McDevitt and Mahler (1986) also delineate a developmental sequence for the self that follows the contours of development in object relations. This notion was explicated in terms of representations by Main et al. (1985), who stated that individual differences in attachment can be understood as individual differences in mental representation of the self in relation to attachment. Children securely attached to the caregiver explore their environment more confidently than those who are not securely attached, accentuating the development of abilities that foster self–recognition. (See Tables 5.3 and 5.4.)

Main (1983) examined the nature of attachment, comparing degrees of attachment to exploratory and social behavior, as well as to cognitive and language development. Her longitudinal study of 40 infant–mother pairs compared attachment behavior, measured in the Ainsworth Strange Situation at 12 months, to other measures exhibited at 20 months (Bayley Scale of Mental Development), and at 21 months (play session). These were correlated with the classifications based on the Ainsworth Strange Situation. Results indicated that securely attached infants had developed aptitudes that lead to enhancement of the ability for self–recognition. For example, they had larger vocabularies than insecurely attached toddlers, gave more spontaneous verbal self–directions, played more readily with both the adults, appeared to take greater pleasure in playing with objects, were more fascinated by a puzzle toy, and had longer attention spans than the insecurely attached toddlers.

The linkage between secure attachment and enhanced ability for self–recognition is clearly shown in a study by Schneider–Rosen and Cicchetti (1984), who examined samples of maltreated children and normal children. The normal sample consisted of 19 infants (mean age, 18 months, 29 days) whose attachments were classified using the Ainsworth Strange Situation. Infants were then tested using the mirror–and–rouge technique to measure visual self–recognition. They were also tested with the Uzgiris–Hunt scales for performance on object permanence. The researchers also evaluated communicative and linguistic skills.

Of the 19 children, two were classified as anxious–avoidant, 14 as secure, and three as anxious–resistant. Over half of the securely attached demonstrated the capacity for visual self–recognition, and there was a significant relationship between this capacity and the quality of the attachment relationship, with 90% of securely attached infants manifesting visual self–recognition. Most of the 19 infants were assessed as functioning at the sixth substage of the object permanence scale. Affective response to the mirror–and–rouge technique among 74% of the sample, took the form of an increase in positive affect (smiling, laughter, etc.); for the remainder, it was either a neutral or negative response.

There remains, nonetheless, some controversy about the relationship between self–recognition and attachment security. Lewis et al. (1985) have suggested that insecure attachment, rather than secure attachment, may promote self–recognition. Their longitudinal study of 37 infants between the ages of 12 and 24 months showed that insecurely attached infants demonstrated a trend toward earlier self–recognition than did securely attached infants. A less responsive environment, according to this finding, served

TABLE 5.3. Development of attachment versus self-regulation.

Phases of development of attachment[a]	Stages of self-regulation[b]
I. Phase of undiscriminating social responsiveness (0–3 months) Capacity to orient to salient features of environment; orienting behaviors of visual fixation, visual tracking, listening, rooting, and postural adjustment when held; primitive behaviors—sucking and grasping; special signaling behaviors—smiling, crying, vocalizing; these behaviors easily disrupted by competing stimuli	I. Neurophysical modulation (0–2/3 months) Neurophysical and reflexive adaptations to environment; some control of arousal states; some organized patterns of functional behavior; protective processes to defend against strong stimuli
II. Phase of discriminating social responsiveness (3–6+ months) Discriminates between and differentially responsive to familiar and strange figures; emergence of differential smiling, vocalization, crying; more active and varied proximity-seeking and contact-maintaining behaviors	II. Sensorimotor modulation (3–9+ months) Intentional motor responses to stimuli; these sensorimotor adaptations guided by both temperament and attachment relationship; differentiation of self-action from others
III. Phase of active initiative in seeking proximity and contact (7–36 months)	III. Control (12–18+ months) Ability to initiate, maintain, modulate, or cease physical acts,

More initiative in promoting proximity and contact; locomotion and voluntary movements evident in attachment behavior; more active and effective greeting responses; following, approaching, clinging, and other active contact behaviors; later: "goal-corrected" behaviors and attachment by age 12 months

IV. Phase of goal-corrected partnership (36+ months)
Inference about attachment figure's "set-goals"; attempts to alter these caregiver actions and goals; reciprocity of increasing sophistication

communications, and social signals; some compliance; intention; appraisal of different features of environment; self-initiated inhibition of prohibited behavior; awareness of social or task demands defined by caregivers

IV. Self-control (24+ months)
Capacity for representational thinking and evocative memory; symbolic representation of objects in their absence; sense of personal continuity and independence; increased awareness of what is acceptable to caregivers

V. Self-regulation (36+ months)
Ability to delay/inhibit action at the request of others; compliance, modulates behavior according to established precepts, based on stored memory of conventions that govern behavior, in the absence of external monitors; elaboration of sense of self; self-conscious behavior; affective memory; increased adaptation to environment

[a] Ainsworth, (1973, pp. 10–13).
[b] Kopp, (1982).

TABLE 5.4. Development of attachment versus self-representation.

Phases of development of attachment[a]	Stages of self-representation[b]
I. Phase of undiscriminating social responsiveness (0–3) months Capacity to orient to salient features of environment; orienting behaviors of visual fixation, visual tracking, listening, rooting, and postural adjustment when held; primitive behaviors—sucking and grasping; special signaling behaviors—smiling, crying, vocalizing; these behaviors easily disrupted by competing stimuli	I. 0–3 months Responses biologically determined and reflexive; developing distinction between self and other in perceptual clues; no emotional experience
II. Phase of discriminating social responsiveness (3–6+ months) Discriminates between and differentially responsive to familiar and strange figures; emergence of differential smiling, vocalization, crying; more active and varied proximity-seeking and contact-maintaining behaviors	II. 4–8 months Emergence of social activity and behavior; consolidation of self-other, self-permanence merges; differentiation of self-action from others; cognitive growth/primary and secondary circular reactions; learns effect on object and social world
III. Phase of active initiative in seeking proximity and contact (7–36 months) More initiative in promoting proximity and contact; locomotion and voluntary movements evident in attachment behavior; more active and effective greeting responses; following, approaching, clinging, and other active contact behaviors; later: "goal-corrected" behaviors and attachment by age 12 months	III. 9–12 months Truly social organism; established and differentiated emotional experience; reflexive imitation; means-ends; emergence of object-permanence IV. 12–24 months Self-recognition and categorical self clearly established, including fixed categories of self-representation (e.g., gender); beginning of representational behavior; empathy and emergence of complex emotional expression, language, complex means-ends, symbolic representation
IV. Phase of goal-corrected partnership (36+ months) Inference about attachment figure's "set-goals"; attempts to alter these caregiver actions and goals; reciprocity of increasing sophistication	

[a]Ainsworth (1973, pp. 10–13).
[b]Lewis and Brooks (1978).

to promote independence that, in turn, fostered early self aware-ness. As the researchers note, however, the existence of early self–awareness does not address the issue of the quality, negative or positive, of the self–concept. This qualification may be particularly relevant for concepts of depression, since infants who learn at a very early age to represent themselves through an insecure attachment may develop a more vulnerable self than those who develop a positive, albeit delayed, representation.

Relationship of Self–Schemata to Depressive Pathology

Depressives, according to Davis and Unruh (1981), make "idiosyncratic cognitive distortions and negative self–statements on the basis of relatively stable cognitive schemata for conceptualizing personal and environmental information" (p. 125). As noted by the researchers, the term *schema* has been used to refer to a structure that stores memory traces and forms a basis for clustering new information, especially self–descriptive infor-mation. Kuiper et al. (1982) defined schema as a "hypothetical construct . . . an organized cluster of stored knowledge, beliefs, and assumptions regarding aspects of the individual and his . . . world . . ." (p. 80). The schema's contents are created and organized by day–to–day experience, and ". . . can be considered a framework . . . against which the person bases perceptions and judgments concerning relevant information . . ." (p. 599). Self schemata have been examined via performances on cognitive tasks. Markus (1977) performed one such study, concluding that the func-tion of self–schemata was to "facilitate the processing of information about the self (judgments . . . about the self), contain easily retrievable behavioral evidence, [and] provide a basis for self prediction of behavior on schema–related dimensions" (p. 63).

Self schemata guide the input and output of information about the self, and are summations of the constancies individuals discover in their social behavior. As with other concepts discussed in this chapter, the emergence of self–schema has been demonstrated to be a developmental process. A model stressing transition and evolution may offer the best description of the role of the self–schema in depression. As the research of Davis (1979) indicates, a negative self–schema need not always appear as a symptom of depression, particularly at the onset. More likely the negative schema will develop over time. This is also implied by the finding that long–term depressives show more strongly organized personal referents than do short–term depressives, and that self–schema for the former appears to play a more significant role in processing information (Davis & Unruh, 1981).

These observations about the prevalence of negative self–schema, par-ticularly in short–term depressives, were also made by Davis (1979). He examined the relationship of the self–schema to the subjective organization of personal information among depressives and nondepressives in order to determine whether or not depressives possess a negative self–schema. His findings indicate that, at least in short–term depressives, stable negative self–referencing is not firmly established. This finding tends to call into question the reformulated Learned Helplessness Model's (Abramson et al., 1978) observation of stable self–referencing among depressives. It would, however, be consistent with the notion that the pattern of the loss of positive self–esteem in depression may proceed gradually, mirroring the loss of the object, particularly as described in Bowlby's stages of protest, despair, and detachment (Robertson & Bowlby, 1952).

Davis and Unruh's findings imply a developmental change as the self–schema mutate through three structural phases: 1) initial strong form with a set of nondepressive referents; 2) addition of depressive referents that weaken the initial form by the overlay of possibly conflicting referents; and 3) emergence of a strong form characterized by a negative set of features. While most research on self–schematas in depression has used adult subjects, Hammen and Zupan (1984) concentrated on applying the self–schema paradigm to children. The researchers studied 61 eight to 12 year olds who were administered a depth–of–processing memory task, the Children's Depression Inventory (Kovacs, 1980), and the Piers–Harris Self–Concept Scale (Piers, 1969a, 1969b). Results showed that children at all ages evidenced superior recall for words linked to self–reference instructions, in comparison to structurally oriented instructions. However, when depressed children were compared with normal children, the depressed children did not demonstrate any content–specific self–schema effects. They recalled more negatively rated words in self–reference than in the structural condition, but the effect was not significant. Depressed children also showed equal recall for negative and positive content self–reference words, while the nondepressed children displayed clear superiority of recall for positive content words.

Nicholls (1978) identified two distinct schematic phases. According to the researcher, the "halo schema" predominates in younger children (under nine years) and is characterized by the child's perception that a positive outcome reflects both high ability and effort—regardless of task difficulty. The "compensatory schema," dominating among older children (10+ years) indicates that the child believes effort compensates for ability and vice versa.

Kun's (1977) research further elucidates the complexity of the child's internal self–schematic development. This researcher identified the "magnitude–covariation schema," fully developed in children age five to six, and related to Nicholls's halo schema. Under the magnitude–covariation schema, according to Kun, children conceive of change in the degree of success as being positively correlated with a facilitative factor—either ability or effort. However, this schema does *not* incorporate the idea of task difficulty, and, in this regard, is similar to Nicholls's halo schema. Kun also identified the "direct compensation schema," prevalent in children of nine years old, in which either ability or effort can compensate for task difficulty; and the "inverse compensation schema," in which ability and effort are not linked, so that high ability compensates for low effort, while low ability can compensate for high effort. College–age subjects displayed this latter schema.

These "self–schema" studies are significant for several reasons. First, research reveals that, as with other developmental processes, not all children progress through the stages of schematic representation at the same pace. That is, individual differences are common, so that some 12 year olds, for example, may evince a halo schema, while some six year olds may display evidence of a compensatory schema. Whenever these individual variations in development are encountered, such variables as temperament and attachment behaviors are implied. In other words, the constitutional predisposition of the individual child, along with the type of attachment bond forged with the caregiver, may affect the development self–schema. Second, as several researchers have pointed out, the younger the child, the more non–realistic the self–schema representation. Weisz, Yeates, Robertson, & Beckham (1982), for instance, used the phrase "illusory contingency" to describe the type of cause–effect relationship revealed by the halo schema and the magnitude-covariation schema, both of which reveal the child's delusions about the amount of control he or she can realistically exert over uncontrollable events. The third element of schematic development significant for this discussion involves the element of self–attribution the child engages in during each phase of development. On the one hand, it may be argued that the illusory contingency of the halo schema acts as a shield for the child, insulating him or her from experiencing failure. That is, while the halo schema dominates, the child experiences his or her ability and effort as being unlimited in potential. It is almost as if the possibility of failure does not exist. On the other hand, illusory contingency may operate in precisely the opposite manner during the phase of the halo schema, convincing the child that failure was due to his or her own effort and ability, rather than to the fact that the task was too difficult. Such a child might attribute the failure to himself or herself.

For these reasons, tracing the evolution of self–schema becomes crucial. A child who is found to possess a tendency for self–attributing failure during the halo and magnitude–covariation schemata may be paving the way for repeated episodes of failure. The by–product of such continual failure experiences, and their concomitant negative affect, may be depressive symptomatology. Once again, then, the importance of studying the developing self for understanding the pathogenesis of infant and childhood depression and depressive–like phenomena is highlighted, for it is within the nurturing soil of the self–concept that the seeds of such phenomena may take root and flourish.

In addition to being viewed as a phenomenon of negative self–attribution, depression can be understood as an inadequate definition of the boundaries between the self and other, or between self and object relationships (Fast, 1976). Fast summarizes some of the implications of what she sees as the ambivalent period between the ages of six and 12 months that have been related to adult depression. For both normal and abnormal development:

Initially all benign experience is within the self–boundary, and all negative experiences outside. . . . At successful resolution, both positive and negative self–representation must be within the self–boundary—but that boundary now excludes both positive and negative representations of other persons and the non–human environment. Depressive symptoms are related to the inappropriate continuation of the primitive good–bad boundary; inadequate establishment of self–other boundaries; faulty development of sense of self, of the ego–alien and of separate–but–related; unstable internal structuring of self and others and the world; and an experienced helpless dependence on another for . . . functioning. (pp. 265–266)

Conclusion

The development of the ability for self–recognition implies a preliminary distinction of the self from others. When, and to what extent, self–awareness is reflected in self–recognition is a matter of conjecture. The literature amply demonstrates that visual self–recognition represents an early precursor in the sequence of self–awareness (Amsterdam, 1972; Dixon, 1957; Lewis & Brooks, 1978; Schulman & Kaplowitz, 1977). Visual self–recognition (measured by mirror recognition) is a culmination of processes that have been tested repeatedly, and the developmental process has consistently elicited common reactions.

Though the dominance of the visual media in eliciting stages of self–recognition is predictable given the verbal and cognitive limitations of infants, it is also apparent that much of our knowledge of self–recognition is limited to studies based on visual self–recognition. Whatever the limitations of such procedures, one can reasonably state that the development of self–recognition is an important precursor to the development of a self–concept.

In comparing the material on the self, self–awareness, self–recognition, etc., with other research literature such as cognitive functioning (evocative memory and representational thought), social orientation, language skills, affective development, empathy, object relations, attachment, and separation–individuation, it is apparent that a crucial transitional period exists that intensifies toward the end of the second year of life. From the psychoanalytic perspective, Mahler and her associates theorize that emotional object constancy is established at about this time (Emde, 1983), and the disequilibrium and struggle of the rapprochement subphase (15–25 months) paves the way for individuation in a normative process.

The work of Amsterdam (1972) and Lewis and Brooks–Gunn (1979) strongly suggests that self–recognition initially develops between the ages of 18 and 21 months for a majority of infants. Kagan (1981) uses cognitive measures of self–recognition and concludes that self–awareness emerges between 18 and 24 months. His linguistic analysis reveals a major increase in self–descriptive utterances during this period. Kagan shows that by the end of the second year, self–awareness, empathy, mastery of goal–oriented behavior (as displayed in smiles of mastery), and self–descriptive utterances are all correlated.

Research on the relationship of attachment to self–recognition suggests that securely attached infants, by the age of 20 months, possess enhanced abilities for self–recognition. Insecure attachment diminishes the capacity for self–recognition. Ainsworth et al. (1978) suggest that the more secure the tie to the mother, the more secure the child is in exploring his or her environment, thereby enhancing the sense of self. Attachment is differentially correlated with the quantity and quality of verbalization at 20 months of age. Securely attached infants use more words and morphemes, while insecurely attached infants verbalize less and make fewer self–directed utterances.

If the self–schema model of depression is accurate, then it has important implications for the study of the development of a depressive cognitive bias, since negative self–schema confers a vulnerability to depression. For nondepressives, the self–schema is positive; for mildly depressed individuals, the self–schema is mixed; for long–term depressives, the self–schema is negative (Hammen & Zupan, 1984, p. 599). Determining at what age the capacity exists to develop schemata is obviously crucial, therefore, in determining when infant depressive–like phenomena can develop.

The development of early depression may also be linked to a faulty patterning of self boundaries during this 18 to 24 month period, according to Fast (1976). Demonstration of this will require determination of self–awareness sufficient to sustain affective states upon which the latter depends (Lewis & Brooks, 1978).

Although behavioral evaluation and phenomenological reporting may allow for inferences about self–esteem, as one researcher (Coopersmith, 1959) cautions, the methods are always context sensitive. Research on self–esteem clearly requires an interdisciplinary and flexible approach, as Harter (1983) advocates. Even with such an approach, many conceptual and methodological problems still confront investigators.

CHAPTER 6

Correlates of Empathy to Depressive Phenomena

The importance of understanding the developmental course of empathy has been recognized only relatively recently, since the publication of Feshbach and Roe's (1968) paper on empathetic responses in children ages six and seven. At that time the authors noted that little was known about the developmental aspects of empathy, its causes, and its social consequences. Not until Hoffman and others formulated a developmental model was a comprehensive link established between empathy and other affective, social, and cognitive realms.

Even less is known with any certainty about how empathy contributes to depression in children or how deficits in the development of empathy may signal underlying depression. Theories related to empathy, such as secondary intersubjectivity (Trevarthen & Hubley, 1978) and affect attunement (Stern, 1985), describe a general process by which a parent's affect informs an infant of the parent's affective state and manipulates the affect of the infant.

Research is only beginning to apply these theories to such major epidemiological phenomena as the high incidence of depression among the offspring of depressed patients (Kashani, Burk, & Reid, 1985; McKnew, Cytryn, Efron, Gershon, & Bunney, 1979; Weissman & Boyd, 1985). While explanations for depressive–like phenomena in infants and children undoubtedly encompass biological as well as environmental factors, the role of empathy in transmitting affects and patterns of behavior between parent and child cannot be ignored as a possible contributing factor in the etiology of these disorders. Hoffman (1984) has noted that even infants can experience empathy, although the way that it is experienced will change with the course of cognitive and affective development. It seems reasonable to assume, then, that empathy may provide a conduit through which a child can experience a depressed parent's affective state.

An investigation of empathy in relation to childhood depression is important, as well, because of empathy's hypothesized connection to prosocial behaviors that may be absent in depressed children. Hoffman (1983) has suggested that empathic distress leads naturally to guilt, and ultimately to altruism and other prosocial behaviors. However, investigators such as Zahn–Waxler, Cummings, McKnew, Davenport, and Radke–Yarrow (1984) have shown that while young children at risk for depression by virtue of their parents' depression appear capable of empathic distress, their behavior manifests the distress in unexpected antisocial behavior. The absence of prosocial behavior in certain circumstances may thus provide an important clue about expressions of childhood depression.

This chapter examines the major components of empathic responses, especially as they may allow for empathic distress and the potential for infant and childhood depression. It also traces the sequence of empathic distress in an attempt to understand how deviations in empathic development reveal themselves in unexpected ways in infant and childhood depression.

Case Report

Kalmanson (1982) presents a case of early psychotherapeutic intervention for a poor black adolescent mother and her newborn son, James. In this case, monthly meetings with a psychotherapist provided crucial aid in reducing the psychological and physical risk that initially appeared inherent in their situation.

At age 19, Wendy had been abandoned by her infant's father. She was ambivalent about the birth, although she discounted abortion as an option, and originally planned to give the baby up for adoption. After the birth, however, she was unable to relinquish parental rights. A social worker led her to an infant–parent program whose central theme was evaluation and intervention "with infants and families where marked disturbances of attachment endanger the infant's normal developmental process" (p. 10). Wendy and her baby entered the program when James was only one week old.

After an initial assessment of their relationship and living situation, predominantly during sessions taking place in their home, the therapist began to assist Wendy with the psychological problems that threatened to interfere with her ability to provide adequate care for James. Wendy proved self–sufficient in getting adequate food and clothing for herself and her infant, and the social worker was able to assist her in finding housing.

Further meetings with Wendy revealed important aspects of her own childhood that influenced her attitudes about raising James. An unstable home life with a mother whose care was unreliable, critical, and abusive, had led Wendy to consider all dwellings and relationships temporary. Kalmanson wrote, ". . . [c]ombined with the impermanence of the physical relationship was an impermanence [in social] relationships" (p.11). The traumatic death of her younger sister at age 15 months had also contributed to Wendy's fears and self–doubts about motherhood and the welfare of her infant. Having been abused herself, she was fearful of repeating this pattern with her child. She manifested her anxiety by attributing malevolent behavior to the infant and making negative comparisons between James and her own father; yet her physical behavior and attention to James was responsive and affectionate in the therapist's presence.

By helping Wendy recognize the relationship between her own unhappy experiences and her current anxiety, as well as her ability to act independently, the therapist was able to alleviate some of Wendy's concern. As their meetings continued, Wendy's attribution of malevolent intent to James decreased.

As James approached 15 months, the age at which Wendy's sister had died of a poisoning accident, she became extremely anxious that some disaster might befall him and also spoke of her desire to have a tubal ligation. By discussing her sister's death, Wendy, while still anxious, became less preoccupied with disaster, and eventually stopped mentioning the ligation. After James's 15 month "birthday" had passed, the therapist was optimistic that Wendy's ability to care for James would continue to improve.

By following the progress of mother and infant almost from birth, the investigators appeared to be able to significantly influence and improve the quality of the parent–infant relationship.

Definitions of Empathy

Empathy can be defined in various ways. A major division in definitions depends on the relative weight one places on cognitive processes (e.g., person perception, being 'aware' of another's thoughts, feelings, intentions, etc.) and affective states (affective responses and reactions to the feelings of others). For example, Feshbach and Roe (1968) defined empathy as "vicarious affective response" (p. 133).

Hoffman also defined empathy as "vicarious affective response," adding that it is an "affective response . . . more appropriate to someone else's situation than to one's own . . ." (Hoffman, 1982b, p. 281). He stressed that while empathy is an affective response, it also contains cognitive and motivational components (1982b), and that "the ability to respond vicariously may depend on the extent to which one can cognitively infer another's affective state" (1977, p. 169).

Hoffman further differentiated between direct and empathic affect: "When a person responds with direct affect, the stimulus event [impinges] on him; when a person responds with empathic affect, the stimulus event [impinges] on someone else" (1982b, p. 281). He stated that empathy, in terms of arousal of affect, can best be defined by whether the arousal is appropriate to another's situation or to one's own: "The focus of the definition is on the *process* of affect arousal rather than on the accuracy of the match or the [cue] type . . . to which the observer responds" (1982b, p. 281).

According to Hoffman, empathy depends not only on the arousal of affect, but also on the level of mental representation that the observer is capable of experiencing (1982b). (See Tables 6.1 and 6.2.) Empathy can be evoked by "expressive cues" or "situational cues," but is likely to be a response to a combination of these factors. Hoffman also suggested that a child's past experience and socialization will influence empathic development (1975, 1982a), and that one can empathize not only with those who process information similarly to oneself, but also with those who process information differently.

Hoffman's theory of empathic development is built, to a large extent, on the notion of a progression in a growing child's overall cognitive sense of others (1982a, 1982b). "How people experience empathy depends on the level at which they cognize others," he wrote (1982b, p. 283), and the development of empathy, as well as empathic distress, must correspond to this developmental sequence. Hoffman (1975, 1984) finds evidence of four stages in this cognitive capacity. Infants during the first year of life cannot distinguish between the self and others; boundaries are fused. By the end of the first year, infants have achieved some sense of person permanence, allowing them to view others as distinct from the self. Hoffman accepts Piaget's and Bell's views that children by this stage can maintain a mental representation of a person in the absence of a presenting stimulus. But sense of the object is still unstable and possibly regressive. Fatigue or extreme emotional arousal may precipitate a return to self–other fusion characteristic of the first year. In the third stage of cognitive development with respect to a sense of others, Hoffman concludes that young children can not only accept the separate existence of others, but can accept that others have internal states specific to their own desires. Hoffman labels this phase "perspective taking." A young child in this stage typically attributes to others characteristics actually appropriate to himself or herself. Research into perspective taking offers conflicting results when considering the age at which changes in perspective occur. For example, Piaget's early research (1932) suggested that not until the seventh or eighth year was a child capable of abandoning his egocentricism and accepting the perspective of others. Hoffman, using different task measurements, however, suggested that two to three year olds are capable of taking the spatial perspective of others, and that even children younger than two can engage in role taking in familiar, highly motivating settings (Hoffman, 1984). (See Tables 6.3 and 6.4.)

"Person identity," the final stage in development of a cognitive sense of others, refers to the ability to accept that others have identities of their own with internal states that go beyond the immediate situation. Hoffman suggests that though children recognize their own names, appearance, and identities by between six and seven years of age, not until between

TABLE 6.1. Empathy versus object permanence.

Stages of development of empathy[a]	Stages of object permanence
I. Global empathy (0–1 year) Prior to person permanence; fusion of self and other; in neonates, specific heightened response to infant crying; global empathic affective response:"as if what is happening to the other were happening to them" (Hoffman, 1982b, p. 284)	I. 0–1 month Reflexive interaction with environment; no active search behaviors; no discernible concept of object permanence (Bower, 1972; Corman & Escalona, 1969) II. 1–4 months "Primary circular reactions"; reflex-based habits; active search behaviors (looking and hearing); no representation of object (Bower & Patterson, 1973; Gratch et al., 1974) III. 4–10 months "Secondary circular reactions"; habit schemes; adjustments to displacement of object; qualified search for disappeared object; developing sense of object permanence (Goldberg, 1977; Meicler & Gratch, 1980; Moore et al., 1978) IV. 10–12 months Increased ability to manipulate environment; active search for completely disappeared objects; enhanced eye and hand coordination; attributes of permanence (Bremner, 1978a,b; Butterworth, 1977; Gratch et al., 1974)

V. 12–18 months
"Tertiary circular reactions"; ability to follow a disappearing moving object; person permanence; libidinal object constancy (Harris, 1975; Ramsay & Campos, 1978; Saal, 1975)

VI. 18–24 months
New cognitive strategies for object representation; maintains a model in physical absence of model; reconstructs complex movements; object permanence, complete, and active search (Bell, 1970; Decarie & Simineau, 1979; Wachs, 1975)

II. Egocentric empathy (1–2 years)
After person permanence; other persons are distinct; although infant distinguishes others as separate physical entities, he/she responds as if he/she has the same feelings; e.g., offers to help in a way that he/she would find comforting

III. Empathy for another's feelings (2–3 + years)
Role taking established; distinguishes others' feelings as separate; responds to broad range of emotions and, with development of language skills, in a variety of symbolic ways; stimulus need not be physically present for empathy to occur

IV. Empathy for another's general life condition (6–9 years)
Person identity established; distinguishes others as "continuous persons with separate histories and identities"; can empathize in accordance with another's general life conditions and not in response to immediate situational stimuli

[a]Hoffman (1975, 1977, 1982b, 1984).

TABLE 6.2. Empathy versus object constancy.

Phases of object constancy[a]	Stages of development of empathy[b]
I. Autistic phase (0–2 months) Consciousness dominated by internal bodily sensations; stimulus barrier (which shields against overstimulation) replicates prenatal state; primary goal is tension reduction	I. Global empathy (0–1 year) Prior to person permanence; fusion of self and other; in neonates, specific heightened response to infant crying; global empathic affective response: "as if what is happening to the other were happening to them" (Hoffman, 1982b, p. 284)
II. Symbiotic phase (2–5 months) Association of mother's features with her actions; stimulus barrier replaced by child/mother symbiosis; rudimentary affective exchanges with mother that are basis for later social relationships	II. Egocentric empathy (1–2 years) After person permanence; other persons are distinct; although infant distinguishes others as separate physical entities, he/she responds as if he/she has same feelings, e.g., offers to help in a way he/she would find comforting
III. Separation-Individuation phase (5–25 to 36 months) A. Differentiation (5–9 months) Discrimination of, and then preference for, mother; first active distancing from mother; quality of attachment relates to degree of stranger and separation distress	

B. Practicing (10–15 months)
   Awareness of bodily separateness; advent of self-produced locomotion; increased affective bond, internal image of mother; low stranger distress; low-keyed in mother's absence

C. Rapprochement (16–24 months)
   Evocative memory and representational thought; increased sensitivity to approval/disapproval; increased separation and stranger distress; ambivalent desires for attachment/separateness

D. Object constancy (25–36 months)
   Libidinal object constancy; mother-concept that can be recalled in her absence, is invested with strong feelings, and portrays her as separate person with both positive and negative attributes

III. Empathy for another's feelings (2–3 + years)
   Role taking established; distinguishes others' feelings as separate; responds to broad range of emotions and, with development of language skills, in a variety of symbolic ways; stimulus need not be physically present for empathy to occur

IV. Empathy for another's general life condition (6–9 years)
   Person identity established; distinguishes others as "continuous persons with separate histories and identities"; can empathize in accordance with another's general life conditions and not in response to immediate situational stimuli

[a]Mahler, (1958); Mahler et al. (1975); Mahler and McDevitt, (1968).
[b]Hoffman (1975, 1977, 1982b, 1984).

TABLE 6.3 Empathy versus self-regulation.

Stages of self-regulation[a]	Stages of development of empathy[b]
I. Neurophysical modulation (0 to 2–3 months) Neurophysical and reflexive adaptations to environment; some control of arousal states; some organized patterns of functional behavior; protective processes to defend against strong stimuli	I. Global empathy (0 to 1 year) Prior to person permanence; fusion of self and other; in neonates, specific heightened response to infant crying; global empathic affective response: "as if what is happening to the other were happening to them" (Hoffman, 1982b, p. 284)
II. Sensorimotor modulation (3–9+ months) Intentional motor responses to stimuli; these sensorimotor adaptations guided by both temperament and attachment relationships; differentiation of self-action from others	II. Egocentric empathy (1–2 years) After person permanence; other persons are distinct; although infant distinguishes others as separate physical entities he/she responds as if he/she has same feelings, e.g., offers to help in a way that he/she would find comforting
III. Control (12–18+ months) Ability to initiate, maintain, modulate, or cease physical acts, communications, and social signals; some compliance; intention; appraisal of different features of environment; self-initiated inhibition of prohibited behavior; awareness of social or task demands defined by caregivers	III. Empathy for another's feelings (2–3+ years) Role taking established; distinguishes others' feelings as separate; responds to broad range of emotions and, with development of language skills, in a variety of symbolic ways; stimulus need not be physically present for empathy to occur
IV. Self-Control (24+ months) Capacity for representational thinking and evocative memory; symbolic representation of objects in their absence; sense of personal continuity and independence; increased awareness of what is acceptable to caregivers	IV. Empathy for another's general life condition (6–9 years) Person identity established; distinguishes others as "continuous persons with separate histories and identities"; can empathize in accordance with another's general life conditions and not in response to immediate situational stimuli
V. Self-Regulation (36+ months) Ability to delay/inhibit action at request of others; compliance; modulates behavior according to established precepts, based on stored memory of conventions that govern behavior in absence of external monitors; elaboration of sense of self; self-conscious behavior; affective memory; increased adaptation to environment	

[a]Kopp. (1982).
[b]Hoffman, (1975, 1977, 1982b, 1984).

TABLE 6.4. Empathy versus self-representation.

Stages of self-representation[a]	Stages of development of empathy[b]
I. 0–3 months Responses biologically determined and reflexive; developing distinction between self and other in perceptual clues; no emotional experience	I. Global empathy (0–1 year) Prior to person permanence; fusion of self and other; in neonates, specific heightened response to infant crying; global empathic affective response: "as if what is happening to the other were happening to them" (Hoffman, 1982b, p. 284)
II. 4–8 months Emergence of social activity and behavior; consolidation of self-other; self-permanence merges; differentiation of self-action from others; cognitive growth/primary and secondary circular reactions; learns effect on object and social world	
III. 9–12 months Truly social organism; established and differentiated emotional experience; reflexive imitation; means-ends; emergence of object permanence	II. Egocentric empathy (1–2 years) After person permanence; other persons are distinct; although infant distinguishes others as separate physical entities, he/she responds as if he/she has same feelings; e.g., offers to help in ways that he/she would find comforting
IV. 12–24 months Self-recognition & categorical self clearly established, including fixed categories of self-representation (e.g., gender); beginning of representational behavior; empathy and emergence of complex emotional expression language, complex means-ends, symbolic representation	III. Empathy for another's feelings (2–3 + years) Role taking established; distinguishes others' feelings as separate; responds to a broad range of emotions and, with development of language skills, in variety of symbolic ways; stimulus need not be physically present for empathy to occur
	IV. Empathy for another's general life condition (6–9 years) Person identity established; distinguishes others as "continuous persons with separate histories and identities"; can empathize in accordance with another's general life conditions and not in response to immediate situational stimuli

[a]Lewis and Brooks, (1978).
[b]Hoffman, (1975, 1977, 1982b, 1984).

ages eight or nine do they have a sense of the continuity of their identities over time. He suggests that somewhere between six and nine years of age the sense of a continuing identity emerges.

Hoffman's theory of empathic development follows similar contours. He outlined four developmental levels of empathic response occurring from infancy through late childhood (1982a, 1982b): global empathy, egocentric empathy, empathy for another's feelings, and empathy for someone's general life condition.

1. *Global Empathy*   Global empathy occurs prior to the development of person permanence during the first year of life; at this stage expressive cues emanating from another may provoke a global empathic affective response—a fusion of feelings and stimuli that originate from the infant and from the incompletely separate other—such that "they may at times act as if what is happening to the other were happening to them" (Hoffman, 1982b, p. 284). The transitional phase from the first to second level occurs as the infant approaches, but has not yet achieved, person permanence. This phase is marked by vague, momentary distinctions between self and other. Thus the infant probably reacts to the affect of others in a global sense (Level 1) or dimly perceives that the affect is a product of the other's emotional state.

2. *Egocentric Empathy.*   Egocentric empathy, the second level, develops after person permanence, when the infant is fully aware of the distinction between self and other, and "is . . . able to be empathetically aroused while . . . being aware that another person . . . not the self, is having the direct emotional experience" (1982b, p. 284). However, the infant is still unable to distinguish fully between his or her own emotional state and that of another. The infant may confuse the two, offering the type of help he or she would find most comforting.

3. *Empathy for Another's Feelings.*   The third level develops by three years of age, coincident with the onset of role taking, wherein the infant becomes aware that the feelings of others are independent of his or her own, and are based on others' needs. At this point an infant is aware of, and can respond empathically to, a broad range of emotions, and can use language skills to empathize through symbolic rather than facial or other somatic expressions. The stimulus need not be physically present for empathy to occur.

4. *Empathy for Someone's General Life Condition.*   By late childhood, as the child gains awareness of others as separate people with separate histories and futures, he or she cognitively and affectively grasps that the feelings and experiences of others may not be confined to the immediate present. Hoffman says of empathy at this final stage of development: ". . . though one may continue to be empathically aroused by another's immediate distress . . . empathic concern is intensified when one knows that the other's distress is not transitory but chronic"

(1982b, p. 285). This may occur among the offspring of depressed parents. Hoffman observes that "children of highly power–assertive or love–withdrawing parents [are] less likely to have appropriate cognitions and affects and more likely to experience deviation anxiety" (1983, p. 266). At this level, the child integrates contradictory situational or expressive cues with knowledge of someone's general life condition.

As children progress through these developmental levels, they become progressively more capable of displaying differentiated empathic responses and become adept at processing information from various sources including: "their own vicarious affective reaction, from the immediate situational cues, and from their general knowledge about the other's life" (1982b, p. 285).

The influence of cognitive development on the development of the evolving capacity for empathic arousal appears quite clearly in Hoffman's description. He is, however, careful to note the bidirectionality of influence, and has suggested (1981) that the ability to be vicariously aroused affectively enhances the development of the "cognitive sense of others" (p. 77).

. . . the ability to be aroused vicariously may not only precede . . . development of the cognitive sense of others, it may actually contribute to that development by alerting the child to affective arousal in others, providing him with initial cues about what affects they are experiencing, and mobilizing his efforts to assess cognitively . . . their condition. . . . (p. 77)

Schachter and Singer (1962) have stressed that emotion is a function both of arousal and of cognition appropriate to the arousal state:

Given a state of physiological arousal for which an individual has no immediate explanation, he will . . . describe his feelings in terms of the cognitions available to him. To the extent that cognitive factors are potent determiners of emotional states, it should be anticipated that precisely the same state of physiological arousal could be labeled 'joy' or 'fury' or 'jealousy' . . . depending on the cognitive aspects of the situation. (p. 398)

Development of Empathic Distress

Hoffman's model of empathy helps explain how young infants and children in certain environments, such as children whose parents are depressed, can develop depressive symptomatology themselves. The vehicle is empathic distress, which unfolds in a pattern similar to empathy in general (Hoffman, 1982a). Progression through the four stages of empathic development makes an individual susceptible to empathic distress, which Hoffman defined as ". . . the involuntary, at times forceful experiencing of another person's painful emotional state. It may be elicited by expressive cues that directly reflect the other's feelings, or by other cues that convey the impact of external events on him" (1975, p. 613).

During Hoffman's first level of empathic development, when the self and the other are still fused, the infant will respond to another's distress as if the unpleasant feelings were partly internal, partly situational, and partly emanating from another. At this global stage, the infant cannot differentiate among the possible sources of distress; sources remain fused. As a result, the infant may act as if another's experience is his or her own, and may, for example, expect to be assuaged himself or herself in response to distress cues from another. Cognitive immaturity may render an infant more vulnerable to another's distress than he or she would be at subsequent stages of cognitive development in which he or she could correctly identify the source of the distress. Indeed, in the earliest stages of life an infant may be unable to insulate himself or herself from the affective states of others, most notably parental depression. With the acquisition of person permanence and the progression to egocentric empathy, for the first time the young child can experience empathic distress and be cognizant that it originates in another person, not in himself (Hoffman, 1982b). When a child has advanced to Hoffman's third level of empathic development and can begin to understand different perspectives, he or she can empathize with complex types of distress, such as another's disappointment or betrayal. Moreover, the young child can feel empathic distress simultaneously with other conflicting emotions.

At the fourth level, empathy for another's plight, the variety of cues to which a child may respond enables the child to experience empathic distress for general rather than specific reasons. For example,

. . . if the image of the model's general life falls short of the [child's] standard of well-being. . . . This fourth level then may involve a certain amount of distancing—responding partly to one's mental image of the other rather than to the stimulus immediately presented by the other. (Hoffman, 1982b, p. 289)

Empathic distress, like empathy in general, therefore, also has both cognitive and affective components sensitive to a child's developmental status. The affective component refers to the ability of the emotional components for arousal. Hoffman (1984) notes that the affective and cognitive components apparently develop through different processes, but despite these differing developmental processes, the affective and cognitive factors interact and "tend to be experienced, not so much as separate states but as a *unity*" (stress added). Empathic distress and/or guilt have been called "hot cognitions," since they are "emotionally charged" (Hoffman, 1984, p. 127).

Though Hoffman (1982a) distinguishes between "empathic distress" and "sympathetic distress," the two "types" of distress display sequential relatedness, the former engendering the latter. Hoffman makes clear the relatedness and distinguishes between the two types in the following manner:

[O]nce people are aware of the other as distinct from . . . self, their own empathic distress, which is a parallel response— . . . a replication of the victim's presumed feeling of distress—may be transformed . . . into a . . . reciprocal feeling of concern for the victim. That is, they continue to respond in a purely empathic, quasi-egocentric manner—to feel . . . highly distressed themselves—but they also experience a feeling of compassion or . . . sympathetic distress for the victim, along with a conscious desire to help because they feel sorry for him or her and not just to relieve their own empathic distress. In short . . . the affective and cognitive components of empathy combine to produce a qualitatively different feeling in the observer. (p. 290)

Two other factors that relate to the child's early response to distress in others may account for how the process of self—other differentiation (which presumably would create a barrier between the self and the other) and empathic distress (which is at least partially egoistic) unite to produce a developmental basis for "sympathetic distress." Hoffman (1984) stated that these aspects "are manifest in the earliest stages of self-other differentiation":

1) the transfer of the unpleasant affect—and the urge to terminate it, associated with the initial global self—into its emerging separate parts ('self' and 'other') and 2) the subjective experience of 'sharing' distress . . . due to the gradual attainment of a sense of the other . . . gives the child the experience of wishing the other's distress to end. (p. 117)

Demonstrations of empathic development, whether in relation to depression or not, have been extremely limited and typically focus on a single age group. For example, Strayer's study (1980) offers insight into the incidence of empathy and empathic behaviors among preschoolers. Fourteen children approximately four and one half to five and one half years of age were observed over an eight week period in natural settings and in a donating experiment for interrelations among empathic behaviors, affective states, and performance in perspective-taking tasks. In 39% of naturally occurring displays of affect observed, such displays were matched by similar affect or evoked an instrumental response indicating empathy. Strayer observed that the empathic responses were spontaneous and not dependent on verbal requests for participation. Happy displays occurred most frequently, and the subjects responded to happy displays significantly more than to other affect displays. Those children who had a higher incidence of happy displays were also likely to exhibit more empathic responses to others; those children with more frequent sad displays were less likely to exhibit empathic behaviors.

Another study (Feshbach & Roe, 1968) examined conditions simulating empathy in a group of 46, six and seven year old first-graders. Empathy was defined as a "vicarious response" (p. 134). The procedure called for each child to view a series of slides with narrative. Following the presentation, the child was asked to state how he felt. Twenty-seven children in the group were presented with the series a second time and asked to indicate the feelings of the central child in the series. Results indicated that children displayed greater empathy for other children of the same sex. Discussing these results, the researchers suggested that the finding is of theoretical significance, since it supports the hypothesis that similarity may promote empathy and that empathy may require a certain degree of social understanding. However, they note that recognition, alone, of another's affective state does not explain *how* empathy will be displayed.

Studies of empathy and empathic distress in early infancy have focused on the reactive newborn cry, a phenomenon associated with infants as young as two days old, who cry at the sound of another newborn's cry. Hoffman suggested that while this phenomenon may signify an "innate precursor of empathy distress" (Sagi & Hoffman, 1976, p. 175), it is not a "mature empathic response" (Hoffman, 1981, p. 130). Simner (1971) determined that a two day old infant's reactive crying is based on the vocal properties of another crying infant. He compared the newborn's reactions to other stimuli, such as loud and intense inanimate, computer-generated sounds, determining that newborns responded differently to various stimuli, with significant response to the cry of other newborns.

Sagi and Hoffman (1976) replicated Simner's results using one day old infants under three experimental conditions: a spontaneous cry of another infant; a synthetic, computer-generated cry (with similar properties such as burst laugh and sudden onset, but still recognizable by adults as a non-human sound); and a period of silence. The infants cried significantly more often when exposed to a newborn's cry than under the other two conditions. The authors noted that this selective response "provides direct evidence . . . for an inborn empathic distress reaction" (p. 175).

Empathic Transformation into Guilt and Its Relationship to Prosocial Action

When empathy is construed as a component of the observer's reaction to another's plight, a tacit assumption is that the observer is innocent. However, when cues from the immediate situation imply that the observer is causing the plight, self-blame may transform empathic distress into feelings of guilt, which Hoffman explained represented the overlapping of empathy for someone in distress with self-attribution responsibility for that distress. As an interpersonal concept, guilt may be defined as "the bad feeling one has about oneself because one is aware of actually doing harm to someone" (Hoffman, 1982a, pp. 297–298).

Hoffman's definition of the guilt arising through empathic distress is conceptually different from other definitions, such as those that refer to guilt as a "conditioned anxiety response to anticipated punishment" (1982a, p. 297), or guilt "which is a remnant of earlier fears of punishment or retaliation that resulted in repression of hostile . . . impulses . . . triggered by the return of the repressed impulses to consciousness" (1982a, p. 297). For empathic distress to create guilt, according to Hoffman, a cognitive sense of others must be fully developed, such that the individual can separate the self from the other and know with some certainty who created the harmful act.

Experimental evidence strongly suggests that the arousal of guilt in adults may actually serve to motivate altruistic and prosocial behavior. Since Hoffman defines empathy as "vicarious affective response to others," empathic distress, by possibly producing guilt and a desire to help a victim, may stimulate prosocial activity. This disposition forms the motivational dimension of guilt, which, like empathic distress, contains affective and cognitive components. According to Hoffman, the affective dimension contains "the painful feeling of dis-esteem for the self because of the harmful consequences of one's action . . ." (1982a, p. 288). The cognitive component of guilt assumes an awareness of the harm that one's behavior might engender, and that one is the agent of the harm that befalls another. This cognitive sense of others requires that causal links be recognized that relate one's actions to change in conditions of the other. Recognition of control over one's behavior represents another crucial dimension of the cognitive component of guilt.

In this model for the development of guilt, empathic distress is viewed as a developmental prerequisite that makes possible feelings of guilt; though later guilt may be virtually independent of its empathic origins, and ". . . although empathic distress may be a necessary factor in the *development* of guilt, it may not, subsequently, be an inevitable accompaniment of guilt" (Hoffman, 1984, p. 125). In examining the linkage between empathic distress and guilt, Hoffman wrote that:

It seems likely . . . that once the capacity for guilt is attained [it] may become a part of all subsequent responses to another's distress, at least in situations in which one might have helped but did not. From then on, even as an innocent bystander, one may rarely experience empathic distress without some guilt. (p. 126)

Investigations have shown that the affective state influences the expression of prosocial behavior, although it is not yet clear whether experience of another's distress leads to prosocial behavior as Hoffman suggests, or to antisocial behavior. An answer to this question is necessary to help clinicians predict how a child's experience of another's distress will be reflected and, conversely, how to interpret both prosocial and antisocial behavior. The implication of the research of Underwood, Froming, and Moore (1977), for example, is that positive affect fosters more generosity than sad affect. This conflicts with the empathy research by Hoffman and others, which suggests that children who experience the negative affect of others not only have a heightened awareness of the needs and feelings of others, but also that this empathic tie to others magnifies prosocial behavior.

It seems possible that certain *extreme* environments may actually inhibit the development of prosocial behavior that Hoffman hypothesizes should emanate from the ability to experience empathic distress. In environments where the child has not experienced empathic responses from a parent, a type of arrest may occur in the infant's empathic development and guilt—accompanied by antisocial, rather than prosocial behavior—may result. Such environments may impair what Hoffman described as the motivational component of guilt, since these children's experiences may prevent them from perceiving a clear contingency relationship between distress in one individual and its alleviation by another. This discrepancy or non-contingency in the environment may result in unexpected and atypical expressions of depressive symptomatology, such as aggressiveness and conduct disturbances. Thus, while empathic distress may function as the medium through which a child can experience depression, lack of reciprocity in empathic interaction between caregiver and child may block what Hoffman views as the developmentally expected outlet for such distress—prosocial behavior. The behavior of children of depressed parents, who are considered at risk for depression (Kashani et al., 1985; McKnew et al., 1979; Weissman & Boyd, 1985), may be explained in this manner. The seemingly contradictory findings of a study on altruism, aggression, and social interactions among children of bipolar parents support this view (Zahn-Waxler et al., 1984). In a normal population, according to Hoffman's model, children would be expected to experience the distress of another and react with altruism. Among the children studied by Zahn-Waxler et al., many of whom were depressed, antisocial behavior accompanied the child's seeming distress.

The researchers compared a sample of seven boys with a bipolar parent with a control group of 10 boys and 10 girls (ages 1–2½ years). Parental diagnoses were based on Schedule for Affective Disorders and Schizophrenia (SADS) and *DSM–III* criteria. Four of the families contained a bipolar mother, and three a bipolar father. Five of the seven bipolar parents had spouses also diagnosed as having unipolar depression, and in the sixth family, the spouse of the unipolar parent was diagnosed as alcoholic and neurotic. Among the control families, all mothers received a normal diagnosis.

The children were studied in the home and in laboratory settings. By the age of two to two and one half, they were observed in structured laboratory observation settings along with a same-age, familiar playmate.

For the peer observations, interactions were assessed under conditions representing and/or evoking conflict, distress, frustration and enjoyment. After one to two months, the peer session was repeated. Among the responses coded during peer interactions were aggression, altruism, social interactions, and emotional expressiveness. After peer session observation, a mildly frustrating situation was established by an unfamiliar female adult to examine interactions between the children and a stranger, in a situation devised to assess aggression and altruism.

Responses coded during the structured situations, for both peer and adult situations, included noncompliance with the adult in a "frustration" sequence. Prosocial and related behaviors to simulated distress were coded in terms of altruism, caregiver role, prolonged physical orientation to distress, emotional concern, and the seeking of guidance or reassurance from the mother.

Results of the study indicated a number of differences between the children of bipolar families and the normal control children. Significantly, the researchers found that the children of depressed parents were preoccupied with the distress of others, suggesting that they are capable of some type of empathy. However, they displaced this affect by exhibiting aggression rather than altruism. In the area of antisocial behavior and aggression, sample children were more intensely aggressive and fought harder in an attempt to retrieve a toy that the adult had requested that they share. This group also manifested significantly higher levels of undirected aggression than the control group. In their reactions to peers, the children from bipolar families showed higher and more intense aggression toward peers during the period following separation from the mother. When these children were the victims of aggression, they tended to be passive recipients of the aggression. Comparing the total altruism scores for both groups, there was an evident differential with the sample children, who demonstrated less overall altruism toward peers, along with less sharing and helping behavior. The sample children were, however, less likely than the control children to seek maternal guidance or reassurance during observations of another's emotional state, supporting the idea that these children may not develop the motivational dimension necessary for the formation of guilt.

Though no differences were evident between the two groups when measuring emotional expressiveness and social interactions during peer play, there was a differential shift in emotions between the two groups. The sample displayed heightened emotionality during the simulation of anger, and lessened emotionality following a fight. The reverse was true for the control group.

Discussing the results of this study, the authors noted several significant differences between the sample and control children at age two. Those with a bipolar parent occasionally were less resilient, had more difficulty in interpersonal interactions, and experienced difficulty in dealing with hostile impulses:

. . . 1) they were sometimes inappropriately aggressive, hitting or grabbing from an unfamiliar adult, whereas control children tended to assume a more realistically cautionary or cooperative stance; 2) [after] separation from their mothers, they [were] likely to aggress against . . . playmates; and 3) they were . . . more inclined to respond to peer aggression with passivity. (Zahn-Waxler et al., 1984, p.119)

Additional findings suggest that sample children did not play or share with their friends as much as control children. Preoccupation with distress following simulations and an intense level of aggression toward playmates following separation characterized the control group. Another maladaptive behavior was observed after simulation of other's fights when diminished capacity for pleasure was noted. The authors commented that such examples suggest how dysphoria and anhedonia could evolve in hostile environments.

Barnett, King, and Howard (1979) also found some impairment in childhood prosocial behavior, as measured in generosity, by those who experienced distress personally. Their findings, although using a normal rather than at-risk population, are noteworthy. The researchers examined the differential effect that self- and other-directed affect has on subsequent generosity among a group of 85 children ages seven to 12 years. The children were asked to describe affect-loaded (happy, sad) or affect-neutral situations that they experienced directly, or that had been experienced by another child, using versions of the mood inducement procedure. Children were told that if they desired, they could share their experimental prize tokens with a less fortunate child. Results included the observation that children who described sad experiences encountered by another child shared significantly more than the children who reported sad incidents experienced by themselves. Older children shared more than the younger children, a finding consonant with other studies, suggesting that sharing is chronologically linked to development.

The authors wrote that, though previous research has disclosed the importance of the negative/positive affect orientation on prosocial behavior, the results of this study indicate that the *source* of the affect is "a crucial qualifying factor. Children who had discussed another child's personal misfortunes donated significantly more prize tokens to others than children who discussed personal misfortunes . . . [These] findings have . . . implications for . . . understanding the mood-altruism relationship and the role of empathy in children's . . . helping behavior" (Barnett et al., 1974, p. 167).

In a study conducted by Zahn-Waxler, Radke-Yarrow, and King (1979), mothers were trained to observe their children and to daily record their children's reactions and their own behaviors when encountering episodes of child-caused distress and distress in others. Situations where distress was simulated by the mothers and investigators were used as well.

Over a nine month period, 16 children from intact families were observed and tested twice. Mothers of these children were trained to detail discrete behaviors in the naturalistic home setting. They reported on the children's reactions to physical or psychological distress in others, i.e., in the children's presence someone expressed anger, fear, sorrow, pain, etc. Incidents in which the child caused the event or in which he or she was a bystander were recorded along with the child's reaction in distress simulations.

When the child caused distress, the mothers explicitly instructed the child that he or she had caused the distress in 40% of the recorded instances. Such explanations link the child's action to the emotional distress of the victim and are mainly affective messages with judgmental overtones. Verbal prohibitions or physical punishment were also recorded. In 32% of the incidents of child-caused distress, the child made reparation. The children of mothers who frequently explained the consequences of behavior (i.e., embellished the "basic cognitive message . . . with mother's intensity . . . judgmental reactions . . . convictions, and disappointments" [Zahn-Waxler et al., 1979, p. 325]) had significantly higher reparation rates than children whose mothers did not elaborate the message.

When the child was an innocent witness to others' distress, mothers were less active in explaining the situation to the child. The only frequent maternal response was providing reassurance. While mothers did not usually model altruism to the child's victims, they did so if the child witnessed the distress. In instances when the child was a bystander, he or she was altruistic in 34% of the cases.

The authors offered several hypotheses concerning the link between maternal behavior, emotional altruism of the children, and guilt induction:

The mother's . . . controlling techniques in disciplinary encounters may leave the child with [anxiety] about the self. Making the child feel responsible for . . . other's . . . grief may result in his continuing to feel responsible for [others'] grief . . . in other situations. The young child is . . . vulnerable to guilt induction since he may be less able to distinguish . . . his causal role from the bystander role. (Zahn-Waxler et al., 1979, p. 329)

Research appears to indicate that parents play a critical role in mediating not only a child's prospects for experiencing empathic distress, but how that distress is channeled.

Zahn-Waxler et al. (1979) suggest an important relationship between a child's prosocial behavior and parental role during distress. Children whose parents are depressed and fail to respond to distress, their own or others, may develop a negative cycle of social behavior, in a sense mimicking their parents' failure to respond empathically. The study of Zahn-Waxler et al. (1979) examined infants ages one and one half to two and one half years old and found a positive correlation between children's altruism and mother's role during distress. "How children cope with emotions of distress in others is significantly related to mother's practices specific to children's encounters with distress" (Zahn-Waxler et al., 1979, p. 327).

Conclusion

Determining the extent to which empathic distress may play a role in early development is crucial to infant and childhood developmental research. Hoffman's work offers insight into the developmental sequence that may lead from empathy to empathic distress. His approach incorporates both affective and cognitive components that are mutually reinforcing and evolve over time. Thus the potential for, and the characteristics of, empathic distress also evolve over time. Infancy may represent the period of greatest risk for the development of depression through empathic distress, since a young infant lacks the cognitive tools to differentiate his or her own affective state from that of others. Faced with the continued distress of others, the infant who has not attained some degree of person permanence may be unable to erect any defense against distress. As the infant's cognitive capacities develop through childhood, the potential for empathic distress from immediate expressional or situational cues may diminish in relation to the possibility of empathic distress from more sophisticated kinds of awareness, such as knowledge of another's general life condition.

Empathic development that has contributed to distress, even depression, in children may take an unusual developmental course leading to atypicalities in symptom expression. Whereas empathy, through guilt, is thought to provide the basis for prosocial action according to Hoffman, certain extreme situations may actually disable the motivational aspect of guilt and lead to antisocial rather than prosocial behavior. Children of depressed parents, for example, who lack parental models of empathic response, may thus experience their parents' affective state through empathic distress, but may respond to their own emotions with aggression and acting out.

CHAPTER 7

The Face-to-Face Interaction Paradigm

The face-to-face interaction paradigm is a dynamic experimental model from which researchers have extracted an abundance of data pertaining to the infant's early cognitive and affective development. Perhaps the most compelling finding emerging from face-to-face paradigm studies is the identification of a mutual regulation system forged between mother and infant in the early weeks of life. Thus, Stern (1974b) referred to the "common goal" shared by mothers and infants, permitting the "maintenance of . . . attention and arousal within some optimal range," while Lester, Hoffman, and Brazelton (1985) commented on the behavioral periodicities modulating mother-infant interaction. Brazelton, Koslowski, and Main (1974) coined the phrase "rhythms of exchange" to describe the interactions of the dyadic model.

These writings suggest that the behavior of mother and infant observed during a face-to-face interactive sequence may be viewed as a separate entity. It is as if caregiver and infant are engaged in a private game of intricate complexity and detail; the face-to-face model allows researchers to eavesdrop on this unique interaction.

Case Report

Marci was a congenitally blind infant. At two days of age she was evaluated on the Brazelton Neonatal Assessment Scale and videotaped during face-to-face interaction with her mother. Although Marci had difficulty controlling her crying, she was eventually consolable by tactile input and by her mother's soothing talk. She would raise her eyebrows, soften her cheeks, and make "ooh" faces. Upon hearing her mother's voice, Marci's movements would soften noticeably. At ten days of age Marci evinced a state of immobility occurring whenever there was auditory input from the environment. Initially her parents interpreted this immobility as a sign that Marci did not want to be disturbed. But Marci's mother soon recognized that the immobility was Marci's means of monitoring the environment. Thus, the mother developed a specific mode of interaction with her child. For example, Marci's mother would touch her infant softly and call her name. The mother's sharp insights into her infant's needs and her readiness to establish harmony was revealed by the comment that "[a] blind child can't hold attention; I have to do that for her" (Als, 1985, pp. 8–9).

When Marci was three weeks old, she and her mother were observed in rhythmic interaction during face-to-face encounters. Marci showed signs of organized attending, alternating with brief periods of disorganization. At two months, however, Marci's previous consolidating behavior ended abruptly. The infant became restless, she was easily upset, and was difficult to control. Disruption of the harmonious mother-infant exchange caused Marci's mother to become depressed. During this period, Marci's mother was encouraged to continue her efforts by the therapeutic team. By three and one half months, in spurt-like fashion, Marci emerged from the disorganization to display a gratifying, more complex level of stability. She oriented easily and smiled for prolonged periods. The "touch and sound" game of the early face-to-face interaction was now expanded to encompass longer time periods.

By four months, Marci's repertoire of responses to maternal cues was more fully developed and included vocalization, smiling, and complex sound and tactile games. Upon evaluation, the exchange was viewed as one of "complex differentiated interaction." Indications of a strong attachment within the dyad were evident. Marci would scream inconsolably when anyone other than her mother interacted with her. Her mother, however, was able to placate the infant by engaging in a playful diaper-changing routine. Marci's developmental progress continued during evaluations at seven and one half, nine, and 18 months. Locomotor activity and vocalization became increasingly more sophisticated. Marci's mother was particularly adept at deciphering her infant's signals.

Parental ability to deal with the brief period of immobility that Marci had displayed at 10 days of age suggested that Marci's parents were eager to establish contact with her. While Marci's progress was impressive, it was the nature of parental response that was notable. As witnessed during the face-to-face sequences, Marci and her parents built a mutually reinforcing system of harmonious interaction (Als, 1985).

Defining the Paradigm

The face-to-face paradigm is foremost a model of intimate exchange, generally involving only infant and caregiver. Thus, face-to-face models investigate dyadic behavior exclusively. Moreover, as its name implies, the paradigm relies on face-to-face interaction and is therefore concerned with behaviors emerging from this confrontational setting. The full spectrum of facial expressions and body movements are the markers researchers use to infer information about the infant's internal cognitive and affective development. Such cognitive barometers as gazing behavior and such affective responses as crying, smiling, or frowning are important variables in face-to-face investigations.

While it is difficult to arrive at an exact definition of the face-to-face paradigm, several researchers have described qualities of the model. Fogel, Diamond, Langhorst, & Demos (1982) identified eye contact as a key component. Patterson (1973) called face-to-face models sequences of behavior which shape mother-infant exchange. Crediting the paradigm with defining the developmental course of interaction, Cohn and Tronick (1983) stated that the model permits prediction of behaviors that allow differentiation between normal and at-risk infants. Labeling the face-to-face paradigm a "reciprocal interaction," Slee (1984) observed that it allows researchers the opportunity to examine the first dyadic communication system. Blehar, Lieberman, and Ainsworth (1977) used the paradigm to chart the "contingent pacing of interaction" between mother and infant.

Virtually all researchers using the model to acquire data on early infant cognitive and affective manifestations, as well as on maternal behavior patterns, have described some form of mutual regulatory system. Finally, the face-to-face model offers the advantage of a continuum of observation, enabling researchers to follow dyads over long periods, and to trace subtle chronological development.

While the face-to-face model provides clues to the developmental milestones of temperament and self-object representation, it should be emphasized that the paradigm creates a particularly ideal model for studying attachment and empathic behaviors. The "rhythms of exchange" formula coined by Brazelton et al. (1974) and the "reciprocal interaction " component identified by Blehar et al. (1977), each suggest ways of re-examining attachment behaviors. The model is also useful, however, for understanding temperament and self. It serves as a vehicle for revealing the mechanisms of affect regulation. Affect regulation, in turn, is suggestive of phenomena subsumed under the rubric of temperament dimensions. In addition, affect regulation has been identified as a prerequisite for the development of "self" by such researchers as Kopp (1982).

Thus, the face-to-face model directly contributes to understanding the role of attachment and empathic behaviors in shaping infant response, while evidence concerning the interplay of temperament dimensions and self-development may also be inferred from the model.

Model for Studying Depressive Dyadic Interaction

The paradigm has been used as an experimental model from which data about depressive phenomena have been collected. Since the face-to-face model is particularly suited to probing early infant capacities, researchers have been able to explore aberrant behavior resembling depression from the first weeks of life onward. Equally significant, because the paradigm requires confrontation between mother and infant, it has focused attention on depressive behavior as a characteristic of dyadic interaction. Such issues as whether depressive phenomena can be elicited by manipulating maternal behavior are appropriately examined within the context of the face-to-face paradigm. These investigations suggest that defects in the interaction between caregiver and infant may be a factor in the onset of depression.

Studies using the face-to-face paradigm to probe depressive-like phenomena include one by Cohn and Tronick (1983) involving 24 mother-infant dyads. Mothers were instructed to interact normally with their infants for three minutes. This sequence was followed by three minutes during which mothers simulated depression. While mothers simulated depression, infants exhibited a distinctive cycling pattern, typified by such negative signals as wariness, protest, and gaze aversion. Responses to simulated depression were indicative of "withdrawal and avoidance," and were in sharp contrast to the organized displays of positive affect shown during normal interaction.

Data from this study are valuable not only because they highlight the different infant responses to normal maternal interaction and simulated depression, but also because descriptions of infant response during simulated depression are reminiscent of the learned helplessness models of depression posited by Seligman (1975). Indeed, investigators have noted that lack of contingent interaction initiates the debilitative path of learned helplessness (Kevill & Kirkland, 1979) and the simulated depression sequence in the Cohn and Tronick study may be an analogue of noncontingent interaction.

Another face-to-face study, conducted by Field (1984a), compared infant response in dyads with a clinically depressed mother to infant response in clinically normal dyads where mothers simulated depression. Field's hypothesis was that infants subjected to repeated bouts of depressive interaction eventually acquire immunity to depression. The findings indicated that the infants subjected to simulated depression attempted to reinstate normal interaction, while the infants of clinically depressed mothers displayed significantly more resigned, passive behavior. Field's initial hypothesis, then, may have validity, since the study revealed marked behavioral deviations among the infants of the clinically depressed mothers.

In an investigation using home videotapes of mother-infant exchange, Massie (1978) discovered that parent-infant interaction was inappropriate from the earliest weeks of life for the majority of children who later developed psychotic pathology. Massie found that the constellation of behavior patterns previously identified as normative during face-to-face interaction—including eye contact, gazing, smiling, vocalizing—was conspicuously absent in cases where psychotic behavior later became evident.

These studies provide further insights into infant depressive behavior and suggest possible etiological factors, as well as diagnostic and treatment guidelines. To appreciate these insights fully, however, it is necessary to assess the basic data accumulated during face-to-face studies.

A brief description of how the developmental lines of temperament (as evidenced through affect regulation), self-object representation, and attachment may be identified within the paradigm is essential. A discussion of data involving the infant's visual-perceptual and affective capacities provides a foundation for hypotheses concerning the infant's internal mechanism, and by inference, the role temperament dimensions play in development. Studies focusing on caregiver response add to the composite picture of dyadic interaction, emphasizing the function of attachment behaviors. In addition, the dyadic system itself is reviewed, with particular focus on gazing behavior and infant responses to strangers. From this review, clues regarding the infant's incipient sense of self may be gleaned.

Developmental Lines That Delineate Infant Depression

General investigations of infant behavior have disclosed several recurrent developmental lines or milestones that have facilitated research efforts to chart levels of maturity. These include: evidence of affect and affect regulation, which correlates with the development of temperament; evidence of imitation behavior, indicating self-object representation; and evidence of attachment, a critical product of infant interaction. The face-to-face paradigm has proven particularly fruitful in clarifying the significance of these milestones.

Affect and Affect Regulation

Izard, Huebner, Risser, McGuinness, and Dougherty (1980) documented the broad spectrum of infant affective capacities during face-to-face interaction, clearly identifying interest, joy, surprise, disgust, anger, contempt, sadness, and fear. In response to events testing "incentive" in 54 infants age one- to nine-months, these affect expressions were identified by the Maximally Discriminative Facial Movement Coding System (MAX).

Field (1977) isolated another aspect of emotional displays, noting that mutual affective regulation provides caregiver and infant with optimal affective stimulus. The mother stimulates the infant sufficiently to maintain an optimal range of arousal. The mother's timing and the infant's optimal state of arousal facilitate mutual engagement (Stern, 1974b).

The message of the face-to-face paradigm is that both infant and caregiver should be encouraged to maintain a reciprocal and contingent interchange, or to modify one that is noncontingent and inappropriate. This conceptualization contrasts sharply with the Learned Helplessness model, which predicts that expectations of non-contingency transfer across tasks

(Seligman, 1975). In contrast, mutual affect regulation may reinforce expectations of contingency and affect displays may represent contingent responses to maternal behavior. In fact, the identification of affect displays in the face-to-face paradigm may have value in predicting future abnormalities of interaction.

Specific affects—such as happiness, fear, or anger—have been related to temperament dimensions. Happiness and pleasure, for example, may be measured by the temperament dimension of "smiling and laughter," whereas anger is evaluated by the dimension of "distress to limitations" (Rothbart, 1981). The connection between affect and temperament is pointed out here because affect displays and signs of affect regulation evinced during the face-to-face paradigm may be categorized as indicative of the temperamental predisposition infants bring into the interactive dyad.

Self-Object Representation

Studies of imitative behavior have been the most common means of assessing infant capacity for self-object representation. In a study of imitation response using happy, surprised, and sad facial expressions, Field, Woodson, and Greenberg (1982) observed the visual fixations of neonates on an adult face. The investigators found that neonates with an average age of 26 hours discriminated among these three facial expressions. The same neonates also demonstrated an ability to imitate the facial expressions, as shown through movements in the regions of the brow, eyes, and mouth.

Another study of imitation, designed by Meltzoff and Moore (1983), presented mouth-opening and tongue protrusion gestures to 40 healthy newborns (ages 42 minutes to 71 hours). Twenty-six of the infants produced more mouth-opening responses to mouth-opening displays than to tongue displays. Twelve produced more mouth-opening responses to the tongue displays, and two produced an equal number of mouth-opening responses to both displays. The authors stated that the infants did not immediately display perfectly matching responses, seeming rather to correct their responses over successive efforts. These findings appear to eliminate the possibility of a rigid and stereotypic, ingrained motor routine in neonates. Thus, imitation behavior observed within the face-to-face paradigm assumes a new dimension: it may be contingent on the development of mutual reinforcing cues communicated between caregiver and infant. Both Field et al. (1982) and Meltzoff and Moore (1983) suggested that what might generate these imitations is the infant's innate ability to compare sensory information gained from visually perceived expressions with proprioceptive information about their own unseen body movements to their internal representations of visually perceived modes, suggesting the incipient development of a sense of self.

In another study investigating the parameters of imitative skills between birth and six months, Fontaine (1984) examined 84 infants ranging in age from 21 to 167 days. The infants were presented with four facial models (tongue protrusion, mouth opening, cheeks swelling, and eyes closing) and with two manual models (opening-closing of the hand and pointing of the index finger). Only the facial models elicited an imitative response.

Imitation behavior, indicative of the developing sense of self, may also play a role in the infant's growing awareness of discrepancy in the environment. Meltzoff and Moore (1983) observed that imitative behavior does not imply a perfect mirroring response. Rather, through repeated, successive attempts, the infant refines his or her behavior until a response resembling the behavior to be imitated is achieved. Imitation may then serve as a prelude for the infant's later awareness of contingency and non-contingency relationships. As is noted in Chapter 8, contingency awareness may be a determinative factor in the etiology of depression.

Attachment Behavior

Studies on the development of the infant's attachment to the people in his or her environment have underscored the importance of the human face as a stimulus for the infant (Bowlby, 1958; Gewirtz, 1961). The face-to-face paradigm, therefore, becomes an ideal method for studying the ramifications of attachment behavior.

Bowlby (1958) described the development of an infant's first relationship through the five behaviors of crying, smiling, sucking, clinging, and following, as innate stimulators of maternal caregiving responses. Robson (1967) added eye contact as a sixth variable. Exline (1982) stated that "the combination of gaze with facial and vocal expressiveness . . . could serve to create in the infant a tie to the mother's face" (p. 168). The face-to-face paradigm presents researchers with a unique opportunity to explore this phenomenon of the early development of attachment behaviors and to isolate aberrations in this developmental line, suggestive of depressive-like phenomena.

Infant's Perspective

The face-to-face paradigm is particularly suited to acquiring information about the infant at a relatively early age (many studies involve neonates just a few hours old). By amassing information on the early visual-perceptual capacities and affective responses of very young infants, researchers are creating a profile of normal and deviant development.

The visual-perceptual faculties in the following studies may be viewed as the basic biological apparatus that infants bring into the dyadic exchange. This biological apparatus is dependent largely on innate, constitutional factors. While these studies outline the typical spectrum of visual-perceptual capacity experienced by most infants, individual deviations from these norms may be attributed to temperament. That is, temperament (i.e., the unique behavioral style of each individual infant) impinges on the biological apparatus. Thus, the behavioral response displayed in part signifies the individual temperamental profile each infant brings into the dyadic exchange.

Infant Visual-Perceptual Faculty

A summary of the developmental course of the infant's discriminatory and preferential visual-perceptual capacities is appropriate when exploring manifestations encountered in the face-to-face paradigm. Several studies have begun to establish the infant's visual-perceptual capacity, have verified infant preference for facial as opposed to non-facial stimuli, and have identified the ability of the infant to discriminate among facial stimuli. Data generated by these studies have enabled researchers to sketch a portrait of normal visual-perceptual capacities during early infant life, often within a few hours of birth. With the articulation of developmental norms of infant capacity, the potential for identifying deviations and pathologies becomes evident. Thus, studies of this type may eventually yield specific diagnostic criteria for infant depression.

Early reports of the central visual acuity of newborns suggested widely disparate estimates of the infant's visual competence, while reports of Snellen acuity at birth have also varied. However, more definitive data on visual acuity were provided when Dayton et al. (1964) used electrooculography in 39 full-term infants with a mean age of one day. Results were obtained in 32 infants and confirmed that some infants may have visual acuity of at least 20 to 150. Summarizing, the authors concluded: "[v]isual acuity in infants is at least 20 to 150 and may be even better. This level of acuity is adequate for a modicum of binocular vision in newborn infants" (p. 869). Active peripheral vision was illustrated by Harris and MacFarlane (1974), who showed that the neonatal visual field runs from a minimum angle of 25 degrees from the center of fixation to the periphery.

A key to understanding infant visual-perceptual capacity was the finding that normal full-term neonates are capable of selective visual attention to patterned stimulation (Fantz, 1963, 1965; Salapatek, 1969). Fantz (1963) reported that infants under five days of age possess an innate ability to perceive form, as shown by their consistent attraction to black and white patterns more than to plain colored surfaces. Moreover, selective visual responses of these infants were clearly keyed more to pattern than to color or reflection, even though the latter variances have frequently been viewed as primary visual stimuli. Other studies have supported this conclusion (Fantz, 1965, 1966; Stechler, 1964; Stirnimann, 1944).

Fantz and Miranda (1975) discovered that infants under seven days old selectively fixed on curved contours rather than straight patterns. The researchers inferred the existence of a general discrimination ability, such that neonates can distinguish form of contour from time of birth.

In another study of infant development, Antell and Keating (1983) evaluated 40 normal, healthy neonates between 21 and 144 hours old to determine how well they could discriminate between two different visual stimulus arrays. One array consisted of two versus three black dots, while the other contained four versus six black dots. These infants could discriminate between the smaller number of dots, but not between the sets containing four versus six or the inverse. This result indicated neonatal ability to abstract numerical invariance in small-set arrays, and may provide evidence of complex information processing during the first week of life.

Relying on the already demonstrated preference of newborns and two month old infants for patterned versus non-patterned stimuli, Adams and Maurer (1984) assessed contrast sensitivity between these two groups of infants. The researchers found that while newborns are far more sensitive to contrast than previously anticipated, two month olds are more sensitive than newborns. Interestingly enough, however, at two months of age increasing contrast did not increase preference among these children. Included in the study were 60 infants between one and five days old. Stimuli took the form of six 2×2 checkerboards, with luminance contrast within each checkerboard. Also employed were plain gray squares with four equal-luminance quadrants matching the luminance of the checkerboards. The neonates were shown both the checkerboards and the gray squares. When the older children were compared with the neonates, greater ability to detect contrasts was noted. While the newborn infants clearly preferred checkerboards over matched gray squares (and the more contrast the better) the two month old infants demonstrated no such preference.

These investigations imply that the infant possesses a rudimentary mechanism for performing discriminatory and preferential functions dating from birth. With age, the infant's visual-perceptual apparatus grows in complexity, becoming an exquisitely tuned instrument for exercising responses to varied stimuli.

Visual-Perceptual Discrimination

The discovery of the infant's visual-perceptual capacity to discriminate, between faces or among the features of one face, has given researchers another diagnostic tool for charting cognitive development from its earliest inception. Evidence of discriminatory capacity implies that the infant is able to discern subtle differences from a very early age. Implicit in the notion of discrimination is the idea that eventually choices can be made and that selection among stimuli may be purposeful. Moreover, studies defining the parameters of the infant's normal potential may suggest deviant discriminatory capacity, a sign of depressive and other pathological phenomena.

Evidence of discriminatory behavior was found within the first weeks of life by Haith, Bergman and Moore (1977). Their study involved 24 infants from three to 11 weeks old. Infants were shown faces of their mothers and a stranger in still, moving, and speaking position. When mothers began to speak, scanning in the eye area intensified among the infants. From this behavior the researchers inferred the presence of an incipient discriminatory mechanism.

Other discrimination trials have shown that infants of three and one half weeks old can fixate on the eyes of a real face (Wolff, 1963). Maurer and Salapatck (1976) reported on developmental changes noted in scanning the faces of six infants at one month of age and six infants at two months of age. Each infant was presented with the faces of the mother, a female stranger, and a male stranger, while the infant's eye movements were observed. Younger infants fixated away from the faces, and looked at strangers more than at the mothers. The older infants fixated on the faces, and spent more time on facial features, especially the eyes. Additionally, the older infants fixated on the eyes more than the mouth when compared with the younger group.

From these investigations it may be postulated that older infants are more apt to look at the discrete details of an object and to choose those features with greatest contrast. It has also been suggested that as they grow older infants tend to invest special meaning in the eyes, since mothers often attempt to establish eye contact with infants. This latter interpretation was made by Robson (1967) and concurs with findings by Ames (1975) that infants look longer at faces with open eyes, and by Ahrens (cited in Mauer & Salapatek, 1976), who noted that infants smile only at faces containing two eyes.

Maurer and Barrera (1981) studied infant perceptions of natural and distorted schematic faces, using visual preference habituation techniques on infants one and two months old. The infants were shown schematic drawings of faces arranged naturally, symmetrically but scrambled, and asymmetrical and scrambled. The older infants were able to discriminate between all three variations, while the younger did not discriminate between any of them. The older infants demonstrated a preference for the faces that were arranged naturally, which was not the case with the younger ones. Thus, by the age of two months, infants may well be capable of recognizing the natural schematic arrangement of the human face.

The two month olds were also able to discern differences between two scrambled faces. Their preference for the normal arrangement of facial features was demonstrated by the fact that they spent more time looking at normal faces than at symmetrically scrambled ones. In contrast, one month olds did not discriminate between different facial arrangements.

Visual-Perceptual Preference

As with visual-perceptual discriminatory capacity, visual–perceptual preferential capacity represents yet another aspect of the infant's early cognitive mechanism. Indications of preferential behavior add a further nuance to understanding the infant's cognitive capacities, because expressions of preference clearly embody the concepts of intentionality and purposefulness. From such studies, the precise age of preferential onset may be targeted, and inferences may be made about the internal and external variables motivating behavior. Finally, just as discriminatory capacity suggested norms of behavior and implicit clues to deviant response, so too do preferential studies alert investigators to both expected manifestations and to variant responses that may signal pathology.

Investigations of the development of preferential capacities have revealed that infants can manifest an active attentional selective process in their visual preferences when looking at certain visual stimuli. In substantiating this phenomenon, Fantz (1973) found that one of the most preferred visual stimuli in one week old infants was a human face.

The finding that four month old infants pay selective attention to a face, rather than to geometric patterns, was demonstrated by McCall and Kagan (1967). Four stimuli were presented on three-dimensional sculpted faces, painted in flesh tones, and labeled "regular," "scrambled," "no eyes," and "blank." Infants were observed through one-way windows and coded independently according to smiling, vocalization responses, and fixation on the stimuli. Smiles were recorded with significantly greater frequency in reaction to the regular face than to the variant faces.

Gibson (1969) noticed that four month old infants undergo a significant transition in facial perception as they begin to discern the invariant relationships that exist between facial features. As this occurs, infants respond more to the configuration of features than to individual features. Cohen, DeLoache, and Strauss (1979) confirmed this with studies demonstrating that by four months of age infants are able to respond to faces as entire entities rather than as isolated features, and that infant responses to face-like stimuli are based on the similarity of the stimulus to the human face.

Caron, Caron, Caldwell, and Weiss (1973) studied how four and five month old infants discriminated between elemental and structural facial features. The infants were first shown a distorted schematic face. Next, the infants were shown an intact face. The study provided clear evidence that for four month old infants, the eyes were a more salient facial feature than the nose or mouth; they perceived both eyes, paired horizontally, as a structured unit; the entire head, including hair and facial contours, was more important than the inner facial pattern; they did not perceptually organize the invariant arrangement of eyes, nose, and mouth as facial elements. By contrast, for the five month old infants, the researchers reported that the mouth had become as salient a feature as the eyes, that the head no longer predominated over the inner facial contours, and that the configuration of the face itself had come to represent a distinct visual entity. The fact that the four month old infants could not discriminate inverted inner faces, the horizontal nose-mouth arrangement, or a scrambled nose and mouth from a normal face, suggests that they are not yet able to perceive faces as distinct entities. These findings corroborate Fagan's (1972) observation that infants do not discriminate between different faces until they are five and one half months old.

Ahrens (cited in Mauer & Salapatek, 1976) observed that through the fifth month of age, two-dimensional schematic representations of the face were effective in eliciting smiles. By six to seven months, infants can discriminate between two faces of the same sex (Cohen, DeLoache, & Pearl, 1977; Kagan, 1976). As infants reach six months of age, they are able to discern two different views of the same person. While infants paid more attention to different representations of a familiar face, they recognized that the two faces had something in common. LaBarbera, Izard, Vietze, and Parisi (1976) used a visual habituation paradigm to demonstrate that infants ages four to six months old could distinguish between joy and anger, as well as joy and a neutral expression in photographs of a single model.

Fagan (1976) exposed infants to photos of faces that were paired with other faces to demonstrate that infants can recognize faces at the age of seven months. In the first two experiments, infants were able to discriminate the face of one man from another, as well as the pose of one face from another. In further experiments, variants of the previously exposed face were employed as a familiar target to determine whether the infants were able to identify it during recognition testing. The infants responded familiarly to a man's face, which they had seen earlier in a different pose. Moreover, the infants were able to discern between male and female characteristics by identifying familiar faces shown earlier in different poses. Nelson, Morse, and Leavitt (1979) established that infants seven months old could discriminate among the photographs of happy and fearful faces of several adults.

Lewis (1969) used a cross-sectional design to study 120 infants, broken into four groups of 15 males and 15 females, and studied at the ages of 12 weeks, 36 weeks, and 57 weeks. As stimuli, he used a normal face, a cyclops face, a schematic face, and a scrambled face. These stimuli were blinded to the independent observers who recorded fixation times. The male infants spent significantly longer periods with these stimuli than the females. Interest in the facial stimuli decreased as the infants, irrespective of sex, grew older. Grouping all ages together, the infants preferred the stimuli in the following order: regular, schematic, cyclops, and scrambled. It is noteworthy that data showed that the most realistic stimulus, the regular face, attracted decreasing interest through the first year of age, while the least realistic stimulus, the scrambled face, attracted increasing interest with age. The infants spent significantly longer time smiling at the stimuli during the second six months than during the first; significantly, more smiling time was given to the regular and schematic faces than to the cyclops and scrambled faces. Vocalization data showed that as the infants grew older, a monotonic increase in vocalization was noted. Throughout the study, age differences showed that facial stimuli produced significantly less fixation, although the same stimuli produced significantly more vocalization and smiling. The realistic faces drew more vocalization and smiling than distorted faces.

The evidence accumulated from these studies confirms a general infant visual–perceptual preference for facial stimuli. Certainly by four months of age infants are capable of responding to facial dimension, prefer regular over scrambled and other aberrant faces, and can discern basic facial expression. The investigations indicate that by seven months infants not only recognize individual faces, but can discriminate between emotional expressions. The responses of infants, who are demonstrably equipped with intricate visual-perceptual capacity, therefore assume a new significance. These responses may be studied, for example, as a barometer of normal development, and may provide many clues for identifying phenomena that portend a depressive reaction.

Affective Response

The relationship between affect and temperament has been noted by several researchers (Buss & Plomin, 1975; Ekman, Friesen, & Ellsworth, 1972; Izard, 1977; Rothbart, 1981; Thomas, Chess, Birch, Hertzig, & Korn, 1963). The following studies discuss affective response to facial stimuli. In reviewing these investigations the role of affect, as a marker of temperament, should be kept in mind.

Investigations of affective response in infants have offered a plethora of data pointing to the existence of an infant apparatus designed to communicate emotional manifestations present in the early months of life. Not only has it been shown that infants recognize and discriminate among a wide range of external emotive behaviors, but that they also react to these affects by exhibiting parallel affective responses, suggesting a complex and rich internal array of affects.

Within the face-to-face interaction paradigm, manipulation of external facial expressions—by the presentation of facial facsimiles, by caregiver facial variation, or by other displays of adult facial patterns—has played a vital role in the methodology of experiments. By observing how external facial expressions can provoke affective and cognitive responses from the infant, researchers have acquired a more profound understanding of the normative emotive exchange that occurs between infant and caregiver. Careful delineation of normal affective reactions may lead researchers to diagnostic clues regarding deviant affect, as well as to a formulation of treatment techniques for affective abnormalities.

Newborn infants can produce all the muscle movements involved in generating characteristic adult facial patterns (Oster, 1978). The presence of facial templates for a number of discrete emotions has been demonstrated. Observing infants one to nine months old, both trained and untrained judges could recognize the characteristic facial expressions associated with interest, joy, surprise, sadness, disgust, anger, and fear (Campos, Barrett, Lamb, Goldsmith, & Stenberg, 1983; Izard et al., 1980).

Polak, Emde, and Spitz (1964) examined the "smiling response" by presenting infants with the real face of the experimenter nodding at a rate of approximately once every two seconds, as well as a life-size color cutout photo of his or her face nodding at the same rate. When the infants were two months to three months old, their smiles appeared more quickly, were stronger, and lasted longer in response to the real face than to the photograph, suggesting that the human face has positive social reinforcing value as the one aspect of an infant's environment that responds directly to him or her.

Young-Browne, Rosenfeld, and Horowitz (1977) studied discrimination of sad, happy, and surprised facial expressions among 24 infants aged three months. Infants were first habituated to a set facial expression, and then another expression was presented to them. After their response to the second expression decreased, a third expression was introduced. Increases in looking time after presentation of new expressions were used as a measure of discrimination. The infants showed significant capacity to discriminate between the surprised faces and the happy faces, and occasionally the ability to distinguish between the surprised and sad faces. Conclusions were based on a comparison of the experiment infants with a control group of 12 no-stimulus change infants.

Commenting on the results of the study, the researchers observed:

. . . the fact that such subtle stimulus changes are even noticed by young infants has implications for the role of facial expressions during parent-infant interactions and for the later association of appropriate emotional responses with different facial expressions. It is now conceivable that facial expressions displayed by parents could come to function as discriminative stimuli for appropriate emotional responses at a very early age. (Young-Browne et al., 1977, p. 561)

Barrera and Maurer (1981) conducted an investigation into facial expressions perceived by infants at three months of age. They broke their study into two experiments. The first used habituation to determine whether the infants could discriminate between smiling and frowning expressions on their mothers' faces. At three months, infants were able to discriminate smiling (happy) faces from frowning (angry) faces, and to recognize the difference between the two expressions, at least when presented by the mothers.

In the second experiment, the same technique was used to assess discrimination between smiling and frowning female strangers. Results indicated that the infants were able to discern between these expressions with the strangers as well. Infants in both experiments discriminated between smiling and frowning expressions. A greater incidence of infant discrimination was noted toward the mother than toward the strangers, however, indicating that discrimination between the mother's expressions might have been easier for the infants.

In addition, Malatesta and Haviland (1982), for example, found that mothers model primarily positive affects, and they observed that positive affect displays may be discriminated earlier because they are more frequently seen and thus less novel. The significance of the negative emotional expressions of the infants cannot be clearly ascertained from the first experiment of Barrera and Maurer. The fear and sadness displays may be less aversive than the anger display and, therefore, not as frequently avoided. Or perhaps fear and sadness, unlike anger, do not signal either a reduction of or break in face-to-face contact.

In conclusion, by using the paired-comparison novelty technique, the researchers demonstrated that five month old infants can discriminate facial displays of emotion by visual means alone, and that the reactions to photographs parallel the infant reactions seen in actual mother-infant interactions.

Nelson and Dolgin (1985) studied the ability of seven month old infants to distinguish facial expressions of four adult models displaying happy and fearful emotions. The researchers showed that the infants could generalize their discrimination of the two expressions across the four models if the happy faces were presented first, but not if the fearful faces were presented first. In a follow-up experiment, 32 additional seven month old infants looked significantly longer at the fearful faces, when poses by the same model were presented simultaneously.

The emotions of joy, anger, and neutral expressions were studied by LaBarbera et al. (1976) in 12 infants at four months of age and 12 infants at six months of age. The mother of each subject sat in front of a translucent screen, holding her infant in such a way that the screen was readily visible. A series of 19 slides was then projected from the rear for each infant. The first, second, and third slides showed neutral, joyous, and angry facial expressions. The four month old infants looked at these images longer than did the older children.

The authors demonstrated in their analysis that the joyous expressions ranked significantly higher in looking time among these infants than did the neutral or angry expressions, with virtually no difference in looking time between neutral and angry. Both groups of subjects in this study were able to discriminate the joyous from the angry and neutral expressions, both groups spent more time looking at the joyous expression than at the other two, indicating that both groups recognized joy as an emotion.

This may be attributable to a perception of positive reward values in the joyous expression or to lack of awareness of, or inability to recognize, the adverse message contained in the expression of anger.

In an earlier work, Izard (1971) gave insights concerning infant affect recognition, which his later findings reconfirmed. He suggested that the biological mechanisms behind particular discrete emotions begin to function when emotion becomes part of the adaptive life of the infant. The recognition of joy as an emotion can become its own self-fulfilling reward for the infant. If that recognition draws the infant into expressions of joy, the recognition can also serve to reinforce bonding between infant and mother by fostering mutually enjoyable experiences. It seems reasonable to conclude from this work that the threats implicit in expressions of anger would require coping responses not yet available to a six month old infant.

Cardiac Response

In addition to measuring cognitive and affective infant response to facial stimuli, a number of studies have used cardiac fluctuation as an indicator of infant response. These studies have generally sought to correlate cardiac changes with other observed criteria, such as visual-perceptual response or affect manifestation. Use of cardiac monitoring within the face-to-face paradigm has significant implications. By broadening the arsenal of diagnostic tools available, cardiac response increases appreciation of the myriad behavioral capabilities of the infant, and provides another means of defining the boundaries of normal and abnormal infant phenomena.

Cardiac response provides the researcher with a tool for probing the internal self-regulatory mechanism of the infant. Also, because cardiac alterations correlate with affective factors and with the degree of environmental receptivity, these measurements may suggest modes whereby temperament (as evidenced through affect), attachment (as evidenced through environmental receptivity), and emerging self (as evidenced through the regulation of cardiac patterns) are interwoven to create a particular infant response.

Finlay and Ivinskis (1984) reported that cardiac changes have often been used to study infant perceptions. Deceleration of heart rate is generally taken to indicate that the perceptual system is becoming more receptive to environmental stimulation (Graham, 1979). In contrast, cardiac acceleration apparently signals a condition of non-receptivity to environmental events.

A normal face, another in which the eyes, nose, and mouth had been rearranged, a face with no eyes, and a blank face were presented to a group of infants by Kagan, Henker, Hen-Tov, Levine, and Lewis (1966). The authors observed that fixation times to the normal and rearranged faces were similar, although smiling and significant decreases in heart rate occurred more often in response to the normal face. Cardiac deceleration was greatest in response to the normal face at four months of age, but by eight months, deceleration was greatest in response to the scrambled face, indicating the older infants were more open to novelty than were their younger peers.

Sophisticated investigations among older infants have suggested that cardiac alterations may also correlate with the expression of negative affect. Vaughn and Sroufe (1979), for example, observed 16 infants, eight to 16 months old, whose heart rates were recorded telemetrically during a face-to-face paradigm. After baseline heart rates were obtained, mothers positioned behind a screen played peek-a-boo with their babies. After an infant showed signs of positive engagement, the mother appeared from behind the screen and called the infant's name while wearing a full-face mask. She then returned behind the screen and repeated the peek-a-boo game. Finally, the mother called the infant's name at the same time as a stranger emerged wearing the same mask. Five seconds later the stranger removed the mask and approached the infant closely.

Each infant showed a crying face prior to the actual onset of crying. At onset, the heart rate was faster in 14 subjects than before crying. The sequence progressed from fixed attention in response to the incongruous event to a crying face and crying. There were clear heart rate accelerations in response to the incongruous event. Heart rate acceleration occurred during the latter part of the attentive phase. The heart rate was 12 beats faster than baseline. Heart rate acceleration following the onset of crying was pronounced in every case, at times by more than 30 beats. The researchers concluded that heart rate acceleration is not only a by-product of crying, but is also associated with negative affect that precedes crying.

Caregiver's Perspective

During face-to-face interaction, caregiver response to infant affect may yield significant clues about the phenomenon of infant depression. Since newborns lack the verbal competence necessary to provide subjective data on their internal state, the researcher is forced to devise objective criteria when assessing infant affective or cognitive response. By contrast, when the responses of a caregiver are considered, the researcher can rely not only on objective criteria, but can incorporate the caregiver's subjective impression as further evidence of the infant's internal mechanism.

By comparing caregiver subjective impressions with an objective assessment, the researcher can examine the role of the caregiver in initiating and reinforcing infant affective and cognitive response. The caregiver perspective then can offer deeper insights into the etiology of infant depression. Indeed, caregiver responses may be deemed vital "markers" in the attempt to delineate the precise boundaries of infant depressive-like phenomena.

Although the face-to-face paradigm yields clues regarding the impact of temperament and self-object representation on infant development, it is in the realm of attachment behaviors (as witnessed by the "contingent pacing of interaction" (Blehar et al., 1977) and "reciprocal interaction" (Slee, 1984) that the model offers its greatest insights. The following studies suggest ways in which infant behavior is determined by the type of attachment bond formed with the caregiver.

In a study designed by Johnson, Emde, Pannabecker, Steinberg, & Davis (1982), the researchers collected data on the frequency with which mothers accurately perceived emotions in their infants. Mothers of 597 infants ranging in age from one to 18 months provided current and retrospective estimates of the onset of infant emotion. Unexpectedly, these young infants displayed a significant number and variety of emotions: a majority of mothers reported observing interest, joy, surprise, anger, and distress in their infants. Moreover, most of the mothers perceived these emotions during the first three months of life, and reported distinct emotions in infants quite early. This study adds data not only on the early emotional development of infants, but also hints that maternal perceptions may play an influential developmental role.

Maternal perceptions of infant affective reactions formed part of a cross-sectional investigation by Johnson and Moeller (1972), involving 611 mothers of infants whose ages ranged from birth to 18 months. Striking among the findings was that the mothers perceived several discrete emotions, including interest, enjoyment, and distress by three months of age. Most of the mothers also identified surprise (69%), anger (86%), and fear (69%) by the same age.

These two studies suggest that three months may be a maturational threshold for a child, at least from the maternal perspective. By this point in an infant's development, the caregiver is then able to identify a significant number and variety of emotional responses in the infant and to discriminate among these discrete emotions.

A longitudinal investigation by Klinnert, Sorce, Emde, and Svejda (1984) explored changes that occur over time in caregivers' perceptions of their infants' emotions. Using 34 mother-infant dyads, the researchers studied the infant target ages of three, six, nine, 12, 15 and 18 months. Emotions were assessed by means of a questionnaire designed to determine whether mothers could isolate these emotions at three month intervals. Available data were limited to the emotions of surprise, fear, and anger.

All mothers identified interest and enjoyment in their infants from the age of three months onward. Ninety-one percent of mothers reported the presence of surprise and anger by that age; 100% of mothers observed these emotions by 18 months. Fear was present in 65% of the infants at three months; 97% of mothers reported this emotion at 18 months.

Overall, the high correlation between the Johnson and Klinnert data has significant implications: the replication of similar results confirms the validity and reliability of caregiver-supplied data on emotional identification. Klinnert's work also allows for the inference that a signal system was established by three months of age whereby infants communicated certain affective states to their mothers through specific behavior patterns, and mothers responded appropriately.

Applying this signal model to the surprise response, for example, it was found that between the ages of three and 18 months facial expressions were the most common behavioral indicators of this emotion, closely followed by motor reactions. The latter reactions were often detected as jumps, although most mothers noticed the Moro reflex or elements of this reflex, such as throwing the arms back or arching the back.

The researchers also discovered that crying was the most common infant signal of fear. As was found with the behavioral responses indicative of surprise, motor reactions were the second most common response. In addition, about half of the mothers commented on red-faced expressions in their infants, while most of the other mothers reported such motor responses as kicking or back arching. Crying was the distinct signal for differentiating between fear and surprise at three months. Clearly then, at this early age, a system is fully in place whereby the infant cries and is soothed by the mother. This aspect of the signal network was continuously observed through the study, and appeared to achieve the goal of physical proximity between mother and infant. The three month olds also used crying to express the affective response of anger, although some mothers distinguished these cries by labeling them as "hard," "loud," or "forceful." At nine months, approximately 25% of mothers reported that their infants expressed anger by intentionally pushing the caregiver away.

Despite variations among certain aspects of emotional behavior observed, it was apparent that the affective signaling system provided continuity between the mothers and infants during the period studied. Embraced within the system of signaling were identifiable affective behavior patterns manifested by the infants. The reports of the mother suggested that facial expressions formed only a part of the signaling repertoire of the infants, indicating that such expressions may be components of a broader emotional network of exchange.

Contingent and reciprocal interactions most likely contribute considerably to the infant's experience, as well as enhance the overall quality of emotional experience. This emotional signaling system may serve as a mechanism through which infants acquire the continuity essential for developing a sense of self. Further monitoring of this signaling system may offer more understanding of how caregiver perceptions may influence, promote, or channel the development of self-object representation in both its normal manifestations and in manifestations suggestive of inchoate depressive phenomena.

Mutual Dyadic Interactive Mechanism: General Dyadic Behavior

As a method of obtaining data about the young infant's capacity for interaction with the caregiver figure, the dyadic model has proven to be a durable and fruitful investigatory tool. Observations of behavior patterns exhibited within the dyadic model led Lewis (1969) to assert that the infant constructs a schema of the maternal face that gradually becomes integrated by three months of age. Accepting the existence of such schemata, Stern (1974b) theorized that a multiplicity of schematic diagrams is created, enabling the infant to maintain an internal assortment of spatial configurations and varying facial patterns derived from the external world.

Studies using this model have also given researchers a telescopic view of the behavioral dynamics that emerge during the infant's primary and seminal relationship. By creatively monitoring play sessions, Stern discerned a rhythmic pattern of interaction between caregiver and infant. The main goal of the interaction was the regulation of perceptual input. Lester et al. (1985) have recently refined this analysis and described rhythmic interaction in the face-to-face paradigm as a series of "coordinated cycles of affective display which may be operationally defined as synchrony." Brazelton et al. (1974) similarly observed the "rhythms of exchange" permeating the dyadic model, and isolated specific infant strategies for coping with unpleasant stimuli, along with counterpart maternal responses to such strategies.

All of these studies used a dyadic or face-to-face interaction paradigm between caregiver and infant. The data gleaned from these investigations create a composite portrait that highlights the astonishing versatility, adaptability, and resilience of the infant's internal mechanism. The dyadic model has also permitted researchers to trace the evolution of the infant's internal mechanism chronologically.

Based on data accumulated from a dyadic model, Lewis (1969) assumed that the infant develops a schema of the mother's face by the age of three months. Stern extended this hypothesis to encompass many different schemata, which develop from interactive play and begin to take form as they integrate into the infant's grasp of the surrounding environment. In Stern's play sessions between infants and their mothers, a simulated game called "pre-peek-a-boo" was played. The infant looks at the mother and smiles, vocalizes, and displays increasing arousal and positive affect, including heightened motor activity. As the game becomes more intense, the infant begins to show signs of displeasure, fleeting sobriety, and moments in which grimaces replace the smiles. This behavior continues to progress, until the infant suddenly looks away sharply, turning the head quickly so that the face of the mother remains in peripheral view as the level of intensity declines. Following this behavior, the infant's gaze returns to the mother as the level of intensity seen earlier begins to increase again, accompanied by smiling, arousal, and renewed positive affect. At this point, the infant again averts his or her gaze from the mother. This process repeats itself until the infant is clearly modulating states of arousal and affect within definite limits, and regulating levels of perceptual input.

Play activity has as its goal the mutual regulation of stimuli in order to maintain the positive affect gained by maintenance of optimal levels of arousal, according to Stern. The infant's contribution to regulating this level of stimulus is primarily through control of gazing. The infant learns how to adapt to novelty and complexity within familiar contexts, partially as a result of face-to-face play in which the caregiver provides ever-changing facial expressions, voice tone, and movements. Through an evolving process in which the caregiver engages, relaxes, and re-engages the infant in response to his or her cues, the infant is able to learn how to maintain organized behavior when faced with increasing degrees of arousal (Brazelton et al., 1974; Stern, 1974b).

Lester et al. (1985) quantified the social interaction rhythms in 20 three and five month old term and pre-term infants and their mothers, by videotaping the caregiver dyads in a three-minute face-to-face paradigm. Each face-to-face interaction may be described as a sequentially segmented, structured system of reciprocally regulated positive and negative cycles of attention and affect. These coordinated cycles of affect display were defined as "synchrony," which was assumed to develop as a consequence of each partner's learning the rhythmic structure of the other and modifying his or her behavior to fit that structure. The researchers identified periodicities in the behavior of each mother-infant dyad at both three and five months. Term infants displayed more coherence than pre-term infants at both ages, and more often led the interaction at both ages.

These results appear to confirm earlier descriptions of rhythmic interaction, previously reported as occurring two to three times a minute (Brazelton et al., 1974). It has been suggested that interactive social rhythms give the infant a structure to form temporal expectations that organize cognitive and affective experiences (Lewis & Goldberg, 1969; Stern, Beebe, Jaffe, & Bennett, 1977). Lester et al.'s work demonstrates that temporal patterning is a fundamental property of early face-to-face interaction between mother and infant, and that by three months of age the sequential nature of this social interaction is made up of periodicities of affective displays. These social interaction rhythms may be evidence of an early communication system, in which the precursors of linguistic structures are learned through repetition of behavioral cycles.

Brazelton et al. (1974) analyzed the behavior of five caregiver–infant dyads considered to be normal, to study intense interactions over short periods of time, ranging from two to 20 weeks. In assessing infant behavior toward the mothers, the investigators discovered four distinct strategies for coping with unpleasant stimuli:

1. Active withdrawal to increase physical distance.
2. Rejection, in the form of pushing the offensive stimulus away with hands or feet while maintaining the original position.
3. Reducing sensitivity to the offensive stimulus while maintaining the original position—yawning, sleeping, presenting a dull appearance.
4. Crying or fussing; this behavior summons parents or caregivers to assist the infant in coping with unpleasant stimuli.

During the brief period of interaction with their infants, mothers behaved in the following ways:

1. Reduced the level of activity that interferes with interaction.
2. Encouraged a more alert, receptive state leading to interaction.
3. Established an expectant atmosphere to encourage interaction.
4. Attracted infant's attention to facilitate message sending and receiving.
5. Provided sufficient time to reciprocate the infant's message and responses.

Each of these behaviors was intentional on the part of the mothers, as signified by the quality of their behavior.

   Within two weeks, there was sufficient evidence to establish differing degrees and durations of attention, as well as interruptions of attention when mother sent unpleasant stimuli. Especially noteworthy was that an interdependence of rhythms appeared to be basic to attachment, as well as communication. The researchers stated,

. . . [w]hen the balance was sympathetic to the needs of each member of the dyad, there was a sense of rhythmic interaction which an observer sensed as 'positive.' When the balance was not equalized . . . there seemed to be a 'negative' quality in the entire interaction. (Brazelton et al., p. 74)

   To establish a temporal structure for face-to-face interaction, Kaye and Fogel (1980) videotaped 37 infants at home with their mothers in face-to-face dyadic play at 6, 13, and 26 weeks of age. The results suggest a typical sequence of mutual responses: the mother greeted the infant's onset of attention with one or more smiles, exaggerated faces, or head bobbing. The infant then responded with a smile, vocalization, wide mouth, etc. With the younger infants, the mothers used touching and posture changing to attract their attention.

   At all ages (6, 13, and 26 weeks), the mothers used facial activity to hold the infant's attention. At six weeks of age a cycle consisted of about 20 seconds attending and 18 seconds of not-attending, compared with approximately five seconds of attending and 12 seconds of not attending at 26 weeks of age. The mean proportion of time during which infants were oriented toward their mothers' faces declined from 70% at six weeks of age to 32.8% at 26 weeks. On the other hand, the infants' period of attention overlapped with the mothers' facially expressive behavior, which increased as the infants grew older. Infants' vocalizations, smiles, and mouth openings occurred at six weeks of age. By 26 weeks these exchanges approached a dialogue in complexity. When the infant was between six weeks and six months of age, mothers' rates of discrete change in facial expression, when they had their infants' attention, increased by approximately 50%; the infants' corresponding rates increased by approximately 200%.

Among the conclusions drawn by the researchers were that interactions begin with eye contact, which peaks around the time that the social smile begins (8 to 12 weeks). The amount of joint attention during face-to-face interactions decreases after the twelfth week of age, when infants become interested in inanimate objects. Moreover, analysis of the contingent sequences following the onset of infant attention revealed that up to six weeks of age, infants rarely initiated expressive greetings. Without the mothers' greetings, infants almost never made contact. By contrast, spontaneous greetings by 26 week old infants became as frequent as those elicited by their mothers.

Dodd (1979) and others have documented the effects of being out of synchrony. Dodd compared the amount of gazing in 10 to 16 week old infants exposed to nursery rhymes. Experimental sessions lasted four minutes, during which the researchers recited nursery rhymes in a bright manner, maintained eye contact for the infants when possible, and changed the stimulus every minute from synchronous to asynchronous, or the reverse.

The tests demonstrated that the subjects paid significantly more attention to synchronous presentations than to asynchronous ones. Thus, even though they could not understand the words that were being said, the 10 to 16 week old infants realized when sounds and lip movement did not correspond.

Tronick, Als, Adamson, Wise, and Brazelton (1978) observed seven mothers and their healthy, full-term infants, between one and four months old, in a face-to-face paradigm. Two contiguous events were studied: three-minute normal interaction, then three minutes of still-face interaction. During the normal interaction the infants oriented toward and greeted their mothers; when later they failed to respond, the infants sobered and looked wary. The infants usually stared at the mothers, gave them a brief smile, then looked away. The infants then monitored the mother's behavior by briefly glancing toward and then away from them. Eventually, the infants withdrew, orienting both their face and body away from the mothers. This sequence was observed in all infants from one to four months old. During the still-face condition, the infants smiled significantly less and had their gaze and head oriented toward their mothers for less time than in the normal condition. This still-face interaction, during which smiling decreased significantly and was replaced by infant wariness and gaze aversion, indicates that even infants as young as one month are capable of distinguishing affect modification in their caregivers. Thus, Tronick's work suggests that these infants possess the ability to recognize discrepancy and to alter affective response in the presence of discrepancy.

From early studies with the face-to-face paradigm such investigators as Stern (1974b) have noted a fascinating phenomenon: the dyad itself may be conceptualized as a separate entity or mutual system within which a delicate equilibrium is maintained by mutual arousal and stimulation. Data that support the existence of this mutual system of interaction include evidence of a particular kind of visual attentive behavior on the part of the infant, manifestations of increasing infant excitation to human stimuli, and verification of his or her physiological ability to control eye movement. In addition, the discrepancy hypothesis, which provides the theoretical explanation of how an organism responds to new stimuli, has enabled researchers to articulate more cogently the rules of interaction operating within the mutual system of maintenance and arousal. The following studies trace the development of these insights as witnessed within the dyadic framework.

Mothers and infants both share a common goal, which Stern (1974a) defined as being,

. . . the mutual maintenance of a level of attention and arousal within some optimal range in which the infant is likely to manifest affectively positive social behaviors such as smiles and coos. This definition of a goal is no different from stating that the object of play is to interest and delight one another. (p. 404)

The maintenance of arousal in which positive social behavior will develop is a goal that both mother and infant achieve through different means. Perceptual input can be controlled from moment to moment in order to influence directly the infant's own fleeting state of arousal. The mother achieves this by bringing to bear all methods available to her to modulate the level, timing, nature, and pattern of stimulation.

In his study of mothers and infants at play, Stern (1974b) realized that by the third month of life, gazing patterns between mothers and infants comprise the "first dyadic system in which both members have almost equal control over and facility with the same behavior" (p. 188). The early development of this system between mother and child has considerable implications. Control of the eyes provides a measure of control over the input of perception and this capacity permits the infant to regulate his or her internal state within given limits at an early age. Importantly, control of the eyes is, in Stern's words, "one of the few effective operations regulating perception that is fully available to the infant during this transient developmental period'' (p.188).

Discrepancy Awareness Hypothesis

The Discrepancy Awareness Hypothesis, as articulated by McCall and McGhee (1977) posits a mechanism whereby the infant utilizes developing cognitive and affective capabilities to respond to new stimuli in the environment. The researchers have defined ''discrepancy'' as the degree of similarity in the gestalts of two stimuli. According to the theory, infant response to gradations of discrepancy is reflected on an inverted U curve. Thus, McCall and McGhee suggest that the perception of a discrepancy that moderately deviates from a familiar, standard stimulus will result in an optimal level of both attention and positive affect; in contrast, familiar stimuli will evoke lower levels of attention and non–positive or neutral affect; while extreme discrepancy will result in low levels of attention, accompanied by negative affect. Moderate discrepancy, in other words, registers on the highest portion of the inverted U model.

As thus conceived, the Discrepancy Awareness Hypothesis presumes that infants possess adequate memory capacity, enabling them to distinguish and discriminate between stimuli, and furthermore, that a process of retrieval from memory storage exists. One of the main issues to be resolved before discrepancy awareness can be verified, therefore, is whether very young infants possess adequate memory capacities. In addition, the type of memory required for engaging in the process of discrepancy awareness may be labeled ''evocative memory,'' rather than ''recognition memory.'' As defined by Nachman and Stern (1984), evocative memory connotes a stored memory unit that may be retrieved and brought to consciousness in the absence of an external presentation of the stimulus; recognition memory, in comparison, refers to the process whereby a stimulus is recalled when it is physically presented to the infant. Confirmations of evocative memory capacity linked to a retrieval process have been reported in infants of nine months old (McDevitt, 1975) and, more recently, the presence of a memory storage system has been established in seven month olds (Nachman & Stern, 1984).

A second assumption of the Discrepancy Awareness Hypothesis is that the theory emphasizes affective displays as prime evidence of the infant's awareness. Signs of affect represent the main tools for measuring or tapping the potential for discrepancy awareness. As such, researchers have dwelled on the qualitative aspect of mood, whether positive (e.g., smiling) or negative (e.g., crying). Significantly, these discrete affective behavioral displays relate to temperament dimensions. Positive affect has been correlated with raised expectancy and increased learning (Masters, Barden, & Ford, 1979; Masters & Furman, 1976). Crying, in contrast, has been linked to "distress to novel stimuli" (Fagen & Ohr, 1985). The suggestion, then, is that the infant's temperament, as revealed through individual variations in expressing affective states, will have a significant impact on his or her capacity to experience discrepancy initially and to respond to the discrepant stimulus subsequently.

The Discrepancy Awareness Hypothesis also assumes that fairly sophisticated cognitive capacities may be inferred from the behavior of very young infants. McCall and McGhee (1977) report that a brief period of attention is exhibited by the infant following introduction of a discrepant stimulus. Kagan (1984) described a similar phenomenon, clearly identifiable during the first year, and labeled it the "period of alerting." Regardless of whether the label of "attention" or "alerting" is used, both of these studies suggest that the infant is engaging in internal cognitive processing.

Elaborating on the actual process that occurs with the introduction of a unique stimulus, McCall and McGhee note that first the infant experiences the stimulus as being "discrepant" to ones he or she has previously encountered. Accompanying this discrepancy awareness are both affective and cognitive correlates, which the researchers term "subjective uncertainty." During the state of subjective uncertainty, the infant scans his or her memory for related stimuli in order to resolve the uncertainty. Indeed, the period of subjective uncertainty may be viewed as a time during which the infant seeks an engram (coded memory unit) with an appropriate cognitive and an appropriate affective component. If the stimulus is moderately discrepant from previously experienced events, the infant will likely be able to resolve his or her state of subjective uncertainty rapidly and display positive affect. But if the event is one of extreme discrepancy, negative affect will result, indicating that an appropriate engram has not been found and that subjective uncertainty has not been successfully resolved.

Positive affect is more likely to occur if the infant is successful in distinguishing between moderately and severely discrepant stimuli in resolving subjective uncertainties. Negative affect occurs more frequently during the infant's unsuccessful attempts to resolve severe levels of subjective uncertainty produced by extreme discrepancies. The presentation of discrepant stimuli, therefore, can result in either successful processing, or in processing that may be characterized as overly effortful and strenuous.

McCall and McGhee reason that positive affect indicates resolution of subjective uncertainty through cognitive comparisons between the new stimuli and appropriate, previously retained engrams. Moreover, positive affect will be patterned on an inverted U curve of subjective uncertainty, which demands the resolution of moderate or greater uncertainty before positive affect can occur. Moderate discrepancy will also evoke positive affect fairly rapidly, owing to a short processing time, while an affective and cognitive response to an extreme discrepancy may take longer, because the infant may remain entrenched in a state of subjective uncertainty.

In addition, McCall and McGhee qualify their theory by noting that negative affect will not occur as a common response to large magnitudes of discrepancy if the special nature of the stimuli does not increase levels of subjective uncertainty. Such an event might occur in situations where discrepancy involves transformations of stimuli normally representing security and safety (a parent's face, for example).

This description of infant response raises a key theme pervading the Discrepancy Awareness Hypothesis. Specifically, the infant appears to derive the highest levels of gratification from, and appears to be internally best equipped to process, *moderate* stimulation. Extremes of stimulation, either because the stimulus is too different or too familiar, result in less than optimal response. With extreme discrepancy, negative affect will be displayed; with overly familiar stimuli, the infant's alerting period will be followed by disinterest. One might, therefore, deduce that infants are innately motivated toward situations in which the stimulus is sufficiently novel; at the same time, however, the infant possesses an internal mechanism programmed to resist extreme or traumatic stimuli.

The role of temperament in infant response is a second theme dominating the Discrepancy Awareness Hypothesis. As noted, the level of discrepancy present in the new stimulus—whether moderate, extreme, or familiar—will evoke affective, cognitive, and behavioral responses, which in part relate to temperament. Significantly, the converse is also suggested: that is, the temperamental predisposition that an individual infant brings to the new stimulus will affect the efficiency with which he or she resolves subjective uncertainty. An infant with a high degree of persistence (a temperamental dimension) will be equipped to exert effort and diligence in scanning his or her memory for an appropriate engram. Such an infant will be more motivated to resolve the subjective uncertainty and to integrate the stimulus into his or her internal schema. In contrast, an infant with a low degree of persistence may become frustrated upon being presented with even a moderate degree of discrepancy, may abandon pursuit of an appropriate engram, and may be more susceptible to the experience of negative affect. Thus, not only will the stimulus determine infant response, but also the infant's temperament will determine how the stimulus will be interpreted. The Discrepancy Awareness Hypothesis, therefore, suggests a mode of interaction between infant and environment; while the stimulus will impinge on the infant, the infant (primarily through the vehicle of temperament) will equally impinge on the stimulus.

Kagan (1974) has theorized on the sequence of events that occur, both cognitively and affectively, when the infant is exposed to a discrepant stimulus. This researcher notes that when the infant is presented with a new stimulus during the first year of life, a discernable sequence of events can be charted. Immediately following presentation of a new stimulus,

Kagan reports that an alerting reaction occurs. After alerting, generally lasting from 10 to 15 seconds, one of three behavioral sequences will follow. The first sequence occurs when the child resumes what he or she was doing prior to introduction of the new event, without displaying emotional response. The second behavioral sequence occurs if the child smiles, laughs, vocalizes, or exhibits excited motor ability. In the third possible behavioral sequence, the muscles of the infant's face become tense, the eyes widen (a combination labeled "wariness") and the infant may turn away and cry. Kagan notes that in order for the infant to respond to the stimulus with either a smiling or a wary response, the initiating event must be a sudden unexpected change or an event that is discrepant from the infant's prior internal experiential schema. Significantly, Kagan stresses that the child's response may be determined by the particular expectations that he or she brings to the event.

In describing the alerting state, Kagan reports that the phenomenon may be viewed as an orientation reaction. During this time, inhibition of motor activity, decreased heart rate, and lowered muscle tonicity occur. If the event is extremely discrepant and cannot be assimilated, the infant will either turn away and redirect his or her activity or display prolonged focusing of attention on the event, accompanied by inhibition of activity and, on occasion, changes in facial expression and crying.

Testing his model in a clinical setting, Kagan studied 140 infants aged seven and one half months, and found that moderately discrepant events indeed produced the most smiling and the least amount of crying. Thus, the researcher concluded that moderately discrepant events are most likely to lead to prolonged attention, excitement, and smiling, although the last response is the least frequent. Moreover, moderately discrepant events are less likely to cause wariness or crying, and thus it may be inferred that moderately discrepant events are relatively assimilable.

Kagan isolates the infant's temperament as a factor that influences the likelihood of favorable assimilation to a discrepant event. The researcher reports that few investigations have found a visual or auditory event that produced smiling in more than 75% of infants tested. In fact, typically 20 to 50% of a random infant group smile at a moderately discrepant event, suggesting that some infants are not easily disposed to smile. Individual differences, therefore, may account for a higher threshold to this reaction. Thus, the operation of a constitutional variable related to the ability to establish and resolve discrepancies is implied.

Tracing the temporal sequence of discrepancy reaction, Kagan has observed that during the first six to eight weeks of life, the child alerts primarily to unexpected changes in physical aspects of his or her environment and, on occasion, cries following this alerting. After approximately eight weeks, the infant alerts with increasing frequency to events that are not merely changes in physical parameters, but are transformations of their own earlier experiences, i.e., psychologically discrepant events.

Kagan's work thus provides valuable data for tracing the sequences of responses that occur during the presentation of discrepant stimuli, and for highlighting the role played by temperamental traits in responding to discrepancy.

If the theorists writing about the Discrepancy Awareness Hypothesis are correct, the infant possesses sufficient capacities in the early months of life to engage in a process of fairly sophisticated discrepancy awareness. Virtually all of the researchers cited have reflected the view that very young infants possess a fairly intricate affective and cognitive repertoire, and furthermore, that the temperamental predisposition of the infant will influence his or her mode of dealing with discrepancy. However, beyond the ability to differentiate between discrepant stimuli and to engage in comparisons (discrepancy awareness), additional cognitive and affective capacities have been established in very young infants. Most notable are the capacities to discern causality and form expectations.

According to Borton (1979), the adult form of the concept of causality includes a component of contingency (causes must be spatially and temporally contiguous) and a component of regularity (causes and effects have always occurred in the same sequence in the past). In a study investigating whether three month old infants are capable of discriminating causal from apparently non-causal physical events, the researcher tested 15 three month old infants exposed to three situations: 1) single-object movement (involving a single object moving across a horizontal track); 2) contact causal movement (one object moved toward a second stationary object, colliding with it, launching off the second object, and leaving the first object stationary); and 3) non-contact between two objects (a first object approaching a second stationary object and stopping short of collision, at which time the second object moves off simultaneously as if having been struck by the first object). Infants were scored with regard to frequency of certain looking patterns indicating disruptive tracking. Data from the study strongly suggested that the infants were sensitive to cues specifying causality in a perceived event. This study was later replicated, suggesting to the researcher that infants of this age are capable of a fundamental understanding of causality in perceived mechanical events.

Expectancy has been described as the readiness for one event as opposed to another. The ability to expect an event implies the use of prior information about a stimulus that speeds response to an identical or related stimulus.

Stern and Gibbon (1978) have specifically explored the topic of expectancy. Describing how expectancies may be initially formed by infants, these researchers have argued that the temporal patterns in which stimuli are presented and perceived will coalesce to create expectancies in the infant. These researchers posit that even from birth the infant is capable of estimating time intervals, of forming temporal expectancies, and of evaluating variations from expected stimuli.

During the earliest months of life, according to these researchers, an interactive social system develops between caregiver and infant. This system is nonverbal, and stimuli derive their value for the infant mainly from sensory properties, including the temporal framework in which the stimuli are presented. Stern and Gibbon also note that affective displays in infants have been intimately linked to the manner in which stimuli are distributed over time. Also, Stern and Gibbon report that accumulating evidence suggests expectancies are formed based on immediately preceding experience. In a study of three mother-infant dyads (involving three to four month old infants), the researchers employed a process of repetitive stimuli. All of the infants demonstrated anticipatory response, even when the time variable between the presentations of stimuli were varied. Indeed, the infants behaved as if they calculated a mean and used it as the point of expectation.

Stern and Gibbon suggest then that by four months of age, if not earlier, attention span is sufficient to enable infants to experience expectation based on the repetition or frequency of stimuli presentation. Significantly, Stern and Gibbon posit that the interactive social system between caregiver and infant represents the vehicle within which expectation develops.

Gazing Patterns Within the Dyadic Model

Stern (1974b) has described gazing as the "first dyadic communication system" in which both caregiver and infant exert virtually equal control over and facility with the same interaction. Studies that elucidate aspects of gazing are basic to the formulation of etiological hypotheses about early infant development. The face-to-face paradigm, because it scrutinizes behavior within a dyadic framework, offers researchers a rare opportunity to investigate the parameters of gazing patterns.

Gazing pattern studies have focused on facial expression and play behavior. Among the most compelling results has been evidence that gazing patterns may be triggered not only by factors emanating from external interactive catalysts, but by an internal mechanism that regulates infant functioning. As observed by Messer and Vietze (1984), increasing attention has been given in recent years to gazing patterns between mothers and their offspring. In a study of two groups of infants, Fogel et al. (1982) employed a structured paradigm using four conditions in the following sequence: normal face-to-face interaction between mother and infant (1.5 minutes); mother leaves the infant alone (1 minute); mother enters and assumes a still-face posture (45 seconds); mother resumes face-to-face interaction (1.5 minutes). The first group of infants, called the "look group" (mean age 10 weeks), were exposed to the same paradigm, except that during the third phase of the study the still face of the mother was triggered by the infant's smile.

Eight categories were chosen to reflect the rates of emotional expressions: gazing at the mother, gaze avoidance, distressed, brow, smiling, crying, shielding (using arms to cover face or body), and pointing (index finger extension directed toward mother). The infants gazed least at the mother during the still-face segment. Gazing at the mother represented 57% of the normal and resumed-interaction segments, but only 45% of the still-face segments. The "look group" showed "distress brow" (wariness) during 38% of their resumption, compared to 7% for infants of the "smile group." Thirty percent of the first group cried during the resumption, compared to 5% who cried in the second group.

The authors concluded that the realm of reciprocal interaction for the infant might be almost entirely in the "mutual exchange, amplification and modulation" of emotional experience, and that the resumption of the mother's contingent behavior results in a restoration of the infant's response patterns. In the context of this paradigm, "the two month old has the ability to remember and to anticipate, as well as to act in ways that reveal genuine emotional involvement" (p. 57).

This study is significant because it suggests a variation on the Strange Situation (Ainsworth, 1969) used to assess attachment in one year old infants. In the Fogel study, however, not only were the infants much younger (10 weeks old) than infants traditionally tested in the Strange Situation, but additionally, the infant's behavior was artificially manipulated. The fact that infants exposed to this sequence were distressed, cried more, and displayed more "fussing" behavior in comparison to the control group, is noteworthy for several reasons. First, the intensity of response caused by the manipulated situation confirms Tronick's theory (Tronick et al., 1978) that even very young infants can identify discrepancy stimuli. Second, the response of the infants was characterized by a high degree of negative affect, suggesting an internal upheaval of the mechanism regulating temperament dimensions. Finally, Fogel's study is significant because it suggests ways in which caregiver behavior that is discrepant or non-contingent to a very young infant may culminate in the phenomenon of insecure attachment, later seen at one year of age in the Strange Situation.

Stern studied 18 infants, 12 of whom were twins, during the third and fourth months of life. Observations were made in the home using a television camera. A full morning was used to videotape all play and feeding interactions as they would normally take place. Two observers were used, one of whom scored whether the gaze of the infants was on or off the mother. The mothers' play with the infants showed that many patterns represented the unusual variants of interpersonal behaviors that take place between adults and infants, such as communicating in "baby talk." Equally notable in the mothers' behavior, apart from the words used, was an exaggeration of other linguistic elements, such as range of pitch, and the speed at which pitch was changed. The rate was most often slow, but sometimes it was unexpectedly rapid.

During interactive play with their infants, mothers also adopted extraordinary facial expressions noteworthy for their degree of exaggeration, long duration, and slow tempo of formation. The mothers would also bring their faces very close to their infants during play, in violation of adult norms respecting interpersonal space. Slowing the tempo and exaggerating facial expressions may help infants maintain the identity of their mothers' faces and establish a stable facial schema.

This striking maternal behavior, as expressed by facial exaggeration and vocalization, may result not so much from the presence of the infants as from the fact that their gaze is focused on the mothers. In itself, the gaze of the mothers was extremely long, when compared to normal adult gaze interaction (Argyle & Kendon, 1967; Exline, Gray, & Schuette, 1965; Kendon, 1967). Under their infants' gazes the mothers are less likely to look away, leading to the assumption that maternal gaze aversion is inhibited significantly while the infants' gaze is focused upon the mothers.

When the mothers addressed their infants, all three of these maternal variations on normal adult interpersonal behavior—vocalization, facial expression, and gazing—took place simultaneously. Stern made the important observation that "mothers who cannot perform these behaviors . . . elicit less 'play' from their infants" (1974b, p.195).

During play interaction, a wide variation appeared in the infants' interest in gazing at their mothers, not only on a day-to-day basis but also within a given day. Even when infants wished to gaze at their mothers, they did not do so steadily, just as when trying to avoid contact they did not gaze away continually. Whether seeking contact or avoiding it, infants alternated between gazing at or gazing away from their mothers, with the only variable being assigned to levels of interest as expressed by durations of gazing or gazing away. This suggests that the incidence of gaze-to-gaze intervals is not influenced by the reinforcement or averting values in the faces of the mothers, since they change greatly from interaction to interaction.

Mothers were more likely than infants to initiate gazing at the infant from a neutral state. When mothers started gazing at the infants, they were more likely to maintain that gaze for a long period of time, at least until the infants responded by returning the gaze. The probability of mothers terminating the gaze was also less than the probability of the infants joining in mutual gazing. When mutual gazing occurred, mothers and infants shifted between gazing states. The mothers held their gaze when the infants looked at them, looked away, and then back. This may be, as Stern has noted, the most noteworthy gesture of the dyadic gazing pattern. As a consequence of this pattern, the infants, not the mothers, establish and break the pattern of mutual gazing in 95% of all mutual gazing patterns studied by Stern (1974b).

Field (1979) studied 36 infants at the age of three months who were ranked into groups according to their gestational ages: 18 term infants with an average of 40 weeks gestation and 18 preterm infants whose average gestational age was 32 weeks. The object of the investigation was the measurement of looking and looking away (gaze alteration behaviors) of the infants, in response to differing levels of facial animation. The faces, in ascending order of animation, were the standard, inanimate Raggedy Ann face; a Raggedy Ann face that could move and talk; a mother's face seen during less animated imitations of her infant's behavior; and a mother's face seen during spontaneous face-to-face interactions. The reactions of the infants to these exposures were videotaped in a laboratory resembling a living room.

Results of these trials indicated that both term and preterm infants spent longer periods of time looking at the dolls' faces than at the mothers' faces. Looking times increased in the order of mother's spontaneous face, mother's imitative face, moving-talking doll's face, and inanimate doll's face. The infants looked at the animated doll's face significantly less than at the inanimate doll's face. The full-term infants spent more time looking at their spontaneous mothers' faces than did the premature infants. The preterm males looked at the spontaneous mothers' faces for less time than did the other infants. Among both term and preterm infants, the tonic heart rate increased significantly during the spontaneous mothers' face situation, and significantly decreased, below baseline, during the inanimate doll's face situation.

As for heart rates among the mothers, those with term infants had a significantly lower heart rate during imitative situations, while those of preterm infants had significantly increased heart rates during the spontaneous situation. The author summarized her findings as follows:

The lesser activity of the imitative mothers and the greater attentiveness and approximately baseline levels of heart rate for the infants suggest that mothers' imitations of infants . . . may have closely approximated the infants' capabilities of information and processing and arousal modulation. (Field, 1979, p. 193)

Comparison Between Healthy and At-Risk Infants

The studies already discussed have clarified some of the dynamics of gazing behavior encompassed within the dyadic framework of the face-to-face interaction paradigm. By combining the perspective of mother and child, researchers have deciphered a dyadic exchange mechanism specific to gazing patterns. As the studies in this section have demonstrated, comprehension of the dyadic exchange mechanism is further enhanced when normal infant-caretaker pairs are contrasted with at-risk infant-caregiver dyads. From such comparison studies, researchers have been able to identify precise behavioral deviations. The significance of these deviations is uncertain at this time. Variations from normal gazing patterns encountered in an at-risk infant-caregiver dyad may be of minimal significance for later infant development or, as is more likely, may be a harbinger of such phenomena as infant depression. Although the definitive diagnostic implications of aberrational gazing patterns within at-risk infant-caregiver models have yet to be documented, researchers should be alert to these deviations among susceptible at-risk populations.

In a study conducted by Field (1977), three groups of infants were observed in a face-to-face paradigm, controlled by 12 infants three and one half months old. The study groups included: normal, full term infants; post-term, postmature infants (average age 16 days, with parchment-like skin and long, thin bodies); high risk, premature infants (gestational age 32 weeks), suffering from respiratory distress syndrome.

Field's findings indicated that mothers of normal infants were less active (66%) during infant gaze than mothers of infants in the postmature group (75%) or the high-risk group (80%). Mothers of normal infants were found to be less active (52%) during group infant gaze aversion, while mothers of the high-risk, premature infants were most active. Infants looked at their mothers only 40% of the time during attention-getting situations; in contrast, they looked at their mothers 79% of the time when mothers imitated infant behavior. Normal infants gazed more than the other two groups of infants. These early interactional styles and patterns of continuity proved to have more important effects than did early separation.

In a 1981 study, Field used a paradigm designed to compare the gaze behavior of four month old normal, healthy, full-term infants with preterm, high-risk infants having a mean gestational age of 32 weeks and a mean birth weight of 1,800 grams. Field found that eight percent of the mothers of the pre-term infants showed more gaze aversion than the mothers of the term infants, and that preterm infants showed more gaze aversion than term infants in all of the animated situations. All infants showed less gaze aversion with their "moderately active" partners (siblings and peers) and during the doll-and-mirror interactions.

Sigman and Parmelee (1974) compared the visual preferences of four month old premature and full-term infants. Preference for mobile stimuli following an habituation procedure was shown by the full term infants but not by the premature infants.

In another study by Field (1982), 20 normal infants from uncomplicated term deliveries were compared with 40 high risk youngsters (20 postterm, postmaturity syndrome infants and 20 preterm, respiratory distress syndrome children). After birth, the preterm group was less alert and attentive to the stimulation than normal term infants. Postterm, postmaturity syndrome infants were hyperactive, easily aroused, and irritable in the Brazelton examination (Brazelton, 1973). At four months, the behavior of these infants was compared in completely spontaneous face-to-face interactions, and their heart rates were recorded. Field found that mothers of the high-risk group verbalized more than mothers of normal infants, and that term infants looked at their mothers more than did the high-risk infants. Heart rates in the high-risk group elevated significantly during spontaneous interaction. Crying was more frequent among the high-risk group. Contingent smiling and vocalization responses were more frequent in the normals. Preterm infants exhibited significantly more sad faces than postterm infants, who in turn exhibited more sad faces than the term infants.

The researchers suggested that infants seem to have specific information-processing and/or arousal modulation abilities depending on their thresholds to stimulation (higher for the preterm and lower for the postterm). Both subgroups have a significant degree of difficulty modulating arousal, as shown by limited attention-affective displays and degree of gaze aversion. These observations imply that the goal of mutually regulating stimulation in dyadic interaction can be accomplished through the synchrony of affective interaction, as well as by arousal modulation and intensity of stimulation.

Infant Attachment and Response to Strangers

The reciprocal nature of caregiver-infant interactions is documented and outlined in preceding sections of this chapter. Beyond the typical rhythmic patterns identified, however, several researchers, including Massie (1978), have probed patterns of disharmony that occur within the face-to-face interaction paradigm. Massie characterized the discrete units of behavior isolated during any given dyadic exchange as "attachment displays." Attachment displays may be viewed as temporal sequences during which the infant either is or is *not* cohesively in rapport with the caregiver. In addition, researchers seeking to illustrate the inverse of healthy attachment have drawn on the well–documented phenomenon of "stranger anxiety" as a manifestation of negative response on the part of the infant. Taken together, the dual concepts of attachment and stranger anxiety have enhanced understanding of the parameters of normal infant development and have yielded some preliminary data on pathological phenomena.

In an investigation of neonatal discrimination between the faces of mothers and strangers, Field, Cohen, Garcia, and Greenberg (1984) reported on 48 normal, healthy infants divided equally between males and females. An equal division was also made between infants exposed to faces alone and those exposed to both faces and voices. The infants were between 22 and 93 hours old (mean 45 hours) when the first face recognition assessment was conducted. A Brazelton Neonatal Behavior Assessment (Brazelton, 1973) was performed, measuring levels of alertness and wakefulness. After these measurements proved satisfactory, infants were placed on rocking chairs in a three-sided enclosure for observation. The enclosure had a trap door on one wall, positioned at a 45 degree angle to the other walls of the enclosure. The inner surface of the trap door was located near the face of the infant and was wired with blinking colored lights that kept the infant's attention focused on the direction of the trap door. When the trap door was opened, the face of the mother or a stranger was revealed. During face/voice presentations, the infant also heard the voice of the mother or stranger.

Each infant was subjected to a visual preference test, a series of habituation trials, and a test to determine the level of discrimination. During the visual preference test, the infant was given four trials during which the face or the face and voice of a stranger was revealed *or* in which infants were confronted by the face and voice of the mother. Both mothers and strangers presented smiling faces, or smiling faces and voices, saying the words, "Hi baby, Hi baby," each time the trap door opened. When the infant looked away, the trap door closed, to be reopened after a two-second interval. While the door was closed, the rocking chair was rocked. After preference trials were completed, the infants were presented with the faces of their mothers or their faces and voices. Habituation was deemed to be attained when the infants completed three successive trials recording less looking time than was observed during the first three trials. The neonates were then subjected to a discrimination test, consisting of two exposures to the face of a stranger and two exposures to the mother.

Tabulating the results of the preference trials, 17 of the 24 infants looked longer at the mothers' faces than at the faces of strangers. In the group exposed to both faces and voices, 21 of 24 infants looked longer at their mothers than at the strangers. A significant preference for the face or face and voice of the mother was suggested.

The face discrimination test revealed that 18 of 24 infants in the face-alone group looked at the stranger's face significantly longer than they looked at the mother, demonstrating the novelty effect of the stranger's face. This phenomenon was more pronounced among female infants than among males. The results indicated that although these neonates had had little association with their mothers, they were at least able to distinguish some facet of their mothers' faces. Moreover, the neonates did not need to "learn" their mothers' voices, which they had apparently learned already, in order to distinguish the mothers' faces. Finally, the infants developed a preference for the novel faces of strangers after being repeatedly presented with the mothers' faces.

The researchers also observed that although periods of alertness and looking times were brief, neonates seemed to have already learned to distinguish mothers from strangers in the first hours of life. This finding may hint at an adaptive process, in that those neonates able to distinguish the faces of their mothers may also receive more nurturing responses.

In another study using a habituation technique, Barrera and Maurer (1981) demonstrated the ability of three month olds to recognize and discriminate faces. All 12 of the full-term infants they tested looked longer at the photograph of the novel stranger to whom they were habituated. The results suggest that even three month old infants can discriminate faces of strangers and recognize which face they were exposed to during habituation, at least if the faces are judged by adults to be grossly different from one another.

Langsdorf, Izard, Rayias, and Hembree (1984) tested 20 mother-infant dyads at three months in the face-to-face and still-face situations, and at twelve months using the Ainsworth Strange Situation. Those infants who averted their gaze during the still-face situation at three months were more likely to seek reassurance from mother during the Strange Situation at 12 months. Duration of gaze during still-face at three months was inversely related to the frequency of checking between mother and stranger nine months later. These results confirmed the hypothesis of Langsdorf et al., that the infant's reactions to still-face perturbations can predict reactions in the Strange Situation later. Moreover, Langsdorf et al.'s work also gives credence to Fogel's findings (1984) that discrepancy awareness will interact with maternal cues to determine the particular kind of attachment bond formed between caregiver and infant.

Blehar et al. (1977) corroborated and built upon previous investigations by Stern that suggested that the goal of early dyadic interplay is to regulate stimulation in order to maintain positive affective levels of infant arousal. These researchers observed 26 mothers and infants longitudinally during the first year of life in an attempt to trace the development of attachment bonds. Of the 26 infants in the study (16 male, 10 female), 23 were retained in the study after being exposed to the laboratory setting, a "strange situation," at 51 weeks of age.

Home visits were conducted every three weeks between the ages of three and 54 weeks, while the mothers performed normal household routines. The investigators noted details of the mother-infant interaction and the behavior of the infants in the presence of visitors. Visitors were asked to participate by attempting to elicit vocalization and smiles during encounters with the infants.

Narrative reports were recorded at intervals of six, nine, 12 and 15 weeks. Earlier records were not included, since eye contact and reactive smiling had not been established at the third week. Face-to-face interactions were recorded when mothers bent over the infants, when they held the infants before them face-to-face, and when one adult helped the infant while another adult face was presented.

Fifty-five percent of the face-to-face encounters were recorded while the mothers were holding their infants, 41% as the mothers bent over the infants, and 4% while a third person held the infants. The great majority (91%) of these encounters were initiated by the mothers, who exhibited unsmiling, emotionless faces in only 19% of the encounters.

In addressing maternal behavior during the interactions, these researchers judged 54% of the episodes to be contingent, 15% to be playful, and 13% to encourage further interaction with the infants. Abrupt actions on the part of the mothers were seen only in 37% of the encounters.

Among the infants, 38% responded to the encounters by smiling and 28% by vocalizing. The infants expressed delight by bouncing up and down in 12% of the encounters. Infant response to visitors differed significantly from response to the mothers on only one measure—bouncing.

Mean developmental trends were computed for between the six and nine week visits, and were compared with those from the 12 and 15 week visits. In the second period the infants vocalized more often and their responses were generally characterized as being more intense than in the first period, during which they often fixed only the faces of the mothers in their gaze. Infants who did not respond in the earlier confrontations were not always those who were unresponsive in the second encounters, while those mothers who were unresponsive in the first encounters remained unresponsive in the later encounters.

Comparing early face-to-face encounters and later attachments, mothers who were earlier deemed anxious about their attachments often presented impassive faces in later encounters and frequently did not respond to infants' efforts to initiate reactions. This finding occurred more among anxious mothers than among those securely attached. Anxious mothers also expressed more abrupt, brief encounter behavior than secure mothers. Mothers later assessed as being securely attached appeared more contingent in their pacing, and encouraged further encounter responses. Secure mothers were also more playful and livelier, although this finding was statistically insignificant.

At the end of the first year, mothers of the four infants who had been classified as "intermediate-security-anxiety" displayed the same behavior as they had shown during earlier encounters. Only one difference was significant: they were not as contingent in their pacing as were mothers of securely attached infants. Overall, infants who smiled and bounced more were later judged to be securely attached. Infants who responded more intensely in their encounters with both mothers and visitors, as expressed by greater levels of vocalization and bouncing, were later judged to be more securely attached than infants in the other two groups. These infants, however, tended only to look at visitors and terminated encounters with visitors more frequently than with their mothers. By contrast, anxiously attached infants showed little difference in demeanor to either the visitors or their mothers. Also they were more likely to be fussy in exchanges with their mothers.

This study indicates that between six and 15 weeks of age, infants grow more responsive to their mothers during face-to-face interaction. Mothers of infants expressing positive responses behaved with playfulness and a contingent interactive pacing. Additionally, the researchers noted that infants who were later considered to be securely attached reacted more positively to mothers than to unfamiliar figures during the six to 15 week period.

Depressive Dyadic Interaction

Although researchers are only in the preliminary stages of acquiring data on infant depressive phenomena manifested during early face-to-face exchange, the studies thus far have revealed a host of compelling insights. As already noted, studies by Stern, Lester, and Brazelton delineated the parameters of normal rhythmic cycling within the dyadic framework. Given findings of typical rhythms replicated over several studies, Cohn and Tronick's (1983) discovery that infants subjected to simulated depression engage in a unique cycle of affective behaviors is noteworthy. Comparing affective displays that emerge when the infant is confronted with normal maternal behavior with the affective responses evinced during periods of simulated maternal depression, Cohn and Tronick readily distinguished two distinctly different patterns of reaction.

This study raises a series of questions that have yet to be fully investigated. For example, are the "negative" affective cycles that Cohn and Tronick discerned in infants encountering simulated maternal depression reminiscent of the responses infants displayed when confronted with a "stranger situation," particularly in infants whose mothers have been assessed as anxiously attached? Moreover, what can be surmised about the infant's internal regulatory mechanism from these data, and equally important, how do these findings contribute to understanding the infant's affective repertoire? Cohn and Tronick have rejected the notion that the Discrepancy Awareness Hypothesis accounts for the unique behavior patterns that they observed in infants exposed to simulated depression. Nevertheless, further investigations into depressive phenomena may elucidate more fully the role of this hypothesis in explaining unusual infant behavioral response. If, as these investigators suggest, the Discrepancy Awareness Hypothesis cannot provide a satisfactory explanation, do hypotheses involving such concepts as imitation or mirroring, infant-maternal attachment, and affect regulation offer more fruitful possibilities for explaining infant depressive phenomena?

The data derived from Cohn and Tronick's study have several other profound implications for the study of infant depression and depressive–like phenomena. Evidence gleaned from the work of this team clearly demonstrates that simulated maternal depression can evoke negative affective states in infants, and more significantly, can impair the infants' capacities for engaging in effective self-regulation. Indeed, infants in the study appeared to have difficulty autonomously disrupting the cycle of negative affective states (consisting of depressed expression, gaze aversion, and protest). The flexibility and fluidity associated with rhythms encountered during sequences of normal interaction with caregivers was markedly impaired. Lester, Hoffman, and Brazelton (1985) have noted that the rhythms of normal interaction provide the infant with expectancies for organizing cognitive and affective experience. If this is the case, then impaired interaction, as witnessed during the Cohn and Tronick study, may also represent an artifact from which infant expectancies emerge. Although the Cohn and Tronick study induced an artificial state of depression by instructing caregivers to simulate depression, studies involving mothers who are clinically depressed (postpartum) have revealed that the infants of such caregivers display a pervasive negative mood (Field, 1984a). It may be inferred, then, that in the latter cases, an initial experience of a negative affective cycle generated negative expectancies which eventually generalized into a mood infusing and coloring all subsequent interactions.

Another investigation, conducted by Field (1984a), involves comparisons of infant-maternal dyads in which the mother was diagnosed as a postpartum depressive with clinically normal mother-infant pairs in which the maternal figure was instructed to simulate depression. Several striking differences were recorded among the two infant groups. Most notably, the researchers reported that the infants subjected to simulated depression exhibited more coping strategies, as if trying to resist cues emitted by the mothers. Such coping behavior—similar to strategies observed by Brazelton in viewing normal, dyadic interaction-suggests an internal regulatory mechanism for affect that the infant may assert when confronted with unpleasant stimuli.

In sharp contrast, however, infants of postpartum depression mothers did not resist the negative cues of the caregivers. They appeared resigned or apathetic to messages, suggesting an acquired immunity to repeated sequences of depression. Moreover, these latter infants engaged in a higher degree of imitative or mimicking behavior than their counterparts who experienced simulated depression. From this preliminary data, it can be inferred that the internal capacities for affect regulation may be markedly different in infants whose mothers are clinically normal, as compared with infants whose mothers are clinically depressed.

In one study using an experimental analogue of maternal depression, 24 infants of three months of age were observed in a contiguous experimental sequence consisting of three minutes of normal maternal interaction and three minutes of simulated depressed interaction (Cohn & Tronick, 1983). The mothers were instructed to interact with depressed or normal expressions. During the depressed interaction, mothers were asked to direct their gaze toward the infant, to speak in an uninteresting monotone, to remain expressionless, and to limit body movements and contact with their infants. Six infant-affective states were coded: looking away, protesting, wariness, social monitoring (gazing toward mother smiling), brief positive (facial expression brightened but duration brief), and play.

When observed in both interactions, infants in a depressed condition spent 50% of their time in protesting or wariness, and their positive responses were brief. A well-organized transition for the depressed infants went from brief positive to looking away. On the few occasions when these infants entered positive moods, they were likely to revert quickly to protesting, wariness, and looking away. By contrast, during the normal interaction, the depressed infants rarely protested or were wary, and made infrequent, brief positive displays. Infants in the normal condition alternated between brief positive, monitoring, and play. Even though 40% of transitions from brief positive led to looking away, normal infants then returned to a positive mood.

The Discrepancy Awareness Hypothesis holds that affective response is a function of current discrepancy parameters. Since the wariness response carried over into the subsequent period of normal interaction, this strongly suggests that discrepancy parameters are not responsible for observed behavior. Three month old infants are not only able to detect the affective quality of maternal interaction, but are also able to participate in the regulation of dyadic behaviors, modifying the affective responses of their partner's affective change (Stern, 1974b; Stern et al., 1977; Tronick, 1982; Tronick, Ricks, & Cohn, 1982). They can organize their behavior in response to the adult's behavior. When faced with chronically inappropriate maternal behavior, infants develop a pattern of adaptation characterized by withdrawal and avoidance, reflecting an experience of helplessness.

Field (1984a) theorized that infants raised by depressed mothers may acquire some immunity to depressed behavior, skewing the results of simulated depression studies. She compared the behavior of infants whose mothers became depressed postpartum with the behavior of infants whose normal mothers simulated depression. Twelve mothers were enrolled in each group, and face-to-face interactions between them and their three-month-old infants were videotaped. All mothers were assessed through the Beck Depression Inventory (Beck, Ward, Mendelson, Mock, & Erbaugh 1969) and the State-Trait-Anxiety Inventory (Spielberger, Gorsuch, & Lushene, 1970).

Baseline and interaction heart rates in both infants and mothers were telemetrically recorded and activity levels were measured as described by Bell (1968) using an actometer attached to each infant. A series of three face-to-face play interactions, each lasting three minutes, were recorded. At the first interaction, which was spontaneous, mothers were asked to play with their infants as they would in a home setting. This interaction was followed by one during which the mothers were asked to appear depressed, by gazing toward their infants without expression and by engaging in minimal body movements and physical contact with the infants. At the third interaction, structured as a reunion, the mothers were again requested to behave naturally. The following infant behaviors were coded: positive and negative facial expressions, frequency of vocalizations and durations of looking away, and looking wary and protesting (Cohn & Tronick, 1983).

The infants of mothers who were not clinically depressed initially showed more frequent vocalizations, protests, and wary looks. These same infants also registered higher heart rates and activity levels. Mothers who were not depressed showed similar behaviors, with more frequent positive facial expressions, fewer negative facial expressions, more frequent vocalizations and lengthier amounts of time gazing and engaging in tactile kinesthetic simulation with infants. Their heart rates were also higher than those of the clinically depressed mothers.

During the depressed interaction, both groups of mothers spent less time providing tactile stimulation for their infants, and this phenomenon was the only repeated measured effect of any significance revealed in this trial. Higher heart rates and activity levels were reported among the infants of nondepressed mothers during the depressed and reunion situations than during the spontaneous interaction situations. Compared with depressed mothers, the nondepressed mothers exhibited positive facial expressions less frequently, negative facial expressions more frequently, and vocalized less often during depressed sequences than during either the reunion or spontaneous interaction sequences. The heart rate of nondepressed mothers was also higher during the depressed situation than during the other two situations.

The great proportion of infant behavior observed appeared to focus on an attempt to restore normal interactions. Failing this, distressed behaviors, such as looking away, wariness and protesting, appear to carry over to the subsequent reunion interactions. The author states, "[t]hese indicate a carryover of affective behavior or the establishment of a 'mood' in the infant" (Field, 1984a, p. 520). The unchanging behavior of the infants paralleled the unchanging behavior of the mothers who were genuinely depressed, in that their behavior was less positive during the spontaneous interaction trials, with minimal changes during depressed interactions.

A comparison of the behavior of both groups of infants suggests a passive/active contrast in coping behavior. The infants of depressed mothers appear to mirror the mothers' behavior, indicating that by experiencing frequent lack of control in their early interactions they have developed a depressed, passive/coping interactive style. While these data imply that a mother's depression can be transmitted to the infant through early interactions, the question remains as to whether depressed behavior results from mirroring maternal behavior or can be ascribed to the minimal levels of stimulation these mothers provide.

The cluster of behavioral responses observed by Field in the infants of mothers who were clinically depressed is reminiscent of behavioral manifestations that Seligman (1975) and others noted in models of learned helplessness. Researchers who have studied this phenomenon have isolated several factors that may contribute to the condition. Environmental variables that may affect the infant's perception of contingency (such as delays between behavior and consequence, less than perfect contingency) and lack of discriminative stimuli (poor signaling of contingency availability) were identified by Watson (1966, 1971, 1972) as potential etiological variables facilitating the manifestation of learned helplessness behavior. By failing to establish normative patterns of interaction with their infants, the clinically depressed mothers in Field's study may inadvertently be interfering with their infants' perception of contingency. Thus, these mothers may be triggering a learned helplessness response. Since learned helplessness is considered an analogue for depression, the infants in Field's study may be viewed as manifesting incipient depressive-like phenomena.

Conclusion

These studies offer a series of creative methodologies for investigating infant depression within the face-to-face paradigm. Cohn and Tronick, as well as Field, all found that an interaction in which depression was simulated could yield valuable insights, while Massie investigated dyads in which the infant was later diagnosed as suffering from pathology. In addition, these studies have illuminated possible relationships between hypotheses involving the etiology of depression. Data from Field's study, for instance, shed new light on the phenomenon of learned helplessness, as one analogue for depression.

CHAPTER 8

Learned Helplessness Paradigm

Depressive disorders present a heterogeneous spectrum of manifestations with respect to etiology, levels of severity, and clinical course. In order to formulate empirical models of depression, theorists have categorized clinical phenomena and hypothesized distinct subsets of depression. Because it emphasizes instrumental learning and implicates interactional failures between caregivers and infants, one theory, Learned Helplessness, may especially illuminate the realm of depression in infancy and childhood.

Seligman, Maier, and Geer (1968), expounding on the Learned Helplessness Theory first presented by Seligman and Maier (1967), stated that when individuals view their actions as irrelevant to subsequent outcomes, they display learned helplessness. The cornerstone of the Learned Helplessness Theory is that after the experience of uncontrollable events major motivational, cognitive, and emotional deficits color the psychological experience of the individual. Some researchers (Abramson, Seligman, & Teasdale, 1978) have postulated that all three deficits, together with negative self–esteem, are essential to comprise clinical depression.

This chapter investigates the possibility of a correlation between learned helplessness and infant and childhood depression. In the course of the inquiry, a set of preconditions for clinically significant learned helplessness is inferred. Moreover, the issue of whether infants are developmentally capable of fulfilling these preconditions is examined. In addition, the implications of discrepancy awareness, contingency awareness, and effectance motivation as prerequisites for developing learned helplessness are explored. Relevant clinical studies are reviewed in order to clarify how learned helplessness might either contribute to or constitute depression.

Case Report

Amy was adopted by the L family when she was five weeks old. According to her adopted parents, she was a physically healthy, but "ugly" baby—in sharp contrast to the family's son, who had also been adopted in early infancy. When Amy was 19 months old, the Ls sought professional help, as a result of what they perceived to be serious problems with Amy's development. The couple described the infant as "irritable" and resistant to affection. In addition, they complained that Amy engaged in prolonged screaming fits. Mrs. L claimed that any slight frustration precipitated such a fit.

The Ls also expressed concern over Amy's lack of verbalization. Significantly, they reported that they "could not understand Amy," because she gave inadequate verbal and non-verbal cues. The infant's parents characterized her as hyperactive and accident prone as well. Moreover, based on the parents' comments, Amy's responses appeared peculiarly inappropriate and discrepant. For example, the Ls said that once Amy had been badly burned when sitting on a campfire, but she had not cried. Amy ate voraciously, but seemed to have no awareness of being full. Nor did Amy imitate her parents or "try to please them." She rarely smiled and, instead, the L's reported persistent gaze aversion behavior.

Based on this parental assessment, the therapeutic team expected a child with severe personality disturbance, perhaps complicated by neurological abnormalities. However, Amy actually presented a radically different clinical picture. The infant's scores were well within the normal range on developmental tests and in diagnostic play sessions, although her responses were sober and unsmiling. Language acquisition skills also appeared normal, but Amy asked permission for every move she made. Contrary to her parents' report, Amy responded sharply to their disapproval during testing sessions. From these observations it was apparent that a distinct pattern of non-communication permeated the relationship between parents and child. Clearly, Amy and her parents were a "mismatch"; their responses to one another were marred by non-contingency.

After this 19 month evaluation, the therapists developed a working hypothesis of the relationship between Amy and her parents. It was believed that although Amy may have been an unusually sensitive infant, her behavior problems were due primarily to inappropriate parental response. Thus, Amy's carelessness for her safety was interpreted as a symptom of abnormal, non-contingent feedback in the nurturing environment.

Amy and her parents subsequently entered therapy. At the 24 month evaluation, Amy was found to have made remarkable progress. She emerged as an energetic, alert child. But these behavior patterns receded when Amy heard her mother approaching outside. At these times she became frightened and retreated to a stiff, dull, non-communicative attitude.

Therapy with Amy's parents eventually revealed that the couple, particularly Amy's mother, were not equipped to deal with the child. Subsequently, Amy was placed with another family, the Bs. In marked contrast to Amy's first mother, Mrs. B displayed an intuitive capacity to match Amy's communications appropriately. Indeed, unlike Mrs. L, who was unable to forge a communicative exchange, Mrs. B commented that "Amy tells us things in so many ways."

Two months after Amy's placement with the Bs, clinic appointments were terminated. It was felt that Amy's move to a nurturing environment had triggered strong recuperative powers in the child. The lack of harmony and non-contingency characteristic of Amy's interaction with her first mother had been replaced by a mutually fulfilling, harmonious parent-infant relationship (Naylor, 1982).

Overview of the Learned Helplessness Paradigm

The Learned Helplessness Paradigm posits that for all animals the psychological impact of the perception that one is powerless to achieve one's goals is manifested in a generalized passivity, symptomatic of motivational, cognitive and emotional deficits (Maier & Seligman, 1976; Maier, Seligman & Soloman, 1969; Seligman, 1975; Seligman, Maier & Soloman, 1971). For humans, the psychological impact includes a self-esteem deficit (Abramson, et al. 1978).

Seligman (1975) investigated whether dogs previously exposed to uncontrollable aversive stimuli had difficulty learning to avoid similar stimuli once the experiment allowed them to do so. Describing one such experiment in detail, Seligman stated:

On the first day, the subject was strapped into the hammock and given 64 inescapable electric shocks, each 5 seconds long and of [moderately painful] intensity. Shocks were not preceded by any signal and occurred randomly. Twenty-four hours later, the subject was given 10 trials of escape avoidance training . . . the dog had to jump over the barrier from one compartment into the other to escape shock. The onset of a signal (light dimming) began each trial, and the signal stayed on until the trial ended. If the dog jumped the barrier during this interval, the signal terminated and the shock was prevented. Failure to jump during the signal led to a shock, which continued until the dog jumped the barrier. If the dog failed to jump the barrier within 60 seconds . . . the trial automatically ended. (p. 23)

The investigators observed that dogs previously exposed to the uncontrollable shock situation showed lingering carry-over effects of the trauma, seeming to give up and passively accept further, similar provocations. In contrast, naive dogs successfully escaped avoidable aversive stimuli. The investigators concluded that uncontrollable trauma apparently interfered with the dogs' ability to learn.

As postulated by Seligman, the Learned Helplessness Theory holds that when exposure to aversive, uncontrollable events teaches an animal that it cannot achieve its goal of escaping from traumatic episodes, major motivational, cognitive, and emotional deficits result in the following sequence. First, uncontrollable events undermine an animal's motivation to initiate voluntary instrumental responses that control other events. Second, the experience of vulnerability interferes with learning, affecting the animal's ability to choose responses that might allow escape from further trauma. Finally, uncontrollable trauma produces intolerable fear, which ultimately yields to depression. A possible mechanism by which fear is subsumed by depression was illuminated by Soloman and Corbitt (1974). According to Soloman and Corbitt, emotions can antagonize each other. That is, one emotion comes to the fore and dominates when another emotion is experienced at intolerable intensities. Soloman and Corbitt regarded fear and depression as opponent emotions.

In the experiment described by Seligman (1975), for example, a dog may experience significant fear in response to inescapable shocks. However, whereas effective action taken against the aversive stimulus might normally allow the dog to avoid the stimulus and alleviate fear, in uncontrollable situations no action is effective. As the shocks are repeated, the fear itself becomes painful. Ultimately the dog's central nervous system deadens the fear; passivity results. Thus, at least one irritant, fear, is defeated. Seligman (1975) stated that, in this manner, the Learned Helplessness Theory is compatible with Soloman and Corbitt's suggestion that emotions act as antagonists to each other.

Clinical Relevance of Learned Helplessness Theory

Seligman and co-workers speculated that, like animals, humans could become passive in situations in which they perceive that they cannot mitigate or control future traumatic events (Miller & Seligman, 1973; Seligman, 1972, 1975). Consequently, Seligman et al. and other researchers conducted investigations into the effects of uncontrollable events on humans (Donovan, 1981; Hiroto, 1974; Hiroto & Seligman, 1975; Kevill & Kirkland, 1979; Klein & Seligman, 1976).

An example of such an experiment is Hiroto's 1974 study, which used noise as the irritating stimulus. In the first phase of the study, subjects in one group were exposed to artificial noise that they could terminate by pushing a button. Subjects in a second group were exposed to uncontrollable artificial noise. Subjects in a third group were not exposed to any artificial noise stimulus. Subsequently, all subjects were exposed to artificial noise that they could control by operating a hand shuttle box. As distinguished from the other two groups, the subjects who received prior uncontrollable noise stimulation failed to use the box to control the noise. Experiments such as Hiroto's demonstrate that learned helplessness is a legitimate phenomenon, blunting the ability to effectively protect oneself from trauma.

Self Esteem Deficit

As first noted by Klein and Seligman (1976) and Bandura (1977), when learned helplessness is applied in humans, the original hypotheses by Seligman and Maier (1967) do not distinguish between personal and universal helplessness. With this criticism in mind, Abramson et al. (1978) reformulated the original theory to incorporate the idea that *attributional style* determines vulnerability to learned helplessness depression.

. . . [O]nce people perceive noncontingency, they attribute their helplessness to a cause. This cause can be stable or unstable, global or specific, and internal or external. The attribution chosen influences whether expectation of future helplessness will be chronic or acute, broad or narrow, and whether helplessness will lower self-esteem or not. (p. 49)

The distinction that the authors drew between personal and universal helplessness in humans led them to describe the fourth key deficit characterizing learned helplessness depression: low self-esteem. Abramson and colleagues defined personal learned helplessness as the belief that one cannot solve soluble problems and that failure is directly attributable to lack of individual ability. On the other hand, perceiving that a problem is insoluble by anyone reflects an attitude of universal helplessness and an attributional style less damaging to one's self-esteem.

The reformulated Learned Helplessness Theory, emphasizing the individual's attributional style, predicted that the attribution that an individual makes about the cause of his or her helplessness determines both the generality and chronicity of the learned helplessness. The investigators suggested that individuals view their helplessness as global if they perceive themselves to be helpless in a broad range of situations. For example, upon failing an algebra test, one might reason either, "I am stupid" or "I am stupid at math." The former provokes global learned helplessness; the latter provokes helplessness only during future algebra tests, a helpless response specific in nature.

Abramson and colleagues further posited that individuals who perceive their helplessness as global typically consider their flaws to be so pervasive that they do not regard any conceivable response as capable of controlling aversive events. Nor do such individuals perceive of themselves as potentially capable in most situations. This attitude dramatically reflects the low self-esteem typical of persons with learned helplessness. Such individuals are prone to develop chronic helplessness deficits that transfer across tasks, because the stability of their low self-esteem convinces them that they will always lack the appropriate controlling responses.

In sum, the reformulated Learned Helplessness Theory states that attributions to internal factors suggest a propensity for learning helplessness. The severity of the psychological deficits resulting from learned helplessness depends on the subtleties of attributional style—that is, whether one sees one's shortcomings as all-pervasive and/or chronic, or as situation specific and/or transient.

Learned Helplessness and Depression

Learned helplessness qualities of personal versus universal, global versus specific, and stable versus transient are likely to have profound clinical ramifications. Seligman (1975) stated that he considered the scope of his original theory to be limited to "reactive depression." However, he postulated that although endogenous depressions are not triggered by an explicit helplessness-inducing event, they may also involve a belief in helplessness. Once he and others had reformulated the original theory, these investigators held that the expectation of helplessness was a sufficient but not necessary condition for depression (Abramson et al., 1978).

Data exist supporting the notion that a continuum of susceptibility to the belief in one's own helplessness underlies both endogenous and "reactive" depression. Raps and co-workers (1982) confirmed the association between attributional style and depressive symptoms predicted by the learned helplessness formulation. These investigators compared the responses of unipolar depressives, nondepressed schizophrenics, and medical patients to task-related outcomes. They found that unipolar depressed patients were more likely to attribute poor outcomes to global and internal-stable causes than the other two groups. The authors suggested that this attributional style not only predisposes individuals to depression, but also maintains depressive symptoms once they are present.

Interestingly, the results of some studies concerning a related phenomenon, "illusion of control," while not directly proving a susceptibility to the belief in one's own helplessness on the part of depressed individuals, suggest that such individuals are far less likely than others to believe they control uncontrollable events. This research points to the pivotal role that perception plays in the theory of learned helplessness.

Langer (1975) coined the term "illusion of control," specifically referring to the perception that one controls objectively uncontrollable and chance events. She defined illusion of control as "an expectancy of a personal success probability inappropriately higher than the objective probability would warrant" (p. 311). The results of her studies showed that certain chance situations cause some individuals to feel inappropriately confident. Langer suggested that the more similar a chance situation is to a skill situation with which an individual feels adept, the greater the individual's illusion of control will be.

The construct of illusion of control is at virtually the opposite end of the conceptual spectrum from the construct of learned helplessness. Illusion of control suggests that bravado, like helplessness, is learned and is a function of the degree of success with which one previously attained goals. Significant to the Learned Helplessness Paradigm is Langer's finding that depressed individuals exhibit no illusions of control.

In sum, the adjustments to the Learned Helplessness Paradigm incorporated by Seligman and colleagues (Abramson et al., 1978) establish a model of depression postulating the following flow of events. The individual perceives of himself or herself as helpless in the face of aversive stimuli and then attributes failure to control such stimuli to internal, stable, and chronic factors. Consequently, he or she expects to always be ineffective in attaining most if not all desired goals and in avoiding failure and trauma. This expectation gives way to fear that is experienced at extreme intensities. To defeat this intolerable fear, the nervous system deadens and responds with a resignation and passivity characteristic of depression.

Similar Models of Depression

By equating depression with a belief that one is helpless, the Learned Helplessness Paradigm is similar to other constructs of depression, particularly those evolved by Bibring (1953) and Melges and Bowlby (1969). Bibring (1953) defined depression as "the emotional expression of a state of helplessness and powerlessness of the ego, irrespective of what may have caused the breakdown of the mechanisms which established . . . self-esteem" (p. 24). Bibring conceptualized that normal strivings are inhibited when their futility becomes apparent. For example, a hungry infant signals the caregiver to satisfy his or her needs. If frustrated, he or she responds with anxiety and anger; however, the infant continues to signal his or her needs. If these needs remain unmet, the exhausted infant senses its own helplessness and becomes depressed. Bibring suggested that experiences of helplessness in infancy are perhaps the strongest factors predisposing individuals to later depression. Like the Learned Helplessness Theory, Bibring's theory implies that continued frustration in achieving prized goals may contribute to depression.

Both Lichtenberg (1957) and Melges and Bowlby (1969) emphasized the affective component of helplessness by proposing that depression is a manifestation of felt helplessness. Lichtenberg specified that helplessness is the perception of a low probability of success in the attainment of one's goals when one attributes probable failure to personal deficits. Melges and Bowlby described helplessness as an affective state occurring when an individual perceives that plans will probably not achieve goals. These researchers went on to describe severely depressed patients as helpless because they assumed failure to be typical for themselves. According to Melges and Bowlby, depressed patients believe that frustration and failures are directly due to a personal incompetence that is insurmountable.

Evidence abounds indicating an association between learned helplessness and depression in adults. However, because learned helplessness implies the presence of complex developmental processes, questions remain as to how susceptible children and infants are to developing this form of depression. Furthermore, because attributional styles have been posited to play a significant role in the development of learned helplessness depression, one must ask whether the very young, who may be cognitively incapable of formulating attributions, can "learn" helplessness in the clinical sense. Therefore, the question of whether the Learned Helplessness Paradigm is appropriate for researching depression either occurring in or deriving from childhood and infancy remains to be answered.

Resolution of this issue depends on the results of investigations into the development of competence. For example, what motivates an individual toward attempting competence and positive self-attribution? Is affect associated with success and failure in early attempts to control the environment? Are infants and young children able to objectively distinguish between their own successes and failures? Are they capable of formulating self-concepts and of experiencing self-esteem deficits?

Learned Helplessness in Adults

Experiments with adults reveal that experiencing helplessness in one task can indeed affect performance on other tasks. Kevill and Kirkland (1979) tested 71 female adults for evidence of learned helplessness and impaired transference learning across tasks. In the first phase of the experiment, subjects were exposed to either a neonatal pain-cry or to a noise signal. The subjects were divided into three groups. The first group could terminate the auditory signal by pressing a button. For the second group, pressing a button provided no relief. The third group was given no button to press. Auditory signals were administered randomly and intermittently.

In the second phase of the experiment, all subjects were presented with 20 anagrams to be solved. As a group, subjects who had earlier had a button to press, but could not terminate the auditory signal, had the least success in solving the anagrams. For them, solving the anagrams required the most attempts and resulted in a greater number of failures. The investigators stated that these subjects' motivation to solve the anagrams was undermined by the recent exposure to uncontrollable events.

Donovan (1981) conducted a similar study, also using adult females as subjects and infant crying as an auditory signal. In the first phase of the experiment, mothers were assigned to one of three conditions. They could escape the auditory signal, they could not escape the signal, or they were not exposed to the signal at all. In the second phase of the experiment, the mothers were exposed to a soluble escape task that consisted of sliding a knob in a box from one side to another. The group of mothers pretreated with inescapable infant crying displayed debilitated escape response. In contrast, mothers in the other groups did not. During his experiment, Donovan also monitored the cardiac responses of all subjects. He found that only the mothers pretreated with the escapable cry exhibited cardiac deceleration when cues led them to anticipate the onset of the cry stimulus. Donovan suggested that the differences in cardiac rate could imply that the mothers' prior experience in controlling an auditory stimulus increased their efficacy in interpreting environmental cues.

Thus, Kevill and Kirkland (1979) and Donovan (1981) produced evidence indicating that lack of contingency—that is, exposure to an uncontrollable situation—blunts the individual's capability to respond effectively in subsequent situations.

Learned Helplessness in Children

In a developmental study of learned helplessness, Rholes, Blackwell, Jordan, and Walters (1980) found that although older children display situation-specific learned helplessness, younger children do not. These investigators assessed the persistence and success exhibited by kindergartners, first-, third-, and fifth-grade children in their attempts to identify hidden figures in drawings. The degree of learned helplessness was assessed following both repeated success and repeated failure experiences at this task.

Following failure, the kindergartners, first-, and third-graders in this study showed no evidence of helplessness on further, similar hidden figure tasks. In contrast, fifth-graders who had failed on earlier tasks appeared to become helpless in measures of both persistence and performance on additional, similar tasks relative to those who had not experienced failure.

The results reported by Rholes and his group, indicating that younger children may not be susceptible to learned helplessness, are corroborated by data reported by Ruble, Parsons, and Ross (1976) and Parsons and Ruble (1977). The first of these studies found that kindergartners' perceptions of their abilities are less affected by success or failure than are the perceptions of seven to nine year olds. The latter study found that the experience of success and failure in older children (11 years) has a greater impact on future expectations for success or failure than it has for younger children. The results of these investigations strongly suggest that learned helplessness experiences may not affect younger children in the same manner as older children.

In a 1973 study, Dweck and Reppucci clearly demonstrated differences in attributional style, self-concept, and performance subsequent to failure among eight year old children. The investigators observed that following success at an achievement task, some children do not attribute their success to internal factors. Following failure, these same children do not perform the response required to succeed at successive tasks, despite the motivation and capacity to succeed. This behavior suggested to the investigators that such children had come to perceive outcomes as independent of their efforts. The investigators categorized these children as "learned helpless." In analyzing the attributional styles of helpless children, the investigators discovered that they take little responsibility for either successes or failures, and to the extent that they do take responsibility, they typically attribute both success and failure to ability rather than to effort. The investigators speculated that since helpless children see outcomes as non-contingent upon themselves, they are less likely to view adverse circumstances as being surmountable through effort. Since these children perceive of themselves as deficient in ability, they view effort as both futile and irrelevant.

On the other hand, Dweck and Reppucci also found that some children do attribute success to their own abilities. These children (categorized as "mastery oriented") do not seem to give up when confronted with failure. The investigators concluded that "two children may receive exactly the same number and sequence of success and failure trials yet react quite differently as a function of whether they interpret the failure to mean that the situation is beyond or within their control" (Dweck, 1975, p. 675).

Realizing that the performance of helpless children deteriorates in the face of failure, Dweck (1975) investigated whether altering children's perceptions that their own inadequacies are at the root of their failures could serve as an intervening factor, mitigating performance deterioration. Indeed, she found that when helpless children between the ages of eight and 13 years were educated to formulate less self-implicating attributions, their performance on achievement tasks either was maintained or improved. These data strongly implicate the role of negative self concept in learned helplessness, and correspond to the work of Donovan in adults, suggesting that a learned helpless response may be reversible.

In a 1980 study, Diener and Dweck attempted to examine more thoroughly the nature of the differences between helpless and mastery-oriented children in perceptions of their success. They administered an achievement task on which fourth-, fifth-, and sixth-graders experienced success, followed shortly by a failure experience. Helpless children typically underestimated their successes and did not view success as indicative of ability. In addition, following success, they did not predict that they would be successful in the future. Moreover, after first experiencing failure, they tended to re-evaluate their prior successes in light of their failures and to show a performance decline resulting from a progressive decrease in the use of effective strategies and an increase in the use of ineffectual strategies. Diener and Dweck also observed that for helpless children failure results in negative affect. On the other hand, failure did not trouble mastery-oriented children. They viewed their failure as neither important nor predictive. Indeed, some mastery-oriented children in Diener and Dweck's study actually became more sophisticated in strategy use when they received failure feedback. Noting that helpless children do not recognize or remember the actual extent of their success, that they view other children as more capable, that they do not view present success as predictive of future success, and that they often ascribe success to external factors and failure to internal factors, the investigators concluded that for helpless children, success is a "less successful" experience than it is for mastery-oriented children.

The above studies offer substantial evidence that children from at least age eight and upward are capable of forming negative self-concepts. Furthermore, they clearly link self-concept, as reflected in attributions for failure, to negative affect and to declining performance in the face of failure. However, these studies did not directly address whether children transfer feelings and manifestations of helplessness across tasks.

Dweck, Goetz, and Strauss (1980) tested children classified as "helpless" to determine whether their attributions for failure affected future performance in other settings. Citing previous studies (Dweck & Bush, 1976; Dweck, Davidson, Nelson, & Enna, 1978; Nicholls, 1975) indicating important sex differences in reactions to failure and in attributional style, the investigators predicted that boys would transfer failure across tasks to a smaller degree than girls. This study, therefore, also attempted to determine the role of sex differences in the incorporation of failure into self-concept.

The investigators found that "at the beginning of the new school year when little immediate evidence of . . . performance capabilities is available and when attention is not directed toward concrete evidence . . . girls tend to be more pessimistic than boys about their future performance" Dweck et al. (1980, p. 451). Furthermore, boys showed a greater resilience to failure. They did not predict failure for themselves at other tasks once they had failed at one. Girls, in contrast, showed persistent pessimism in response to failure. Failure at one task typically caused them to predict failure for themselves at other tasks.

Thus, phenomena characteristic of a learned helplessness response have been experimentally identified in children. The next step is a review of documented evidence pertaining to manifestations of learned helplessness in young children, and ultimately, in infants.

Learned Helplessness in Infants

As of this date, no means of examining the attributional style and self-concept of pre-verbal infants has been devised. However, studies have been conducted testing infants for evidence of diminished learning consequent to the experience of uncontrollable events. Some investigations seem to have disproved learned helplessness in infancy, while others seem to have demonstrated that infants can, in fact, learn helplessness.

Ramey and Finkelstein (1978) introduced evidence that argues against a hypothesis that helplessness can be learned by young infants. The investigators exposed three month old infants to 10 minute sessions of non-contingent stimulation. Subsequently, these infants readily learned a task in which visual stimulation was contingent on their control; in other words, these infants did not seem to suffer a cognitive deficit from previous experience with non-contingent stimulation.

Gekoski and Fagen (1984) assessed the effects of prior non-contingent experience on subsequent learning in three month old infants. They exposed infants ranging in age from 10 to 12 weeks to a non-contingent mobile. For some infants the mobile continuously rotated; for others the mobile was static. Infants were exposed to their non-contingent mobiles for 12 minutes each day for seven days. Then they were tested in a 15 minute conditioning session with a contingent mobile that bounced in response to a kicking action. The investigators found that the infant's ability to learn that the bouncing mobile was contingent had not been impeded by prior exposure to non-contingent stimulation, and the investigators concluded that "at three months the infant's ability to acquire a contingent relationship is unaffected by prior non-contingent exposure" (Gekoski & Fagen, 1984, p. 2231).

But in light of evidence that the younger the child, the less vulnerable he or she is to learned helplessness, it is noteworthy that Finkelstein and Ramey (1977) also provided evidence indicating that infants may be able to learn helplessness after all. After three days of familiarization with a non-contingent stimulus, six month olds were exposed to the same stimulus, which was now contingent. After four days of familiarization to a non-contingent stimulus, nine month olds were exposed to a different stimulus that was contingent. Neither group learned to control the stimulus. Considering that neonates have demonstrated instrumental learning (DeCasper & Carstens, 1981), Finkelstein and Ramey's results are suggestive of a cognitive deficit predictive of learned helplessness.

Furthermore, DeCasper and Carsten's 1981 study provided perhaps the most dramatic evidence suggesting that infants might learn helplessness. They demonstrated that 15 minutes of non-contingent auditory stimulation given anywhere from four to 24 hours prior to a conditioning session impaired neonates' ability to learn that appropriately spaced bursts of non-nutritive sucking could trigger the same stimulus.

The results of the above-cited studies are contradictory. Some demonstrate cognitive impairment; some do not. Therefore, the implications regarding infancy and learned helplessness are unclear. However, even if the studies just reviewed had uniformly demonstrated cognitive impairment in infants, their implications for learned helplessness would still be ambiguous. Although evidence of diminished learning suggests cognitive impairment (and cognitive deficits are fundamental to the Learned Helplessness Paradigm) cognitive impairment might actually serve as a protective mechanism, shielding the infant against learning helplessness. By way of explanation, a review of the basic sequence of events posited by Seligman and colleagues (Abramson et al., 1978) is in order.

The Learned Helplessness Paradigm proposes that uncontrollable events result in the perception of past or present noncontingency, that produces self-blame, which in turn produces the expectation of future noncontingency. Having learned to always expect noncontingency, the individual becomes depressed. Therefore, this paradigm, rather than requiring diminished learning, actually demands that the individual retain the ability to learn. Specifically, the individual must learn to expect future noncontingency and to attribute failure to internal deficiencies. That is, the individual must "learn" to be helpless. Studies failing to demonstrate diminished learning therefore may *not,* in fact, fail to demonstrate learned helplessness. In essence, studies demonstrating diminished learning may actually demonstrate the acquisition of a defense against helplessness. This hypothesis points to the importance of evaluating attributional style, rather than task performance, in assessing learned helplessness.

As mentioned, with respect to learned helplessness depression, the paradigm specifies that depression results from deficits of self-esteem. While this section provides evidence of situation specific learned helplessness in children, a review of the empirical data regarding children's ability to formulate negative self-concepts produces no indisputable evidence that young children and infants are capable of self-attributing their failures and of incorporating failure into self-concepts. The ability to self-attribute failure may indeed be developmentally dependent (Nicholls & Miller, 1985; Stipek, 1981a; 1981b; Stipek & Hoffman, 1980; Stipek, Roberts & Sanborn, 1984; Weisz, Yeates, Robertson, & Beckham, 1982). If so, the inability of young children and infants to attribute task-related failure to internal causes may explain why clear-cut instances of learned helplessness in infants and children are difficult to obtain experimentally. Nevertheless, a review of cognitive, motivational, and affective capacities charted through the developmental milestones of temperament, attachment, and self-concept may shed further light on the implications of the Learned Helplessness Paradigm for the study of infant depression.

Temperament Capabilities as Factors Influencing Learned Helplessness

Temperament has traditionally been defined as individual variation in behavioral style. While temperament is ultimately affected by external factors, most researchers agree that it is largely a concept emphasizing constitutional or intrinsic traits manifested from early infancy onward. To assess how temperament may contribute to the etiology of depression in early infancy and to explore how temperament dimensions may serve as a "screen" through which to evaluate infant behaviors, it is useful to articulate the connection between temperament dimensions and the constructs of various learning theorists.

For example, the New York Longitudinal Study (Chess & Thomas, 1985; Thomas, Chess, Birch, Hertzig, & Korn, 1963), a seminal investigation focusing on infant temperament, isolated the following temperament dimensions: *intensity of reaction* (defined as energy level of response), *threshold of responsiveness* (defined as level of stimulation needed to evoke a response), and *attention span and persistence* (defined as ability to continue with activity in the face of obstacles). Rothbart and Derryberry

(1981) coined similar semantic phrases to identify traits of temperament. In their model, *activity level* (gross motor activity), *distress of limitations* (fussing, crying or other displays of distress), and *duration of orienting* (vocalization or gazing behavior at objects for extended periods of time) were noted. Finally, Rowe and Plomin (1977) focused on the temperament dimensions of *emotionality, activity,* and *attention span-persistence*. Although temperamental traits are referred to by different appellations, these researchers concur on the basic constitutional components that comprise the construct of temperament. (See Table 8.1.)

Most pertinent and revealing to this discussion of learned helplessness is the fact that several learning researchers have devised theoretical constructs that appear to presuppose the existence of temperamental dimensions, thus underscoring the role of temperament in shaping infant behavior and/or learning capacity. The following studies discuss McCall and McGhee's Discrepancy Awareness Hypothesis (1977), Watson's Theory of Contingency Awareness (1966) and its implications for investigating the phenomenon of learned helplessness, White's concept of effectance motivation (1959), and Yarrow and colleagues's construct of mastery motivation (Yarrow et al., 1983). Each of these researchers has presented a perspective for interpreting early infant learning capacities and significantly, the concepts are reminiscent of concepts in the area of infant temperament research. Thus, one way of highlighting the constructs of the learning theorists is to evaluate them in terms of the temperament dimensions noted above.

The Discrepancy Awareness Hypothesis

McCall and McGhee (1977) formulated the Discrepancy Hypothesis to explain the mechanism whereby cognitive and affective capabilities are used by the very young infant to respond to new stimuli in the environment. According to this theory, a *moderate* level of stimulus discrepancy will evoke both optimal attention and positive affect, while familiar or extremely discrepant stimuli will evoke low infant attention, accompanied by negative affect. The Discrepancy Hypothesis posits that infants possess sufficient evocative memory to distinguish between stimuli, and further, that a developed process of retrieval from memory storage exists.

The Discrepancy Hypothesis is noteworthy to this discussion because the theory stresses discrete affective displays that relate to temperament dimensions. Thus, qualitative aspect of mood, whether positive (e.g., smiling) or negative (e.g., crying), has been particularly reported on by researchers studying discrepancy awareness in infants. The implication of these studies is that the infant's temperament, displayed through individual variations in the expression of affective states, will have a significant impact on his or her capacity to both experience discrepancy initially and to respond to the discrepant stimulus subsequently.

TABLE 8.1. Temperament dimensions correlated with learning factors.

Temperament dimensions	Learning factors
Rhythmicity[a] Persistence[a]	In 2–3-month-olds, both increased conditioning; rhythmicity provides structure from which to perceive predictability
Rhythmicity[b]	In 3- and 5-month-olds; provides structure for organizing affective/cognitive experience
Persistence[c] Exploration[c]	At 6 and 12 months, correlated with later developmental competence Positive affect correlated with social competence not task competence
Activity level[d]	In 3–4-month-olds, 55% cried in response to violation of learned expectancy
Distress to limitations[d] Duration of orienting[d] Distress to novel stimuli[d]	Formed within group correlation with activity level for infants who cried Correlated with crying response to learned expectancy Correlated with crying in response to learned expectancy
Activity level[e]	In 6-month-olds, correlated with crying in response to learned expectancy
Persistence[f]	In review of research in mastery motivation, the primary measure for mastery was persistence
Positive affect[g]	Increased or raised expectancy
Positive affect[h] Active tempo[h] Negative affect[h] Passive tempo[h]	Increased learning and measures of interest, involvement, arousal Increased learning and measures of interest, involvement, arousal Decreased learning and measures of interest, involvement, arousal Decreased learning and measures of interest, involvement, arousal

[a] Dunst and Lingerfelt (1985).
[b] Lester et al. (1985).
[c] Yarrow et al. (1983).
[d] Fagen and Ohr (1985).
[e] Rothbart and Derryberry (1981).
[f] Morgan and Harmon (1984).
[g] Masters and Furman (1976).
[h] Masters et al. (1979).

The Effectance Motivation System

White's (1959) insights about intrinsic motivation toward competence can shed some light on the appropriateness of the Learned Helplessness Paradigm for studying depression occurring or originating in childhood and infancy. White observed that much of human behavior appears to be directed toward having effects upon the environment, regardless of whether the behavior ultimately satisfies a physiological need. He posited a behavioral system, the sole aim of which is the experience of efficacy or mastery. White proposed that the "effectance motivation system" reflects an intrinsic and universal motive to attain competence, defined as the capacity to interact effectively with the environment.

According to White, the effectance motivation system operates even in very young infants. Moreover, the theory implies specific motivational, cognitive, emotional, and self-esteem capabilities for infants and children.

1. *Motivation*   White proposed that infants are intrinsically motivated to learn, which they manifest by exploring the environment. Early learning experiences and the acquisition of new skills are doubly rewarding: the increased and inherently pleasurable competence new skills bring is matched by the mobility the skills afford infants in furthering their explorations. Therefore, even though activities such as attention, perception, and exploration may be independently motivated, they function ultimately in the service of competence.
2. *Cognition and Behavior*   In suggesting that pleasure is always derived from effectance, White tied emotion closely to cognition. Furthermore, in stating that the effectance motivation system gives impetus to all learning, he suggests that even very young infants strive to learn and are emotionally affected by learning.
3. *Self-Esteem*   White's approach to effectance motivation suggests that self-esteem is rooted in the experience of efficacy (White, 1963). He explained that although parental praise and encouragement figure in the quality of an infant's self-esteem, the infant's own experiences of efficacy and sense of competence regulate the development of self-concept.

Significantly, the components of White's effectance motivation system bear resemblance to several of the temperament dimensions noted above. The "intrinsic motivation to learn" may represent another form of articulating such temperament dimensions as intensity of reaction, threshold of responsiveness (Thomas et al., 1963), attention span and persistence (Rowe & Plomin, 1977), and duration of orienting (Rothbart, 1981). Moreover, by emphasizing that the experience of efficacy propelling the child to learn is largely intrinsic (and therefore constitutional), White's theory clearly alludes to the role temperament may play in the development of both competence and learned helplessness. Nevertheless, White's notion of an effectance motivation system was strictly theoretically based. Thus, investigations conducted by strategists which attempt to make White's theory operational carry the burden of establishing whether it is empirically sound and whether the main inference of White's theory, that infants and young children can learn both competence and helplessness, carries evidential weight.

Empirical Support for Effectance Motivation Construct

Harter's efforts (1974, 1977, 1978, 1982; Harter & Pike, 1984) to make White's model of effectance motivation operational succeeded in providing empirical support for White's basic tenets. Her adjustments to White's construct indicate that effectance motivation can be observed at different developmental levels, and that the Learned Helplessness Paradigm may be appropriate for studying depression occurring or originating in childhood.

To translate White's effectance motivation construct into researchable hypotheses, Harter (1978) dissected the construct into components, correlates, and mediators, and then theorized from a developmental perspective.

1. *Components*   The degree to which her subjects derived pleasure from social reinforcement (Harter, 1974, 1977) suggested to Harter that from infancy onward, individuals require positive reinforcement to encourage and sustain their mastery attempts. Harter proposed two sources of intrinsic motivation. One was White's effectance motivation construct, which Harter agreed was biologically programmed. Harter thus concurred with White that individual behavioral styles (temperament) are fundamental to effectance motivation. The other source had experiential roots and could be determined: 1) by the values imparted by caregivers to children, affecting the internalization of mastery goals; and 2) by the amount of social reinforcement that children received, determining the nature and strength of their self-reward system.

2. *Correlates*   White (1959) originally proposed that successful encounters with the environment are, by nature, rewarding. According to White, mastery and the belief that one is competent are experienced pleasurably. Harter gave credence to White's position, but added that both intrinsic and socially dependent reinforcement combine to produce positive affect.

3. *Mediators*   Harter explained:

with regard to the child's sense of control, a reinforcement history which rewards the child for independent mastery attempts provides an incentive for such performance . . . the combination of perceived competence or high self-esteem and internal perception of control should in turn enhance the child's feelings of efficacy or intrinsic pleasure. As such, these perceptions should serve as important mediators by maintaining, if not increasing, the child's effectance motivation. (Harter, 1978, p. 57)

Harter's most significant contribution to White's arguments, therefore, was the inclusion of socially dependent reinforcement as a factor motivating children toward competence.

In discussing his construct of effectance motivation, White specified that self-esteem is rooted in efficacy (1963). Based on her 1978 refinements to White's construct, Harter derived scales to assess hypothesized domains of self-esteem (Harter, 1978; Harter & Pike, 1984). Harter conceptually and operationally defined self-esteem as "perceived competence" and experimentally isolated three domains of self-esteem (1978): cognitive, social, and physical. In 1978, she developed "the perceived competence scale for children," an instrument through which these three domains of self-esteem could be assessed.

In a 1982 study, Harter used this scale to test a hypothesis that perceived competence is positively related to the strength of one's effectance motivation system. Three hundred third- through sixth-graders were individually tested for perceived competence on all three of the scale's self-esteem domains. In addition, the subjects were tested for extrinsic versus intrinsic motivation in the classroom. The findings revealed a clear correlation between perceived cognitive competence and intrinsic motivation. Harter concluded that children as young as eight years old can make meaningful differentiations among all of the self-esteem domains assessed by the scale.

The Learned Helplessness Paradigm stipulates that low self-esteem plays an important role in an individual's vulnerability to depression. Therefore, valid application of the paradigm to the childhood years requires that children be capable of forming self-concepts. Harter's 1982 findings (that perceived competence is directly related to the effectance motivation system and that young children are cognitively capable of forming self concepts) lend credibility to the suggestion that White's effectance motivation system facilitates application of the Learned Helplessness Paradigm to childhood depression.

White's theories were further buttressed by the results of a series of investigations initiated by Yarrow at the National Institute of Child Health and Human Development (Caplovitz, Morgan, & Mardashi, 1982; Flagle, 1982; Harmon & Culp, 1981; Harmon et al., 1982; Jennings, Connors, Sankaranarayan, & Katz, 1982; Jennings, Yarrow, & Martin, 1984; Messer, Yarrow, & Vietze, 1982; Morgan et al., 1977; Morgan, Harmon, Malpiede, Culp, & Renner, 1982; Morgan, Tolerton, Renner, & Harmon, 1981; Vietze, McCarthy, McQuiston, MacTurk, & Yarrow, 1983; Yarrow et al., 1983). The investigators attempted to determine whether indivdual differences in mastery motivation in infants and young children influence later competence. The findings of these studies are relevant to this review of learned helplessness and depression for two main reasons. First, Yarrow and colleagues considered the concept of mastery motivation to be a derivative of White's concept of effectance motivation. Therefore, the fact that they successfully developed measures of mastery motivation in infancy lends empirical support to White's seminal theory and, by implication, highlights the role that temperament may play in influencing the infant's ability to learn. Second, Yarrow and associates demonstrated that individual differences in mastery motivation showed some continuity across infancy, and that individual differences in mastery motivation strongly correlate with individual differences in later competence (Harmon & Culp, 1981; Jennings et al., 1984; Messer et al., 1982; Morgan et al., 1977; Yarrow et al., 1983). In other words, Yarrow and colleagues found a direct relationship between motivation and competence, a relationship central to the Learned Helplessness Paradigm.

The Yarrow group developed three indices with which to measure mastery motivation in infants. Their primary measure was persistence in task-directed behavior. High persistence was equated with high motivation. By focusing on "persistence," a dimension isolated by both the NYLS (Thomas et al., 1963) and Rowe and Plomin (1977), the researchers were tapping into temperament measurements to evaluate motivation. The investigators also correlated persistence with a second measure, causality pleasure, which they defined as the positive affect shown during or immediately after achieving the goal of the task-directed behavior. The investigators did not observe infants in all the studies exhibit causality pleasure; however, because White considered such pleasure a key component of effectance motivation, the Yarrow group included it among their measures.

Notably, the investigators reported that "some kinds of mastery behavior on some kinds of tasks are significantly related to overall developmental competence early in infancy, whereas other mastery behaviors on other tasks are neither contemporaneously related to nor predictive of later functioning" (Yarrow et al., 1983, p. 170). They concluded from this observation that motivation is not necessarily a precursor of competence; neither is competence necessarily a precursor of motivation. Rather, the relationship between the two constructs is reciprocal. "Competence is necessary for mastery, and mastery motivation is necessary for the development of skills" (p. 170).

By demonstrating a correlation between mastery motivation and competence, the Yarrow group studies supported White's contentions. However, their data called into question White's speculations about the relationship between motivation and learning. The issues of how motivation affects learning, and how learning affects motivation, were specifically addressed by Watson.

Contingency Awareness

Watson's (1966, 1971, 1972) theoretical work provides new possibilities for understanding how the theory of learned helplessness might be applied to infancy, since he specifically addressed the effect of contingency awareness on early learning. Moreover, Watson's theory suggests ways in which temperament may contribute to the development of infant depression, as well as how temperament dimensions may be used to chart the etiology of these phenomena. Watson defined contingency awareness as "an organism's functional knowledge that the nature of the stimuli received is sometimes affected by the nature of the behavior the organism is emitting" (1966, p. 123).

According to Watson's definition, contingency awareness allows one to perceive the possibility of achieving goals. By extension, contingency awareness can supply both the motivation and cognition necessary to initiate efforts toward goals. The construct also allows one to perceive the effect of one's strivings and thereby to experience whatever affective ramifications of success and failure are within one's emotional repertoire. As is evident, contingency awareness paves the way for significant motivational, cognitive, emotional, and self-concept repercussions. Watson proposed that an organism possessing a high degree of contingency awareness is, in essence, ready and equipped to learn. Presumably, one might assume that an organism possessing a high degree of contingency awareness is equally susceptible to the learning of helplessness. Watson (1966) posited that for an infant, the reward value of a stimulus is raised if the stimulus has previously been perceived to be contingent on the same or even some different response.

Watson (1972) proposed that infants of two to three months old are capable of perceiving contingencies. In fact, he posited that whenever infants perceive the occurrence of a new stimulus, they begin a process called "contingency analysis." Regardless of whether the stimulus is positive or neutral, infants will attempt to determine whether a contingency exists between the stimulus and their own behavior. If they are able to ascertain a contingency, the stimulus will gain new meaning and will elicit exhibitions of pronounced positive affect from the infants. (See Table 8.2.)

Watson described the playful interaction between infant and caregiver, in which the caregiver consistently presents the same clear response to a repetitive infant behavior, as both universal and functional. This interaction he termed "The Game" and noted that participants in The Game smile and coo continuously at each other during The Game's course. Watson cited these manifestations of pleasure as evidence that contingency awareness itself evokes positive affect. Beyond teaching the infant contingency relationships, The Game ensures that "we are normally guaranteed to begin vigorous smiling and cooing at fellow species members" (1972, p. 327). Indeed, the behavioral reciprocity typified in Watson's Game can be viewed as a form of prelinguistic language evolution, crucial to the infant's subsequent acquisition of verbal communication.

Although Watson believed that the enjoyment infants derive from The Game establishes that they are capable of perceiving contingencies and of learning, he suggested that infants' learning capabilities are limited by two factors (1972). First, specific behaviors have specific recovery times.

TABLE 8.2. Self-representation versus learning factors.[a]

Stages of self-representation[a]	Learning factors
I. 0–3 months Responses biologically determined and reflexive; developing distinction between self and other in perceptual clues; no emotional experience	I. Contingency awareness is present from birth (Blass et al., 1984; Mast et al., 1980; Papousek, 1961, 1967, 1977, 1981); effectance motivation at birth (Morgan et al., 1977; Morgan & Harmon, 1984; Yarrow et al., 1983); early mother contingent responding related to later vocalizing and learning (Lewis & Goldberg, 1969); early mother contingent responding related to later child competence (Clarke-Stewart, 1973; Goldberg, 1977; Sroufe, 1979)
II. 4–8 months Emergence of social activity and behavior; consolidation of self-other, self-permanence emerges; differentiation of self-action from others; cognitive growth/primary and secondary circular reactions; learns effect on object and social world	II. Contingency awareness is present by 3 months (DeCasper & Carstens, 1981; Fagen, 1980; Fagen et al., 1984; Haith, 1979; Hunt & Uzgiris, 1964; Izard, 1978; Watson & Ramey, 1972) Transference of learning across tasks at 3 months (Fagen et al., 1984; Finkelstein & Ramey, 1977); at 2–3 months, vocal interactions relate to symbolic/communicative ability (Papousek & Papousek, 1984); at 4–5 months, intrinsic motivation may exceed gratification of other drives (Papousek & Papousek, 1975, 1979); at 3 and 5 months, mother contingent responding related to greater periodicity and coherence of interaction (Lester et al., 1985); at 6 months, infants show more pleasure in social interactions than with objects (Yarrow et al., 1983); at 6 months, infants who are most competent show most persistence (Yarrow et al., 1983)
III. 9–12 months A truly social organism; established and differentiated emotional experience; reflexive imitation; means-ends; emergence of object permanence	III. At 12 months, mastery motivation can be established (Morgan et al., 1977; Morgan & Harmon, 1984; Yarrow et al., 1983)
IV. 12–24 months Self-recognition and categorical self clearly established, including fixed categories of self-representation (e.g., gender); beginning of representational behavior; empathy and emergence of complex emotional expression, language, complex means-ends, symbolic representation	IV. Self-awareness begins at 24 months with assessment of abilities

[a]Lewis and Brooks (1978).

Second, young infants of two to three months old have very short memory spans. If the memory span is briefer than the time it takes an infant to recover from and repeat a behavior, the infant will be unable to perceive a contingency between his or her behavior and the external event. For example, within The Game an infant might lift an arm and immediately the mother might kiss it. But unless the infant can lift an arm again quite quickly, causing the mother to repeat the kiss, the infant will not learn that lifting the arm and having the arm kissed are contingent.

Later data provided by a 1984 study (Fagen, Morrongiello, Rovee-Collier, & Gekoski, 1984), however, demonstrated 24-hour memory retention in three month old infants, while a 1981 study (DeCasper & Carstens, 1981) provided evidence that neonates can learn contingencies and retain learning for as long as 24 hours. Moreover, Davis and Rovee-Collier (1983) not only established that two month old infants are capable of learning a contingency in two training sessions, but further demonstrated that memory of the contingency could be retrieved nearly three weeks after the initial experience. These data challenge Watson's assumptions of memory deficits in two month old infants and suggest that memories acquired in the early weeks of life are retained, although they may be submerged. Furthermore, by contradicting Watson's view that early infant learning is limited by memory span, these later data highlight the potential of early experiences—either pleasurable or traumatic—for subsequent learning capability.

Regardless of whether Watson was correct in judging infants' abilities to perceive contingencies, his contention that young infants can learn contingencies and derive pleasure from learning raises several fascinating questions. For example, can learning to perceive and master one contingency facilitate an infant's ability to perceive and master other contingencies? That is, can infants transfer learning across tasks? If so, at what age does this capability appear? Does learning consistently affect emotion? Conversely, how does emotion affect learning? The answers to these questions may reveal ways in which the Learned Helplessness Paradigm may or may not be applicable to infants.

Although Watson tested his theories experimentally, he typically used small samples and thus the reliability of his results may not be fully representative. However, numerous independent empirical studies have demonstrated that young infants are capable of learning.

Watson's initial study was conducted in collaboration with Ramey (Watson & Ramey, 1969). The study included four experiments with eight week old infants. In the first experiment, infants were exposed to a mobile for 10 minutes a day for two weeks, starting in their eighth week. Pressing their heads on their pillows caused the mobiles to turn for one second. Control group infants were familiarized with either a stabile or non-contingent mobile. Over the two week period, the infants who had contingent mobiles significantly increased the number of times they pressed their heads against their pillows, triggering their mobiles to turn. Furthermore, the mothers of the infants with contingent mobiles almost unanimously reported that their infants smiled and cooed when they had caused the mobiles to turn. Mothers of the infants in the two control groups did not report the same phenomenon. The results of this study indicate that eight week old infants are capable of instrumental learning and suggest that contingency awareness is pleasurable.

Prior to Watson and Ramey's investigations, Hunt and Uzgiris (1964) affixed mobiles to infants' cribs so that if the infants jiggled, their mobiles moved. The investigators reported that a few infants were clearly able to control their mobiles. These results seem to corroborate Watson's argument that infants can perceive contingencies. Furthermore, Hunt and Uzgiris observed that when controlling their mobiles, infants smiled and cooed.

Investigators have also been able to demonstrate that neonates are capable of both instrumental learning (manifested in perceiving contingencies and controlling a stimulus) and classical conditioning (in which two stimuli are learned to be contiguous). Furthermore, in both studies cited below, the investigators found that affect correlated strongly with learning.

DeCasper and Carstens (1981) tested neonates for their ability to learn that appropriately spaced bursts of non-nutritive sucking could trigger a vocal music (singing) stimulus. These investigators found neonates with a mean age of 53 hours to be capable of perceiving contingencies and adjusting their behaviors in order to control the stimulus. In addition, they found that prior experience of a non-contingent stimulus interfered with learning.

The investigators determined that infants who were exposed first to contingent singing learned to space their sucking bursts so as to produce more singing. In contrast, infants exposed first to non-contingent singing did not learn the subsequent contingency. Furthermore, the infants first exposed to contingent singing reacted with negative affect (fidgeting, crying, and long periods of no response) to non-contingent singing, whereas non-contingent singing was not upsetting to infants exposed to it first. Apparently the disruption of an already perceived contingency was upsetting.

Blass, Ganchrow, and Steiner (1984) showed that infants as young as two hours can extract predictability from related events. Like DeCasper and Carstens, Blass and colleagues found a strong correlation between learning and affect. Infants in the study's experimental group were stroked gently on their foreheads during 18 two minute conditioning trials. Immediately after the stroking they received an intra-oral delivery of sucrose. Infants in one control group were stroked randomly and then given sucrose during each of the 18 trials. Infants in another control group received sucrose in each trial but were not stroked.

Immediately after the 18 trials, all infants experienced nine, one minute extinction trials in which they were just stroked. The investigators found that only infants in the experimental group presented evidence of classical conditioning. These infants emitted more head-orienting and sucking responses during the stroking sessions, and exhibited a classic extinction function to head stroking during the extinction trials. Furthermore, seven of the nine experimental infants cried during the extinction trials, whereas only one of the 16 control group infants cried during extinction.

While DeCasper and Carstens found disruption of an established contingency to upset neonates, Blass and colleagues found that disruption of an established contingency provoked tears. Therefore, while the results of the DeCasper and Carstens study support both a contingency view of learning and the Learned Helplessness Paradigm, both studies present possibilities for modification of Watson's theory. Watson addressed positive affect in relation to contingency and to learning. Neither of the above-cited studies produced evidence of positive affect associated with learning. However, both of the above studies demonstrated that negative affect correlates with the disruption of a learned relationship.

A series of experiments conducted by Finkelstein and Ramey (1977) supplies evidence that infants can indeed transfer learning across tasks. In the first experiment, all infants (mean age eight and one half months) were familiarized with an array of colored lights that they could activate by pressing a panel. Then one group of infants was exposed to a pleasant audiovisual stimulus that they could activate by executing a pulling action with one arm. A second group of infants was exposed to a non-contingent audiovisual stimulus. The investigators measured the total number of arm-pulls executed by all infants in the second phase of the experiment. As opposed to the non-contingent group, contingent group infants increased the frequency with which they executed the appropriate arm pull movement over the first three sessions. The investigators concluded:

[I]nfants who received prior contingent stimulation . . . [became] more competent and efficient learners in new situations . . . the observed transfer to the more complex discrimination-learning tasks suggests . . . infants who received prior experience learning to control stimulation were subsequently better able to determine the relation between their behaviors and environmental events. (Finkelstein & Ramey, 1977, p. 818)

A third experiment attempted to determine whether contingent stimulation enhanced contingency learning or merely elicited a range of non-specific responses. The investigators presented infants with a two-phase experiment, the second phase of which tested for discrimination learning.

Subjects were four and one half month old infants. In the experiment's first phase, half of the infants received an audiovisual stimulus contingent upon vocalizations. The other infants received no audiovisual stimulus. Only the group receiving contingent stimulation increased the number of vocalizations.

In the second phase of the experiment, all infants were observed during conditioning and extinction periods. Infants were presented pleasant audiovisual stimulation that they could control by manipulating a lever.

The investigators reported that only infants who previously had received contingent stimulation learned to discriminate conditioning and extinction periods.

This segment of Finkelstein and Ramey's study (1977) most dramatically reveals that contingency awareness can facilitate the mastery of complex unrelated learning tasks. Significantly, this last experiment, showing highest order learning, was conducted with the youngest subjects. The results of the experiment appear to strongly endorse Watson's contention that even young infants are capable of learning.

Fagen and Ohr (1985) sought to determine the effect of violation on learned expectancies in early infancy. Their study involved 110 infants of approximately three months, trained to use a crib mobile containing 10 objects by means of foot kicking. Subsequently, infants were exposed to a mobile containing only two of these objects as a model violating the previously established expectation. The researchers found that 55% of the infants cried after exposure to the second mobile. This study reaffirmed earlier findings that during conditioning trials, infants develop reward expectation habits that influence future interactions in similar circumstances. In explaining why only 55% of the infants cried when their expectations regarding the second mobile were violated, the investigators postulated that in response to disrupted contingencies, temperamental differences may be a significant factor for understanding interaction between infant and caregiver.

An implicit motif of each of these investigations is the notion that temperament dimensions strongly influence the infant's learning capacity. By suggesting that learning is due to "intrinsic motivation," White implied the significance of the temperamental component. Furthermore, the theories of Watson and others, indicating that contingency awareness is experienced pleasurably and that disruption of perceived contingencies results in infant distress, indicate that temperamental affective dimensions are vital components of the early learning experience of the infant. Thus, the preceding section suggests two hypotheses: 1) the temperamental variations that each infant brings to the learning situation influence his or her ability to learn either contingency or noncontingency and to respond to these experiences with either pleasure or distress; and 2) temperament dimensions suggest a vehicle through which to assess and perhaps predict the infant's susceptibility to the learning of competence or, in contrast, to the experience of learned helplessness.

Attachment Behaviors as Factors Influencing Learned Helplessness

Attachment refers to an affective tie between infant and caregiver and to a behavioral system flexibly operating in terms of set goals (Sroufe & Waters, 1977). Attachment behaviors are pertinent to a discussion of how learned helplessness may develop in infancy for several reasons. It is generally through the attachment relationship that the infant first encounters contingency and non-contingency experience. Such experiences shape infant response to his or her environment and influence the learning of either competence or helplessness. Manifestations of caregiver response to infant temperament displays will be reflected in the type of attachment formed by the dyad. Furthermore, attachment behaviors provide clues to the development of the "self" of the infant and may yield data about preliminary self-attribution capabilities. Attachment behavior, therefore, can be used to assess the motivational, cognitive, affective, and self-esteem deficits posited by the Learned Helplessness Paradigm and, as well, such behaviors may provide tools for tapping the infant's level of competence or learned helplessness.

When viewed through the Learned Helplessness Paradigm, the data discussed previously on the development of competence can be construed to imply that in at least three realms (motivational, cognitive, and affective) even newborns are susceptible to acquiring a clinically significant learned helplessness. Papousek and Papousek (1983) introduced the additional factor of the infant-parent interaction as a process influencing the infant's potential to learn helplessness. These researchers suggest that maladaptive parent-infant interactions, by blunting the infants' abilities to perceive contingencies, might force them to learn that important events are *not* contingent upon their behavior. By depriving infants of situations most conducive to acquiring a sense of competence, maladaptive interactions may also make the likelihood that infants will encounter satisfying contingency experience remote. (See Table 8.3.)

Seligman and colleagues (Abramson, 1977; Abramson et al., 1978) specified that self–concept plays an important role in the development of learned helplessness. As discussed above, Harter (1978, 1982; Harter & Pike, 1984) operationally defined self-concept as perceived competence, segmented into three skill domains: cognitive, social, and physical. Her isolation of the social domain allows consideration of the infant's earliest social environment—parent-infant interaction—as one arena in which infants might come to perceive of themselves as incompetent.

A compelling example of the ramifications of early parent-infant interaction is provided by Tronick, Als, and Brazelton (1977), whose study evaluated integrative processes as manifested in neonatal behavior. Comparing physiological responses for premature and normal term infants, the investigators isolated three developmental phases, including an initial period of alertness after delivery. Next, a period of depression and disorganization, lasting for 24 to 48 hours, occurs in infants with uncomplicated deliveries and lingers for three to four days if infants have been compromised by medication given mothers during delivery. Finally, neonates experience a "curve of recovery to optimal function," occurring several days after birth. The researchers also observed that two basic forms of regulation color early interaction patterns. These regulatory mechanisms

TABLE 8.3. Secure attachment correlated with learning factors

Secure attachment (study)	Learning factors
Arend et al. (1979)	Increased ego-control (a competence construct, "the disposition or threshold of an individual with regard to the expression or containment of impulses, feelings, and desires")
	Increased ego-resiliency (a competence construct, ability to respond flexibly, persistently, and resourcefully, especially in problem situations; implies the ability to modulate ego-control in situationally appropriate ways, i.e., neither impulsively nor rigidly)
	Increased task competency, compliance, curiosity, and positive affect at 24 months
Belsky, Garduque, & Hrncir (1984)	Increased executive capacity (capacity to execute in a self-initiated manner highest level of functioning)
	Increased attention to environment, exploration, sophistication of play at 12 and 13 months
Frodi & Thompson (1985)	Increased task-oriented persistence, mastery-related behavior, and competence during play assessed across the entire second year
Hazen & Durrett (1982)	Increased competence in environmental adaptation—exploration, flexibility, spatial task ability (i.e., integrating and making spatial inferences) at 30–34 months
Londerville & Main (1981)	Increased compliance, cooperation, obedience, and evidence of more internalized controls at 21 months
Matas et al. (1978)	Higher levels of competence (as measured as composite of positive affect, enthusiasm, responsiveness, and compliance), cooperation, task effectance, and persistence independent of development quotient; stable predictor of adaptive behavior at 2 years
Sroufe et al. (1984)	Predicted affective regulation or flexible emotional modulation (e.g., ability to signal and modulate negative affect effectively) at 4–5 years
	Also predicted levels of self-control and adjustment to others
Sroufe (1983)	Predicted competency in 4–5-year-olds
Sroufe, Fox, & Pancake (1983)	Increased positive attention-seeking behaviors at 4–5 years (e.g., seeking help for cognitive and physical tasks)
Sroufe & Waters (1977)	Flexible goal-oriented response repertoire
Waters, Wippman, & Sroufe (1979)	Peer competence and ego-strength effectance at 3½ years
	Increased positive affect and exploration
	Social adaptation; more smiling and vocalizing toward others

involve the infant's endogenous biorhythmic patterns and parental response in the form of specific extrinsic cues relating to neonate rhythms. If the exogenous parental cue was in harmony with the neonate's endogenous rhythms, entrainment occurred, and the researchers characterized the infant as being ready to learn. Not only does this study provide clues to the incipient development of such phenomena as effectance motivation and contingency awareness, but it also highlights the dominant role of parental interaction in shaping these developmental trends.

In analyzing the fundamental components of earliest parent-infant interaction, several researchers have emphasized the importance of attachment and have postulated specific infant goals during the interaction. Goldberg (1977) cited White's (1959) "feelings of efficacy" as the goal for both parents and infants. Goldberg proposed that the extent to which parent and infant each provide the other with contingency experience determines the extent to which they experience feelings of efficacy. If a parent neglects to provide an infant with sufficient contingency experience, the infant may feel enormous frustration in an attempt to achieve a prized goal.

Goldberg posited that readability, predictability, and responsiveness on the part of infants encourage caregivers to participate in parent-infant interaction and that adults feel effective with easily "read" infants because they can recognize the infants' signals. Predictable infants allow their parents to reliably anticipate their behavior—that is, to make use of prior contingency perceptions about their infants. Responsive infants react to stimulation provided by parents with short latencies and appropriate behavior. Such infant behavior provides immediate gratification of the parent's contingency needs. But Goldberg pointed out that whenever parents are confronted with an infant of limited competence (i.e., an unreadable, unpredictable, or unresponsive infant), the potential risks of interactive failures are high.

Izard and Buechler (1981) hypothesized that the concept of "synchrony," previously discussed by a number of investigators (including Lewis & Goldberg, 1969; Sander, 1969; Stern, 1974b; Thoman, 1975), earmarked parent–infant interaction as a source of mutual, contingency-based pleasure. They described synchrony as "effective, coordinated, mutually responsive mother infant interation. The notion is that appropriately sensitive mothers act or react in synchrony with their infants" (Izard & Buechler, 1981, p. 360).

These investigators proposed that mothers provide young infants with affective synchrony in two ways. First, in loving games reminiscent of Watson's "The Game" construct, mothers playfully interact with infants, mirroring their responses. Second, when infants are angry or distressed, mothers respond quickly and sympathetically to their needs.

According to Izard and Buechler, infants learn contingency when they realize that their emotions affect others. The investigators further posited that awareness of affective contingencies requires that infants perceive that different emotional signals evoke different responses from the parent. Therefore, "unless it can affect the caregiver differently, depending on the particular emotion it is signaling, [the infant] may not develop a sense of itself as a causal agent in social intercourse. It may develop a sense of social impotence that leads to social incompetence" (1981, p. 362).

Brazelton, Koslowski, and Main (1974) followed the interactive behavior of members of five mother-infant dyads when the infants were between two and 20 weeks old. In this study, rather than attempting to "prove" synchrony, Brazelton and colleagues described the significant behavioral components of mother-infant interaction. The investigators discovered "cycles" characterizing the fluctuating interaction between infants and mothers. When infants withdraw their attention from their mothers, mothers tend to respond in like manner. When infants return their attention to their mothers, mothers return attention to their infants. Noticing the usually consistent harmony that mothers engineer with their infants, the investigators considered both mutual attention and inattention to reflect synchrony as long as the baby's needs are met. However, they reported that occasionally synchrony between mother and infant degenerates into dys-synchrony.

Brazelton and co-workers described two significant ways in which mothers' behaviors can disrupt synchrony. Although following the infant's cues for attention and withdrawal produces synchrony, steadily bombarding the infant with attention produces dys-synchrony, as does trying to impose the mother's attentional rhythm on the infant.

Butterworth and Jarret's descriptions (1981) of a capacity for mutual visual referencing, and their postulation of the existence of an inborn potential for "shared visual reality" within the mother-infant dyad, bear striking similarities to the Izard and Buechler concept of synchrony. In an investigation involving six month old infants positioned opposite their mothers, the researchers replicated earlier findings (Scaife & Bruner, 1975) demonstrating that these infants spontaneously gaze in the direction of their mothers. Jones (1985), in a study involving 15 to 18 month old infants, identified a mechanism that maintains "mutual monitoring" between mother and infant, and stipulated that this mechanism is dominant to exploratory mechanisms. The researcher noted that even situations engendering high levels of exploratory behavior did not undercut the dominance of attachment behavior mechanisms, as manifested by a frequency of looks and trips to the mother. This study highlights the compelling influence of the interactional dyadic exchange on the young infant.

Stern, Hofer, Haft, and Dore (1985) proposed that "affect attunement" is the process by which the interaction between parent and infant is instrumental in the infant's developing sense of self. The parent draws conclusions about the infant's attentional and affective state from his or her overt behavior, and then performs an overt response. The infant understands the parent's response as having to do with his or her own original affect experience. Therefore, affect attunement "allows an infant to perceive how he is perceived" (p. 1).

Stern and colleagues proposed that the quality of the parent's response to the infant's affective experience influences the infant's sense of self. When response is attuned to the infant's original experience, both infant and parent assimilate a shared affect state. When response is not attuned, parent and infant assimilate that they are not in harmony. However, more experimental support exists for the suggestion that infants assimilate lack of harmony than for the suggestion that infants appreciate attunement.

In an investigation conducted by Stern and colleagues with 10 normal, white, middle class mothers and their infants (five boys, five girls, age 8– 12 months), the play interactions of the dyads were videotaped, and occurrences of attunement were noted. Interestingly, when mothers either responded not at all to their infant's play, or responded to infant behavior in a way judged to reflect attunement, for the most part, infants took no note of the mother. For example, if an infant energetically banged a toy on the floor and the mother either ignored the infant or rhythmically jostled the infant, the infant typically continued the banging undisturbed. However, when mothers perturbed attunements (for example, if the mother jostled the infant too energetically or not energetically enough), infants almost always interrupted their behavior.

The attunement concept bears similarities to that of synchrony, and somewhat subtler similarities to Watson's contingency awareness. Keeping these concepts in mind, the fact that infants responded to virtually any discord between their behavior and their mothers' behavior can be interpreted to indicate that discord is notable to infants. Discord might suggest to an infant that the mother's affect and behavior are not contingent upon his or her own affect and behavior. The fact that attunement seems less remarkable than nonattunement to infants suggests that infants may harbor illusions of control (Langer, 1975) about their mothers' behavior. Any disruption of this illusion captures the infant's attention. Moreover, the suggestion that infants find the disruption of perceived contingencies notable is reminiscent of findings reported by DeCasper and Carstens (1981), indicating that the disruption of perceived contingencies provokes negative affect in neonates, as well as of findings reported by Blass et al. (1984), suggesting that disruption of perceived contingencies results in negative affect in neonates.

Stern and colleagues concluded that by allowing an infant to recognize a shared affect state, attunement causes infants to develop a sense of mental "self" in addition to a sense of physical "self," and to perceive a mental "other" in addition to a physical "other." If, in fact, attunement reinforces illusions of control, lack of attunement might teach lack of control and, by extension, helplessness.

Development of Self

As detailed in Chapter 5, experimental results obtained by Dixon (1957), Amsterdam (1972), and Lewis and Brooks-Gunn (1979) indicate that while infants between the ages of seven and nine months can visually recognize themselves, not until age 20 to 24 months are they aware that they have stable physical features. At this later age they begin showing other conscious signs of self-recognition, including self-admiration and embarrassment.

One researcher has managed to surmount the barrier posed by the verbal incapacities of infants. By summarizing the pertinent literature, Kopp (1982) arrived at a portrait of the developmental course of self-regulation in infant behavior. Kopp suggested a four-stage sequence of development. At approximately three months of age, infants engage in *sensorimotor modulation*. This phase, according to the researcher, signifies the infant's ability to master voluntary motor acts and to alter acts in response to events. In all likelihood, Kopp notes, the ability to modulate sensorimotor acts reflects individual differences related to biological predisposition, as well as to caregiver sensitivity. Thus, implicit in Kopp's framework is the notion that temperament, as evidenced through biological predisposition, and attachment behaviors, formulated through caregiver sensitivity, play a crucial role in contributing to the infant's evolving capacity for self-regulation. Furthermore, the researcher comments that during the sensorimotor modulation phase, internal cognitive organization begins, and the infant develops an incipient awareness of his or her own actions.

Kopp postulates that, by nine months of age, a more sophisticated *control* phase replaces sensorimotor regulation. Characteristic of this phase is sharpened infant awareness of social demands by caregivers, as well as compliance and self-initiated inhibition of prohibited behavior. During this period, generally stretching from nine to 12 months, the infant displays evidence of initiating, modulating, or ceasing physical acts. Kopp infers that the infant is now capable of expressing intent, and differentiating environmental stimuli, and possesses an elementary awareness of what is acceptable to the caregiver. In short, the control phase suggests intentional modifications of behavior with cognizance of caregiver expectations.

Kopp then suggests that a period of *self-control* is observed, during which self consciousness becomes apparent, as the infant begins to recall positive and negative sensations and to monitor these sensations. Again, this phase within the development of the self evokes constructs previously referred to in discussing the role of temperament and attachment behaviors as milestones of infant development. Thus, pleasurable affect is linked to contingency awareness, while distress is shown to be the affective aftermath of the perception of disrupted contingency. Moreover, harmonious interaction between infant and caregiver, described variously as "synchrony," "rhythmicity," and "affect attunement," results in displays of pleasurable affect; tampering with caregiver-infant exchange provokes negative affect.

Finally, Kopp suggests that the infant progresses to the phase of *self-regulation* at approximately 24 months. This phase, she observes, is not different from the earlier period of self-control in kind; rather, self-regulation connotes a difference in the degree of modifying behavior in which the infant may engage, and indicates that numerous contingency rules have been cognitively incorporated. (See Table 8.4.)

Kopp's schema is noteworthy to infant researchers for two main reasons. First, her theory suggests that the development of the self is an evolutionary or cumulative process. Second, Kopp's hypotheses allude to the factors of temperament dimensions and attachment behaviors as seminal ingredients relentlessly shaping the manner in which self-regulation will ultimately emerge.

The following studies in this section focus on investigations into self-concept using children as subjects. These studies rely primarily on verbal ability to yield evidence of the emerging self. While such investigations are invaluable in determining how self-concept develops, nevertheless, it should be borne in mind that verbal comments may indicate the outcome of a sophisticated process that began during the early months of infancy.

Piaget (1932), Heckhausen (1967, 1981), Veroff (1969), and Kagan (1978) found that by age three children can describe themselves and view task related outcomes as reflective of their abilities. These capabilities and the associated concept of self develop further with maturation. Considered together, data obtained by Broughton (1978) and Guardo and Bohan (1971) suggest the following developmental sequence. Young children conceive of the self in strictly physical and material terms. Later, beginning at approximately age eight, they are capable of perceiving their "inner" (i.e., cognitive and psychological) self.

Keller, Ford, and Meacham (1978), in contrast to Broughton and to Guardo and Bohan, found that children as young as three years old describe themselves more in terms of activities than in terms of physical or material attributes. Secord and Peevers (1974) noted that third-graders not only conceive of themselves in terms of activities, but also color their self-perceptions by comparing their own competence at selected activities to the competence of others.

Although evidence suggests that children generally acquire a stable sense of self by age two, begin to recognize that successes are linked to capabilities by age three years, and begin formulating concepts of how they compare to others by age seven or eight, the nature of children's self-understanding does not necessarily correlate strongly with more objective assessments of their capabilities. Ample experimental evidence exists to show that the ability to correctly associate outcomes and ability develops with maturation. For example, Piaget (1930) observed that children younger than six or seven years old display illusions of control over events that are uncontrollable. Considered in the context of this examination of

TABLE 8.4. Self-Regulation versus learning factors.[a]

Stages of self-regulation[a]	Learning factors
I. Neurophysical modulation (0 to 2–3 months) Neurophysical and reflexive adaptations to environment; some control of arousal states; some organized patterns of functional behavior; protective processes to defend against strong stimuli	I. Contingency awareness is present from birth (Blass et al., 1984; Mast et al., 1980; Papousek 1961, 1967, 1977, 1981) Effectance motivation at birth (Morgan et al., 1977; Morgan & Harmon, 1984; Yarrow et al., 1983) Early mother contingent responding related to later vocalizing and learning (Lewis & Goldberg, 1969) Early mother contingent responding related to later child competence (Clarke-Stewart, 1973; Goldberg, 1977; Sroufe, 1979)
II. Sensorimotor modulation (3–9+ months) Intentional motor responses to stimuli; these sensorimotor adaptations guided by both temperament and attachment relationships; differentiation of self-action from others	II. Contingency awareness is present by 3 months (DeCasper & Carstens, 1981; Fagen, 1980; Fagen et al., 1984; Haith, 1979; Hunt & Uzgiris, 1964; Izard, 1978; Watson & Ramey, 1972) Transference of learning across tasks at 3 months (Fagen et al., 1984; Finkelstein & Ramey, 1977) At 2–3 months, vocal interactions relate to symbolic/communicative ability (Papousek & Papousek, 1984) At 4–5 months, intrinsic motivation may exceed gratification of other drives (Papousek & Papousek, 1975, 1979)

III. Control (12–18+ months)
Ability to initiate, maintain, modulate, or cease physical acts, communications, and social signals; some compliance; intention; appraisal of different features of environment; self-initiated inhibition of prohibited behavior; awareness of social or task demands defined by caregivers

At 3 and 5 months, mother contingent responding related to greater periodicity and coherence of interaction (Lester et al., 1985)

At 6 months, infants show more pleasure in social interactions than with objects (Yarrow et al., 1983)

III. At 12 months, mastery motivation can be established (Morgan et al., 1977; Morgan & Harmon, 1984; Yarrow et al., 1983)

IV. Self-Control (24+ months)
Capacity for representational thinking and evocative memory; symbolic representation of objects in their absence; sense of personal continuity and independence; increased awareness of what is acceptable to caregivers

IV. Self-awareness begins at 24 months with assessment of abilities (Kagan, 1981)

V. Self-Regulation (36+ months)
Ability to delay/inhibit action at request of others; compliance; modulates behavior according to established precepts, based on stored memory of conventions that govern behavior in absence of external monitors; elaboration of sense of self; self-conscious behavior; affective memory; increased adaptation to environment

[a]Kopp. (1982).

the Learned Helplessness Paradigm, Piaget's observation raises the question of whether infants' and children's self-concept is sufficiently skewed in their favor to render perceptions of failure at tasks an improbable and atypical occurrence.

In 1980, Weisz used a card game experiment to compare evidence of illusory contingency in kindergartners and fourth-graders. Within the experiment, an experimenter drew cards blindly from a shuffled deck. The children were told that each time they drew a yellow card from the deck they would win a chip. The experimenter controlled all winnings. Children were asked to predict winnings of other children who differed from them in age, intelligence, effort, and previous practice at the task. Whenever a child based a prediction on age, intelligence, effort, or previous practice, the experimenter scored the prediction as evidence of illusory contingency. Weisz found that younger children revealed many more illusory contingencies than did older children.

Weisz and colleagues considered the apparent developmental trend of the tendency to draw illusory contingencies to be their most significant finding. In discussing the trend they referred to Nicholls's (1978) data suggesting that differing age groups infer causal attributions according to distinct logical structures or schemata.

Nicholls described the *halo schema*, whereby a child (age nine and younger) perceives ability/effort and outcome to correlate positively. In other words, children believe that a positive outcome reflects both high ability and high effort. Likewise, they believe high effort and high ability to unfailingly predict positive outcome regardless of task difficulty. Furthermore, they see high effort as reflecting high ability. Therefore, the correlation between high effort and high ability might convince children who try hard that success at any task is a foregone conclusion. In describing the attributional style of older children, Nicholls referred to the *compensatory schema*, whereby a child believes that effort can compensate for ability and vice versa, so that success can be obtained when low ability is compensated by high effort.

Weisz and co-investigators discovered that younger children are more prone than older subjects to overestimate the degree to which outcomes are contingent on human attributes and behavior has been complemented by the results of other research (for example, Kun, 1977; Nicholls & Miller, 1985). Weisz and associates suggested that "it seems likely then that young children will . . . overestimate their capacity to exercise control and that they will . . . [exaggerate] that capacity" (Weisz, Yeates, Robertson & Beckham, 1982, p. 905).

The investigators concluded that children's relative immunity to perceptions of failure might protect them somewhat from learned helplessness. Oddly, Weisz and associates did not speculate that children's tendency to overestimate their own control might have serious ramifications for offspring of depressed or otherwise incompetent mothers. The fact that illusions of control are typical of the young child could be interpreted as increasing the likelihood that children and infants will feel responsible for the limitations and failures of their parents. One might infer that children of a depressed parent may interpret any maladaptive interaction between themselves and the parent as proof of a global, stable, and chronic personal inadequacy.

As observed by Weisz, illusions of control are tied to causal schemata, which greatly influence causal attributions. Because attributional style in turn influences self-concept, a further examination of causal schemata and attributional style is appropriate.

Kun (1977) examined the development of causal inference schemata by eliciting causal attributions for task-related success or failure for hypothetical people. The ages of Kun's subjects spanned a far wider range than did the ages of the subjects of Weisz and associates (1982) or Nicholls (1978), and thus Kun was able to identify three causal inference schemata. Kun interviewed children ages five to twelve, as well as college students. Subjects employing the first of Kun's identified schemata, the *magnitude-covariation schema,* conceived of degree of success as positively relating to a change in the degree of a facilitative factor, either ability or effort. This schema does not incorporate the idea of task difficulty. In fact, it is identical to Nicholls's halo schema, in assuming that ability and effort are interchangeable. Kun found this schema to be fully developed in children age five to six years old.

Subjects employing the second schema, *direct compensation* perceived that if a change in task outcome remains invariant, change in the strength of task difficulty is positively related to a change in the strength of either ability or effort. In other words, at more difficult tasks, individuals who either try harder or have more innate ability can succeed as well as they would if the task were simpler. This schema, incorporating the idea of task difficulty, but still linking ability to effort, was also found in children age five to six years old. However, Kun observed that it was more prevalent in children up to age nine.

The third schema, *inverse compensation,* is identical to the compensation schema proposed by Nicholls. Subjects employing the inverse compensation schema perceived that if a task outcome remains invariant, change in the magnitude of ability is negatively related to a change in the strength of effort. In other words, high ability can compensate for a lack of effort, and high effort can compensate for a lack of ability. Like the magnitude-covariation schema, this schema does not consider task difficulty. However, unlike the magnitude-covariation schema, it does not link ability and effort. This schema was not found in five to six year olds, but was evident in children as young as nine years. It predominated in the college-age group when subjects in this group were explaining success, but not failure, at hard tasks.

Nicholls and Miller (1985) attempted to replicate the findings presented by Weisz et al. (1982). However, whereas Weisz and colleagues had relied strictly on attribution theory to simply define causal schemata concerning luck and skill, Nicholls and Miller sought to determine qualitative conceptual and behavioral changes resulting from the causal schemata concerning luck and skill. Specifically, Nicholls and Miller examined children's causal attributions and investigated whether at the ages when luck and skill become conceptually differentiated, a decline would be evident in the amount of effort exerted in luck-dependent tasks.

Their subjects were drawn from kindergarten, second-, third-, fourth-, fifth-, and sixth-grade classes. An experimenter familiarized each child with a pair of luck and skill tasks and then asked each child to predict whether increased effort would have improved the performance of hypothetical persons on these tasks. Next, for a set of two luck and two skill tasks, each child was asked to attribute the cause for hypothetical persons' successes and failures. Finally, a second experimenter told each child that he or she was to attempt to complete tasks similar to the ones just discussed. The experimenter presented six new luck or skill tasks, all of which ensured failure on the part of the child. Then the experimenter presented six new skill tasks, all of which were simple enough to virtually ensure success. After each child had completed the last of the tasks, he or she was asked why performance had been better on the second set of six tasks than on the first set.

The investigators distinguished four gradations of differentiation of luck and skill.

1. Luck and skill per se are undifferentiated and not the basis for distinguishing luck and skill tasks. Tasks are distinguished in terms of apparent difficulty. Effort is expected to improve outcomes on both tasks, but the skill task is seen as requiring more effort or as more difficult because of the complexity of its stimuli. The luck task, having no stimuli to compare, is seen as easier or as requiring less effort.
2. Skill and luck outcomes are partially differentiated, but the basis for the distinction is not articulated. Effort is expected to improve performance on both tasks, but the skill task is seen as offering more chance to do well through effort.
3. Skill and luck outcomes are partially differentiated, and the basis for the distinction is explicit. The skill task is seen as offering more chance to do well through effort because it is possible to compare stimuli on it but not on the luck task. Effort is, nevertheless, expected to improve performance on the luck task.
4. Skill and luck outcomes are clearly distinguished. It is seen that there is no way for effort to affect outcomes on the luck task, whereas effort is presumed to affect outcomes on the skill task (Nicholls & Miller, 1985, p. 78).

The higher a subject's grade level, the more likely he or she was to differentiate correctly between luck and skill outcomes. Responses to the question concerning the main reason that hypothetical others either succeeded or failed reflected the age trend demonstrated by Weisz et al. (1982).

Younger children adopted a halo schema; older children reasoned according to a compensatory schema.

The investigators categorized the children's explanations for why they succeeded at more of the final six soluble tasks than at the first six insoluble tasks. Two distinct categories of explanation emerged: responses implying that skill-related factors were responsible for increased performance, and responses attributing poor outcomes to luck and successful outcomes to skill-related factors. For the most part, kindergartners' responses fell into the first category. All other children's responses fell into one or the other category depending on whether the first set of six tasks that they had attempted had been luck or skill dependent. The investigators concluded that causal attributions and levels of differentiation both show age related decreases in illusions of contingency.

The above discussed experiments indicate that naive schemata and illusory contingency are typical of children, particularly those younger than nine years of age. Furthermore, because a marked developmental trend is apparent, with illusory contingency and objectively erroneous causal schemata being virtually universal among young children and less prevalent among adults, the suggestion that infants are even more deluded than children about the amount of control they can exert over uncontrollable events is implied. It should be noted, however, that other investigators (Karabenick & Heller, 1976) have found that illusory contingency and erroneous causal schemata may become more pronounced with development. Furthermore, Surber (1980, 1981) has suggested that the age variations appearing in contingency awareness and causal attributions in essence simply reflect individual rather than developmental differences.

As stated above, information about infants' attributional styles is unobtainable at this time because of lack of verbalization studies. However, the trend data reported by Kun (1977), Weisz (1980, 1981), Weisz et al. (1982), and Nicholls and Miller (1985) suggest that children's difficulty in objectively perceiving the association between task outcome and ability may only hint at the difficulty infants encounter. Children's reluctance to recognize that failure at tasks reflects on their competence has been well documented. The question arises as to whether vulnerability to learned helplessness depression follows the same developmental trend as vulnerability to illusory contingency and consequent self-enhancing attributions. The answer to this question may lie in whether illusory contingency can, in fact, adversely affect self-concept in situations causing children to confront task-related failures.

Contingency and Self-Concept: Attributional Style

As mentioned, Weisz and associates (1982) reasoned that illusory contingency invariably acts as a shield, protecting children from developing helplessness. However, Weisz ignored the possibility that illusory contingency may also function in precisely the opposite way, by convincing a child that the failures of significant others, such as parents, result directly from the child's failure to control non-contingent events. Thus, illusory contingency may actually enhance the child's susceptibility to learned helplessness. Furthermore, Weisz and associates did not address whether illusory contingency might cause a child to self-attribute the cause of mal-adaptive parent-child interactions.

These speculations reflect back to discussions of the possible negative impact of contingency motivation on an infant's or child's self-esteem with regard to unsatisfactory parent-child interactions (Brazelton et al., 1974; Goldberg, 1977; Izard & Buechler, 1981; Lester et al., 1985; Stern et al., 1985). In addition, the question of whether an inflated contingency awareness can threaten self-esteem also arises.

According to Seligman and associates (Abramson et al., 1978), self-concept is reflected in attributional style. Attributions of success to internal factors indicate high self-esteem; attributions of failure to internal factors indicate low self-esteem. Attributions of success to external factors can also result in low self-esteem.

The hypotheses of Seligman and associates about the relationship be-tween attributional style and self-concept are poorly supported by em-pirical data concerning children. However, research by Weiner (1974) and Weiner, Russell, and Lerman (1978) did demonstrate that attributing suc-cess in achieving goals to internal factors elicits positive emotions such as feelings of pride, self-confidence, and self-esteem, whereas attributing failure to internal factors elicits a corresponding negative emotion.

Weiner and colleagues (1978) used a multiple-choice questionnaire to ask children (mean age, 8.4 years) to identify the emotions they would be most likely to feel in response to failure as well as success. This study revealed clear, direct relationships between internal attributions for failure and emotions of sadness, hopelessness, and shame, as well as for the self-concept related emotions of incompetence and resignation. However, be-cause the questionnaire tested children's responses to hypothetical failure situations only, it did not address the questions of whether children, who as a group put faith in illusory contingencies, spontaneously perceive their task related failures and whether they attribute such failures to their own abilities.

In a later study, Weiner, Graham, Stern, and Lawson (1982) explored how affective cues might be used to infer causal attribution. In the first part of the experiment, children from age nine to college age were given the affective reactions of a teacher toward a failing student. Affects pro-vided included anger, pity, guilt, surprise, and sadness. Subjects were then asked to infer the cause of the student's failure. In this age group, systematic linkages were made between the following affect-attribution pairings: anger-lack of effort; guilt-poor teaching; surprise–lack of effort. Moreover, the college age students linked pity with low ability. Next, subjects five to nine years old were tested only for the affects of anger and pity. Findings revealed that the youngest children in this group associated anger with lack of effort, while only the older children (9 years) linked pity with lack of ability. The researchers noted that the impact of individual ability cues on self-esteem increases with age. For example, pity does not function as a cue for five year olds, but does have this function for nine year olds. With cognitive growth, children adopt increased criteria to evaluate personal competence. Affect communication and inferred attributions may be among emerging criteria guiding self-perception and self-attribution of failure.

Studies conducted by Stipek and associates (Stipek, 1981a, 1981b; Stipek et al., 1984; Stipek & Hoffman, 1980) offer some insight into whether children readily recognize their own task-related failures and attribute their failures to internal causes. Stipek and Hoffman (1980) asked children aged three to eight to make causal attributions for their performance on a motor task, as well as for another child's performance at the same task. The investigators found that although children as young as three are able to make realistic judgments about performance, as well as to make objectively sensible causal attributions, they are far less likely to be critical of their own performance and abilities than of another child's. This study demonstrated cognitive capability to perceive failure and to understand the reasons for failure. Simultaneously, however, it demonstrated that children are reluctant to exercise these capabilities in relation to their own performance, suggesting that illusory contingency may be a coping mechanism adopted and shed at will.

Stipek (1981b) examined children's perceptions of their own and their classmates' ability. She determined that children in kindergarten and first grade form perceptions entirely unrelated to their teacher's more objective assessments. In fact, not until second and third grade did children perceive their own and their classmates' ability in ways resembling their teacher's perceptions.

Masters (1972) examined whether seven year old children rewarded themselves contingently or non–contingently after being exposed to a success or failure experience. An increase in the amount of self-rewarding behavior following a success experience was observed by the researcher. However, self-reward following failure increased only when it was non-contingently administered or during a task unlike the one during which failure had been experienced. Masters postulated that by age seven children have internalized a complex system dictating the conditions under which they may engage in self-gratification. This system incorporates such factors as the contingency with which self-gratification is to be received, prior success or failure experiences, and similarity of a current task to a previous task that resulted in success or failure. The researcher concluded that children of this age have learned that self-reward should be contingent upon success. Nevertheless, if circumstances permit discrimination between a current situation and a prior experience of failure, such a distinction will be made and increased self-gratification will occur.

From the data demonstrating that confronting a child with his or her failures can, in fact, force the child to acknowledge failure and to experience negative affect and performance deterioration, one might infer that parents who consistently draw a child's attention to past or present failures can similarly force the child to incorporate failure into his or her self-concept. Healthy parent-child interactions are considered the training ground for effectance (White, 1959, 1963) and contingency awareness (Watson, 1966, 1971, 1972; Papousek & Papousek, 1975, 1977). As both effectance and contingency awareness have been demonstrated to be intrinsic and highly valued goals, possibilities may abound in maladaptive interactions for infants and children to blame themselves for interactional failures.

In order to pave the way for a logical mapping of the Learned Helplessness Paradigm in the childhood and infancy years, the above sections argue that children and infants of all ages are capable of instrumental learning, and that beginning at about three months, and possibly much earlier, infants can transfer such learning across tasks. This section offers evidence that children as young as three years have developed functional self-concepts that allow them to perceive task outcomes, to attribute those outcomes to their own capabilities, and to respond affectively to those outcomes. Moreover, the section suggests that parent-child interactions may offer opportunities to experience failure.

Affect and Locus of Control Beliefs

The literature presented thus far has demonstrated that for older children, and possibly for young children and infants, uncontrollable outcomes can cause negative affect and diminished self-concept, ultimately leading to passive behavior and depression. However, as Abramson and Sackeim (1977) pointed out, such studies demonstrate situation-specific helplessness, rather than a global expectation of personal helplessness.

Research concerning the relationship between affect and locus of control beliefs, although not directly investigating learned helplessness, may be of aid in examining the Learned Helplessness Paradigm. Locus of control refers to the domain, either the external social world or the internal psychological world, perceived as the prime force motivating outcome. Seligman (1975) observed that a person with an *external* locus of control believes that reinforcements occur in his or her life by chance or luck, and are beyond his or her control. In contrast, a person with an *internal* locus of control believes that he or she controls his or her own reinforcers and that personal skill can be used to master the environment. Hiroto (1974) found that "externals" have a tendency to become helpless in an experimental situation more readily than "internals."

It may be suggested that embedded within Kopp's (1982) concept of self-regulation is the notion that the infant begins to distinguish between "external" and "internal" domains of control at approximately 24 months, the age at which self-regulation crystallizes. And the capacity for differentiating between internal and external realms may initiate the concomitant ability to control internal affective and behavioral responses, as well as the ability to self-attribute these responses.

Adults and Locus of Control

Natale (1978), gathering evidence showing that depressives believe outcomes to be non-contingent upon their responses, demonstrated a strong relationship between affect and locus of control beliefs. Natale investigated the influence that induced elation and depression have on locus of control beliefs in nondepressive adult females. Each subject completed an attitude survey (Rotter's 1966 Locus of Control Scale). After the survey, subjects read a series of 60 self-referent statements aloud, a mood-induction technique initially set forth by Velten (1968). For one group of subjects, elevated mood was induced. Another group experienced induced depression. A third group's mood was not artificially altered. After the mood induction procedure, each subject again completed the attitude survey.

Natale hypothesized that depression would prove to be associated with external locus of control beliefs, while elation would prove to be associated with internal locus of control beliefs. His hypothesis was supported by the results of the experiment. Relative to other subjects and to their own pre-test scores, artificially depressed subjects scored higher on a scale of external locus of control. On the other hand, artificially elated subjects received lower scores relative to other subjects and to their own pretest scores. Subjects whose moods had not been altered scored similarly to their own pretest scores. Natale's experiment, therefore, revealed a direct relationship between affect and locus of control beliefs. Furthermore, it showed that locus of control beliefs are at least partially contingent upon effort.

Alloy, Abramson, and Viscusi (1981) studied the influence of induced mood on illusions of control. Citing an earlier experiment (Alloy & Abramson, 1979), demonstrating that depressed subjects have more realistic ideas about how much control they exert over objectively uncontrollable events than do nondepressed persons, the investigators examined the relationship between realistic judgments and depression. Using the Velten (1968) technique, the investigators induced depressed mood in nondepressed college students and induced elated mood in depressed college students. Then, by asking students to judge how much control they had over the onset of an objectively non-contingent light, they assessed the impact of the transient moods on the subjects' susceptibility to illusions of control. Depressed students for whom elation had been induced made inflated estimates of their control. Naturally nondepressed subjects for whom depression had been induced made realistic estimates.

These experiments, using adult subjects, revealed that negative affect prompts individuals to believe themselves incapable of controlling events. Therefore, the data offer support for the above-posited cycle whereby negative affect resulting from the expectation of uncontrollable events reinforces the expectation of uncontrollable events, allowing situation-specific helplessness to burgeon into more generalized feelings of helplessness. Studies conducted with children, however, although they show a directionality between positive affect and feelings of control, do not point to a directionality between negative affect and expectations of lack of control.

Children and Locus of Control

Moore, Underwood, and Rosenhan (1973; Underwood, Moore, & Rosenhan, 1973) found a distinct correlation between affect and altruism as well as affect and self-gratification. They discovered that inducing positive affect in children increases their tendency to donate money to other children. In contrast, inducing negative affect reduces children's tendencies to donate money. Furthermore, they found that both positive and negative moods incline children to generously reward themselves. These same investigators, along with Mischel, Ebbesen, and Zeiss (1973), proposed that positive affective states encourage individuals toward behavior compatible with, and reinforcing of, the affective state, and that negative affective states encourage behaviors that have a probability of countering the affective state.

Using the affect induction procedure developed by Underwood et al. (1973), Masters and Furman (1976) induced positive, neutral, or negative affect in 24 preschool children. Subjects' anticipated success or failure on two skill-related tasks was then measured to determine whether affective states influenced expectancies for success. The investigators found that positive affect correlated highly with elevated expectancies. Significantly, however, negative affect did not appear to reduce expectancy of success. Nor did negative affect influence locus of control beliefs.

Masters and Furman concluded that positive affective states elevate expectancies for success, while negative affective states are ineffective in altering expectancies, a conclusion also drawn by Mischel, Ebbesen, and Zeiss (1971, 1973). Therefore, although they demonstrated that for preschool children belief in internal locus of control is at least partially contingent upon positive affect, they also demonstrated that belief in external locus of control may not be contingent upon negative affect.

When considered alongside the results of experiments using adult subjects, Masters and Furman's data suggest a developmental trend in the relationship between affect and locus of control beliefs. Just as young children and infants appear to be relatively immune from attributing task-related failure to internal factors (Kun, 1977; Nicholls & Miller, 1985;

Weisz et al., 1982), they may also be relatively incapable of anticipating task-related failure.

However, while Masters and Furman showed that negative affect may not influence young children's expectations about control, evidence from an earlier study in which Masters was a principal investigator (Masters, Barden & Ford, 1979) indicated that negative affect does, in fact, impede children's learning. In experiments with four year old children, Masters et al. discovered that induced positive affective states enhance learning, whereas induced negative affective states retard learning dramatically. The investigators obtained ratings of children's facial expressions in order to confirm that positive and negative affect induction procedures had indeed evoked their respective happy and sad moods. Also, affect induction was followed by a learning task. The four learning measures in the study included: 1) total time to mastery; 2) number of trials to mastery; 3) total number of errors; and 4) mean amount of time spent on each problem.

A multiple regression analysis revealed measures of expressed happiness and sadness to significantly relate to all four measures of learning. Children for whom positive affect had been induced succeeded at the task in less time, required fewer trials in order to complete the task, made fewer errors, and spent less time on each problem than did children for whom negative affect had been induced.

At first glance, the Masters and Furman (1976) data appear to have contradictory implications for the Learned Helplessness Paradigm. The former study seems to support Weisz and colleagues' (1982) suggestion that young children and infants are relatively invulnerable to learning helplessness. The latter study, by showing cognitive deficits resulting from negative affect, appears to support the idea that even the very young can learn helplessness. However, as pointed out in the discussion of learned helplessness in infancy, because they refer to the consequences of a particular variable (in this case, affect) on learning rather than on attributional style, the investigator's conclusions actually remain inconclusive with regard to learned helplessness. To elaborate, considering that for the Learned Helplessness Paradigm, learning helplessness is the key to developing expectations of incompetence and to subsequent depression, the finding of Masters and colleagues that negative affect simply impedes learning can also be interpreted as suggesting that negative affect prohibits infants from learning helplessness.

One manner in which an *internal* locus of control may, ironically, function as a factor increasing the likelihood of depressive affect may be derived from the model of empathic distress. As Hoffman (1982a), has noted, when cues from a situation imply to the observer that he or she is causing the plight of another, self-blame may convert ordinary empathic distress—or vicarious affective response for another—into feelings of guilt. These feelings of guilt, according to Hoffman, embody both empathy for someone in distress and self-attributions of responsibility for that distress. Since both Hoffman (1981) and Simner (1971) have identified incipient forms of empathic distress in newborns, and Barnett, King, and Howard (1979) and others have traced empathic development in children, it may be hypothesized that a child with an internal locus of control who experiences high levels of empathic distress or whose empathic distress is repeatedly reinforced by caregivers may engage in a negative self-attribution process culminating in depression. Thus, the negative self-esteem component necessary for the development of full-fledged learned helplessness would be present in such cases.

In sum, Abramson and Sackeim's (1977) criticism of the empirical data often cited in support of the Learned Helplessness Paradigm (that evidence of a mechanism by which individuals transform a situation–specific helplessness into a global helplessness was lacking) has been answered. Empirical evidence suggests that, in fact, negative affect exacerbates beliefs in external control (Alloy et al., 1981; Natale, 1978). Even when no objective measures of negative affect associated with aversive, uncontrollable stimuli have been recorded, the expectation of uncontrollable, aversive stimuli has been shown to be not only self-reinforcing but self-aggravating (Pervin, 1963).

However, just as studies following learned helplessness in children and infants have produced conflicting results, an experiment concerning the relationship between negative affect and external locus of control beliefs (Masters & Furman, 1976) produced no correlation, while Masters et al. (1979) demonstrated that negative affect retards learning. Thus, the Masters et al. data remain open to interpretation. In addition, the empathic distress model suggests that in some instances an internal locus of control may function to increase vulnerability to negative self-attribution, a prerequisite of depressive-like phenomena under the Learned Helplessness Paradigm.

Conclusion

This Chapter raises the issue of whether learned helplessness, a clinical subset of depression posited by Seligman et al. (1968), may be encountered in children and infants. According to Seligman, full-fledged learned helplessness implies acquisition of motivational, cognitive, affective, and self-esteem deficits. Thus, in order to pinpoint the clinical presence of the syndrome, it must be established that infants are developmentally capable of experiencing such deficits.

As pointed out, although even young infants may be superficially "mature" enough to acquire emotional, cognitive, and motivational deficits in the face of uncontrollable events, their sense of self may not yet be stable; nor has it been experimentally demonstrated that their self-concepts include estimations of their abilities. A large body of data indicates that young children and infants may simply not attribute task-related failures to internal causes. Finally, the results of studies concerning the relationship of affect to locus of control beliefs and to learning can be interpreted to imply that even if infants and young children were able to acquire situation-specific learned helplessness, it would be unlikely to escalate into a more global learned helplessness depression.

However, in contrast to data suggesting that infants and young children do not attribute blame for failures to themselves (Stipek, 1981a, 1981b; Stipek & Hoffman, 1980), a study conducted by Stipek et al. (1984) showed that when confronted with their task-related failures, four year olds experience negative affect. Ruble et al. (1976) demonstrated that five year olds recognize failure when forced to, and that their performance expectations decline consequent to the recognition. Therefore, some evidence suggests that by at least age four, children whose parents or peers call attention to their failures might be susceptible to acquiring situation-specific learned helplessness depression. Considering that parent-infant interactions constitute the largest part of early social experience, a clinically significant learned helplessness specific to situations involving the parent would almost by definition be both simultaneously situation specific and global.

As noted in the discussions of effectance motivation, contingency awareness, and contingency-related affect with respect to parent-infant interaction, maladaptive parent-child interactions offer an arena in which infants and young children can be consistently reminded of their shortcomings. Additionally, children's tendencies toward illusions of control might encourage them to accept an unrealistically large portion of the blame for interactive failures. The results of studies investigating the relationship between attachment and mastery provide insight into the validity of these speculations.

Sroufe (1979), for example, discovered that the security of the attachment between parent and infant encourages the infant toward exploration, and he suggested that as a result of a secure attachment, the infant develops a sense of effectance in the social and nonsocial realms. Bridges, Grolnick, Frodi, and Connell (1984) reported the results of a longitudinal investigation into the relationship among mastery motivation, attachment, and maternal variables such as control style. At 12 and 20 months, mother-infant dyads were observed in the laboratory playroom. Infants' mastery motivation was assessed using the Yarrow group's persistence, competence, and affect indices. Attachment was assessed via the Strange Situation (Ainsworth & Wittig, 1969). The mother's control styles and manifestations of support for the infant's autonomy were observed, and their childrearing attitudes were documented in interviews. The investigators determined that at age 12 months, infants of mothers who were sensitive and supportive exhibited secure attachments and strong mastery motivation.

In sum, evidence indicates that young children and infants do not readily attribute task-related failures to internal causes, and therefore probably do not easily develop learned helplessness depression. Thus, the data suggest that young infants appear "primed" to shield or immunize themselves from experiences of helplessness. Studies on effectance motivation and contingency awareness indicate that infants possess an intrinsic readiness to learn, and are attracted to the pleasurable affect encountered when contingency is experienced. Indeed, when effectance and contingency are thwarted, most infants will respond by emitting distress signals. Individual differences in degree of motivation and development of contingency awareness may be attributed to temperamental predisposition. Nevertheless, most infants appear to possess at least a threshold capability propelling them toward mastery-oriented experience. In addition, data on early infant attachment behaviors strongly indicate that infants gravitate toward harmonious interaction with the caregiver and seek to establish a rhythmic or synchronic pattern of exchange that is experienced pleasurably. Finally, Kopp has suggested that the incipient self draws on experiences of efficacy and contingency played out within the parent-infant interaction to establish a regulating mode of behavior. In addition, studies of self-concept in children indicate that self-attribution of failure experiences is avoided. Instead, children rely on a sophisticated schema of illusory contingency or illusion of control to avert confrontation with negative experiences.

Nevertheless, while this research indicates a degree of invulnerability to helplessness, and suggests the mechanisms whereby an infant may circumvent the possibility of falling prey to this form of depression, the reverse may also be argued. That is, it may be inferred that in an infant whose capacities are repeatedly thwarted or misinterpreted, a deviation from normal development can occur. If, for example, the infant's intrinsic behavioral style is that of the temperamentally difficult child, the caregiver may frustrate, rather than nurture, response. Such an infant may experience less gratifying contingency experiences during parent-infant interaction. Subsequently, this infant's self-regulation schema will represent the incorporation of a high degree of non-contingency, as well as contingency, experience. An infant of this type may fail to perceive that he or she can control, regulate, or modify contingency experience to yield pleasurable affect and may, instead, begin to perceive that his or her behaviors provoke non-contingency resulting in negative affect. During the period of early childhood, such a child may express degrees of illusory contingency or illusions of control comparable to those of other children, but in his or her case, the culmination of the process of self-concept has resulted in the belief that negative results or failure experiences are self-attributional. In other words, such children may engage in illusions of control, but the construct will serve to exacerbate the non-contingency experiences, rather than shield against experiencing helplessness.

Although this scenario is hypothetical, two significant points emerge. First, Seligman's Learned Helplessness Paradigm should not be viewed rigidly. That is, while Seligman notes that self-esteem is mandated before learned helplessness can be present, it is important to remember that self-concept is not an isolated entity arising at a precise point during infant development. Rather, self-esteem may be viewed as the ultimate outcome of an intricate process in which innumerable contingency and non-contingency experiences have converged. Thus, the precursors of fully developed self-esteem and the capacity for self-attribution may be identified in early infancy. Second, learned helplessness implies the presence of specific developmental capacities, such as the ability to learn, the ability to experience contingency, the ability to regulate behavior, and, finally, the ability to self-attribute. The cumulative portrait emerging from studies discussed in this chapter strongly suggests that these capacities emerge from the complicated interplay of temperament dimensions, attachment behaviors, and precursory self-regulatory mechanisms. Although it may not yet be possible to diagnose clinical learned helplessness in an infant, various detours from the normal route of development can be identified in the first months of life, and such deviations may serve as signposts, warning clinicians that the probability of depression may be likely in particular cases.

CHAPTER 9

Correlates of Neuroendocrinology to Depressive Phenomena

The study of depression and depressive manifestations has been facilitated by isolating the specific behavioral continuities and discontinuities that correlate with these aberrant phenomena. Yet another paradigm for approaching the study of depression involves the isolation of specific neuroendocrine correlates that may be associated with these behavioral continuities and discontinuities. By identifying such neuroendocrinological correlates and following them within a developmental framework, a previously unexplored method of diagnosing pathogenesis and categorizing depressive disorders in infants and children may be created. Furthermore, the importance of using dysfunctional brain conditions (primarily biochemical in nature) as a means for deriving etiologies of psychiatric disorders is especially appropriate in the area of depression, where chemical treatment with pharmacological agents has achieved noteworthy success (Biederman & Jellinek, 1984; Brown & Mueller, 1979; Bunney & Davis, 1965).

The demonstration of elevated levels of adrenalin in cats frightened by a barking dog (Cannon & de la Paz, 1911) was the first experimental observation that emotional reactions are reflected in endocrine activity (Mason, 1975). The principal neuroendocrinological models to emerge regarding depression have been the biogenic amine theories, which include the catecholamine (dopamine and norepinephrine) hypotheses (Garver & Davis, 1979; Maas, Dekirmenjian, & Jones, 1973; Schildkraut, 1965) and the indoleamine (serotonin) hypotheses (Åsberg, Thoren, Traskman, Berllsson, & Ringberger, 1976; Maas, 1975; van Praag, 1982). In addition to these substances, acetylcholine (ACH) (Janowski, El-Yousif, & Davis, 1974), adrenocorticotropic hormone (ACTH) (Carroll, 1972; Sachar, 1974, 1975), growth hormone (GH) (Garver, Hirschowitz, Fleishmann, & Djuric, 1984; Puig-Antich et al., 1984; Sachar, Finkelstein, & Hellman, 1971), thyroid-stimulating hormone (TSH) (Ehrensing et al., 1974; Kastin, Ehrensing, Schalch, & Anderson, 1972; Prange, Wilson, Knox, Alltop, & Breese, 1972), and luteinizing hormone (LH) (Altman, Sachar, Gruen, Halpern, & Eto, 1975) have all been studied in varying degrees with regard to neuroendocrine disturbances present in affective disorders. Recently, the endogenous opioids (endorphins and enkephalins) have also received a great deal of attention (Costa, Fratta, Hong, Maroni, & Yang, 1978; Herman & Panksepp, 1978; Lal, Miksic, & McCarten, 1978; Willer, Boureau, Dauthier, & Banora, 1979).

Clearly, no single abnormality in neuroendocrine function is likely to be responsible for the myriad clinical and biological phenomena comprising depression (Ettigi & Brown, 1977; Garver & Davis, 1979; Iversen, 1982; Schildkraut, 1978). Instead, a clear discussion of this topic requires an ordered factorial conceptualization of depression and depressive-like phenomena, since this perspective not only mirrors but readily blends with the hierarchical organization of brain structures and endocrine function (Berntson & Micco, 1976; Rothbart & Derryberry, 1981; Tennes & Mason, 1982).

In one particular developmental or hierarchical model, depressive illness is viewed as a final common pathway that "is the culmination of various processes that conceivably converge in those areas of the diencephalon that moderate arousal, mood, motivation, and psychomotor function" (Akiskal & McKinney, 1975, p. 290). Within this paradigm, the specific nature of the depressive syndrome in a given individual derives from an interaction among several factors: 1) genetic predisposition (Arimura, Saito, Bowers, & Shally, 1967); 2) personality traits that may modify the reactivity of the organism to stress (Gershon, Dunner, & Goodwin, 1971); 3) compromised developmental milestones, such as affective development in infants with handicaps (Greenberg & Field, 1982; Suomi, Seaman, Lewis, Delizio, & McKinney, 1978); 4) psychosocial stressors at any point during the life cycle, such as object loss (Bliss, Migeon, Branch, & Samuels, 1956; Parkes, 1964); and 5) physiological stressors which can affect limbic function, such as childbirth, viral diseases, and hypothyroidism (Zwerling et al., 1955).

Personality traits modifying reactivity to stress are of particular importance with regard to the developmental correlates of depression for two reasons. First, personality traits modifying reactivity to stress have received a great deal of theoretical and experimental attention through the study of temperament. Second, an insufficient ability to cope with stress can predispose certain individuals to depression. The nature of these constitutional differences is largely dependent upon both the factors influencing neuroendocrine development (Ganong, 1963; Guillemin & Rosenberg, 1972) and the endocrine system itself.

Case Report

Provence (1980) cites a case of intervention involving a mother, Mrs. A., and her infant, Carla, age 12 months, who manifested organic failure-to-thrive symptomatology. Mrs. A presented at the outpatient clinic concerned about her infant's poor weight gain and feeding problems; Carla's failure to thrive had been called to the mother's attention by a pediatrician when Carla was about five months old. The infant was selective about solid foods and what she did eat was not nutritionally adequate. Although the pediatrician arranged extensive studies for Carla at age 10–11 months, her poor weight gain could not be attributed to any precise physical cause.

Based on an in-clinic visit and subsequent meetings at Mrs. A's home, a nurse-practitioner assigned to the case learned that Mrs. A was extremely anxious that Carla would die. The mother's fearfulness appeared to be related to the death of her own mother two years earlier, and her concern that she would be unable to sustain another loss. The nurse also found that Mrs. A had begun to unsuccessfully force-feed Carla with the help of a friend. The infant's response was regurgitation and passivity or apprehension at mealtimes. Apart from feedings, the relationship between mother and infant appeared intimate, and although small for her age, Carla "did not appear ill or malnourished" (Provence, 1980, p. 5).

Carla's motor activity was relatively low. She was found to prefer her mother to unfamiliar persons, but was unable to make such discriminations appropriately. Carla was responsive when not being fed, and would willingly engage in social play.

After evaluating the case with a mental health consultant at the clinic, the decision was made for the nurse to continue visiting Mrs. A, since she seemed to trust the nurse and hoped she could provide assistance. It was decided that a discussion of the possible relationship between Mrs. A's anxiety over Carla and her own mother's death would not be constructive at that time.

Instead, a series of visits were planned in which the nurse would work to help alleviate Mrs. A's anxiety and devise strategies to make feeding time less tense. Alternative feeding techniques would also be initiated, including allowing Carla to engage in some self-feeding. The nurse further assured Mrs. A that she would be available for assistance as long as she was needed.

Mrs. A responded well to these suggestions, and permitted both the nurse and some friends and relatives to assist in feeding Carla—something she had not been willing to allow in the past. Over a course of weeks, the situation improved steadily and Carla gained weight.

Of this situation Provence wrote that intervention allowed the nurse practitioner to deal with a problem "important to both the physical and mental health of the infant" (p. 9), suggesting that the roots of failure-to-thrive symptomatology lie in an interplay of psychiatric and organic factors.

Interactions Between Internal States and External Events

Contributions of Temperament

The value of a developmental approach to the understanding of depression, in which higher level control mechanisms incorporate preexisting lower level processes, becomes evident when the concept of temperament is used as an investigative tool. Within the construct of temperament, which Derryberry and Rothbart (1984) define as "constitutional differences in reactivity and self-regulation," the term *constitutional* connotes the essential biological makeup of the individual; *reactivity* is defined as the functional state of the somatic, endocrine, autonomic, and central nervous systems; and *self-regulation* is meant to encompass processes occurring at a higher level whose purpose is to modulate the reactive state of these four neuroendocrine systems (Derryberry & Rothbart, 1984, p. 132). Thus, the developmental organization of temperament may be reflected in the neuroendocrine process. Significantly, it has been suggested that neuroendocrine function may, in some cases, coalesce to create a "final common pathway" culminating in depression and depressive–like phenomena (Akiskal & McKinney, 1975; Berntson & Micco, 1976; Rothbart & Derryberry, 1981).

In order to approach the study of depression within the developmental context of endocrinology, it is necessary to isolate the neuroanatomical structures involved. All neuroendocrine structures have the same basic processes of integration. Interaction of biological processes in living organisms is mediated by two types of chemical signals: neurotransmitters and hormones. The operation of these signals is not restricted to the nervous or endocrine systems, and the signals interact by means of "transducing" neurons. The first and most typical neuron is the endocrine-neural transducer, which transforms hormonal signals into changes in firing rate. By *firing rate* is meant the rate at which the presynapse neuron stimulates the postsynapse neuron. A second type of neuron is the neuroendocrine transducer that translates neural activity into hormonal output. Examples of the neuroendocrine transducer are the hypothalamic magno- and parvicellular systems, which produce neurohypophysial (vasopressin, oxytocin) and hypophysiotropic (TSH, ACTH, LH, FSH, GH) hormones (Cardinali, 1983).

The specific focal point for the study of affective states is the limbic system, whose structures have generally been defined in terms of their relationship to the hypothalamus (Papez, 1958; Slusher & Hyde, 1969). Iversen (1982), Carroll (1972), Mason (1968a, 1968b, 1968c, 1968d, 1968e), Starkman and Schteingart (1981), and Iversen and Koob (1977) have cautioned that a unitary concept of limbic function has yet to be developed. Nevertheless some useful generalizations can be articulated. A superimposition of the internal and external states of the organism occurs within the complex of limbic circuitry (Berntson & Micco, 1976). Regarding the external state, all incoming sensations are processed via limbic cortical areas (amygdala and hippocampus); with respect to the internal state, the hypothalamus and its brain stem extensions regulate autonomic and homeostatic functions and modify endocrine function by way of the pituitary (Guillemin & Burgus, 1955; Schally, Arimura, & Kastin, 1973). Another major research finding is that the limbic system expresses or manifests itself in both affect and motivation (Ganong, 1977; Nauta, 1979).

The limbic system functions according to hierarchic principles. One example is that of the hypothalamus, which reacts to external stimuli by emitting corticotropin-releasing factor (CRF). CRF triggers the secretion of adrenocorticotropic hormone (ACTH) by the pituitary. ACTH then acts on the adrenal cortex, causing the release of cortisol, which is the principal glucocorticoid secreted by the adrenal cortex (Anders, Sachar, Kream, Rolfwang, & Hellman, 1970; Goodman & Gilman, 1970; Tennes & Carter, 1973). The level of cortisol is controlled in turn by a negative feedback loop wherein high circulation levels of cortisol inhibit release of CRF (Yates & Maran, 1974).

The hierarchically controlled distribution of cortisol provides a physiological correlate or paradigm for assessing the personality of the individual, in that the model describes, to some degree, reactivity to stress (Krieger, Allen, Rizzo, & Kreiger, 1971). In turn, the framework of temperament is well suited to incorporating the principles underlying cortisol distribution as they become known. As yet, the temperament construct is not sufficiently refined to accurately isolate individual differences in neuroendocrine function.

However, a major step toward identifying neuroendocrinological differences that can be integrated into the framework of temperament was taken by Tennes, Downey, & Vernadakis (1977). Urinary cortisol secretion rates were determined in 20 infants during eight hours for three days. All infants were 11–13 months old. Baseline cortisol levels were obtained on the first day. On the second day, stress was induced by separating the mother from the infant for one hour. During the third day, the child was provided with stimulation in the form of novel toys and socialization for one hour.

Infants who responded with fear or anxiety when the mother left were found to have higher cortisol levels than those who did not react fearfully. Of equal importance was the fact that the fearful/anxious infants had chronically higher levels of cortisol than the other group.

Another pertinent result emerging from this study was the fact that there were two measurably different fear/anxiety groups. One group responded to separation from the mother with easily quantifiable affective reactions such as crying or displaying physical movements aimed at retaining the mother. Members of the other group, in contrast, became immobilized, exhibiting a passive withdrawal that was suggestive of physiological and psychological regression. Members of this group had lower levels of cortisol both chronically and in association with the stress event than did those who reacted overtly. Therefore, the level of neuroendocrine functioning as measured by cortisol urinary excretion rate may be used to predict two different types of behavioral reactivity to stress.

Another finding in this study further illustrated the nature of temperamental differences as reflected in neuroendocrine function. During a play session, the infants were categorized in relation to their response to the toys as being either "happy," "indifferent," or "fearful." Those infants who were happy or indifferent had cortisol levels comparable to the control levels, whereas infants who reacted to the toys with fear showed levels analogous to the separation anxiety levels. The infant's reactions observed in this study are analogous to responses commonly seen in similar stress situations in Ainsworth's Strange Situation Procedure (Ainsworth & Wittig, 1969). Infants whose attachment is termed *resistant* or *ambivalent* (Group C) commonly showed a reluctance to explore and play with toys, and distress at being separated from the mother, either actively or passively. The consonance of Ainsworth's findings with Tennes et al.'s (1977) study suggests that there is a positive correlation between certain affective states and cortisol levels.

Overall, Tennes et al. (1977) concluded that, by one year of age, cortisol levels are associated with *psychological* variables. While this study illustrates the potential value of using physiological measures to identify and elucidate aspects of temperament and its relation to affective states, Posner and Rothbart (1981) have suggested that the converse is true as well. Specifically, studying the development of temperament by behavioral means may provide a useful method for identifying developmental psychoendocrine events. This method is admittedly complex but there is a general consensus that the temperament construct serves as a useful heuristic model (Diamond, 1957; Rothbart & Derryberry, 1981; Thomas & Chess, 1977; Tennes & Mason, 1982).

Relatively little is known about the maturational events occurring in the brain, but many temperament theorists would agree that the infant's innate reactive and regulatory capabilities continue to develop after birth (Rothbart & Derryberry, 1982; Thomas & Chess, 1984). A number of highly organized reflex patterns have been documented in the newborn infant, such as the Moro, Babinski, and tonic neck reflexes. These reflex reactions soon begin to disappear as higher level systems mature and exert their effects. This receding process has come to be known as "inhibitory maturation," and recent studies of the early-stage monoamine systems have found that the development of these systems slowly counterbalances the neonate's initial excitatory tendencies in the areas of motor activity and spontaneous motility (Pradhan & Pradhan, 1980). Moreover, a number of studies have implicated serotonin as a primary early *inhibitor* or *modulator* (Lidov & Molliver, 1982; Pradhan & Pradhan, 1980), exerting an effect as early as the fifteenth day of life in rats, for example (Mabry & Campbell, 1974). Serotonin, a complex amine, has been isolated in the human brain and has been recognized as being structurally similar to lysergic acid diethylamide.

Measurement of the endocrine correlates of general behavioral states is complex, since the emotional manifestations of a neonate are generally restricted to whether or not he or she is awake or asleep, quiet or crying (Tennes & Mason, 1982). Nevertheless, primitive as these states may be, Anders et al. (1970) have found that higher levels of cortisol appeared in association with 20 minutes of crying than occurred after 20 minutes of sleep. This finding was confirmed by Tennes & Carter (1973). Thus, the strongest statement that can be made on the basis of these studies is that an adrenocortical response can be elicited by negative emotion manifested as crying. However, these were simple exploratory studies that did not investigate the causes of crying or differentiate between individual variations in the threshold of emotional arousal.

Unfortunately, in terms of the neonate, both temperament constructs and developmental psychoendocrinology are constrained from making inferences about the links between affective states and brain function, due to the fact that the infant's affective repertoire is still in the stage of rapid evolution. Despite this difficulty, as the neuroendocrine system rapidly matures, behavior becomes more differentiated and consequently more easily measurable.

Biogenic Amine Theories of Depression

Historical Background. Prior to the 1950s, no effective pharmacological treatment for depression was available (Charney, Menkes, & Heniger, 1981; Coppen, 1967; van Praag, 1977). However, it had been noted serendipitously for some time that a small but persistent fraction of hypertensive patients receiving reserpine, an alkaloid of rauwolfia, developed severe depressive reactions (Achor, Hanson, & Gifford, 1955; Faucett, Litin, & Achor, 1957; Freis, 1954; Jensen, 1959). Eventually the evidence relating reserpine and depression became very strong: 1) a higher incidence of depression was documented in patients treated with reserpine than in those treated with other antihypertensive agents; 2) the depressive effect of reserpine was dose dependent; and 3) when taken off reserpine the depression normally cleared, and if a high dose of reserpine was reinstituted, the depression commonly recurred (Bunney & Davis, 1965).

The dramatic depressogenic effect of reserpine triggered a flurry of investigations into its neural action. In the years following, it was discovered that reserpine and related compounds were responsible for a significant reduction in dopamine, norepinephrine, and serotonin in peripheral tissues, as well as in the brain itself (Bunney & Davis, 1965; Carlsson, Lindvist & Magnusson, 1957; Jensen, 1959; Pare & Sandler, 1959). This discovery was of primary importance in disclosing a biochemical bridge between monoamines and behavior.

Concurrently, an association between amine metabolism and mood disorders was suggested by the observation that iproniazid, a chemical congener of the antituberculosis agent isoniazid, occasionally produced mood elevation in treated patients (Pare & Sandler, 1959). Hydrazine compounds, such as isoniazid, were known to inhibit the enzyme monoamine oxidase (MAO) (Zeller, Barsky, Berman, & Fouts, 1952), whose major function had been reported to be the inactivation of biogenic amines (Coppen, 1967; van Praag, 1976). When derivatives of iproniazid were synthesized and found to inhibit MAO and to alleviate depressed mood, there was growing recognition that there might be a relationship between amine metabolism and mood disorders (Randrup & Braestrup, 1977; van Praag, 1978). This argument received more support from the finding that imipramine, an effective antidepressant, was capable of blocking the reuptake of catecholamines (norepinephrine and dopamine) into sympathetically innervated tissues (Charney et al., 1981; Rosenblatt & Chanley, 1965; Schildkraut, 1978; Sette, Raisman, Briley, & Langer, 1981).

Catecholamine Hypothesis of Affective Disorders. Schildkraut (1965) was the first to offer a formulation relating catecholamines to depression. The catecholamine hypothesis of affective disorders proposed that depressions are associated with a deficiency of catecholamines, particularly norepinephrine, at functionally important sites in the brain. Conversely, manias may be associated with an excess of catecholamine (Brodie, Murphy, Goodwin, & Bunney, 1971; Brown & Mueller, 1979; Bunney, Murphy, Goodwin, & Borge, 1972).

The interdependence among hormones has been supported by steadily mounting evidence (Mason, 1968a, 1968b, 1968c, 1968d, 1968e, 1975). However, Schildkraut and others are quick to point out that the catecholamine theory by no means accounts for all the endocrine activity in the brain that may be associated with depression (Coppen, 1967; Garver & Davis, 1979; Puig-Antich et al., 1984; Schildkraut, 1978). However, for our purposes, discussion will be limited primarily to these theories. There is a broad consensus that these theories are of growing heuristic value (Kelley & Stinus, 1984; Schildkraut, 1978; van Praag, 1977, 1982). Therefore, they will be of greatest use in the effort to forge a bridge between depression and the influence of early neuroendocrinological development in the infant.

Indoleamine Hypothesis of Affective Disorders. The indoleamine hypothesis of affective disorders posits a deficit in brain serotonergic function in patients with affective disorders. This directly contributes or predisposes the individual to symptoms of depression (Murphy, Campbell, & Costa, 1978; van Praag & de Haan, 1980). One potential correlation, gleaned from the development of temperament, is the relationship between the onset of "inhibitory maturation" (referred to above) and the appearance of serotonin in the brain (Lidov & Molliver, 1982). The fact that serotonin appears as a major modulator of behavior in rats as early as 15 days after birth at least lends additional support to its importance in terms of development (Mabry & Campbell, 1974). A variation in its concentration or the time of its appearance in the undeveloped brain might easily have pathological consequences for the child and/or adult, since any one of the highly plastic neonatal brain systems may be easily, even permanently, influenced by aberrations in any of the other systems (Bronson, 1982; Dorner, 1983). Investigations involving serotonin suggest that depression may be linked both to low levels of the substance itself and to defects in the neuronal transport mechanism.

Dysregulation Hypothesis of Affective Disorders. Calling attention to the fact that the catecholamine and indoleamine theories are far from adequate in explaining affective disorders, Siever and Davis (1985) have proposed an alternate system derived from the bioamine theories. The bioamine theories are based on the assumption that the neurotransmitter systems involved are either overactive or underactive in affective disorders. In an attempt to clarify what seem to be inconsistencies in these theories, Siever and Davis have attempted a reformulation based upon operational dynamics of neurotransmitter systems. These dynamics predominantly involve time-dependent and stimulus-dependent regulation that is mediated by multiple, hierarchically arranged control systems. Rather than simply observing the level of activity, abnormalities in biogenic amine neurotransmitter systems can be viewed as a malfunction in regulation or buffering of these systems. Such dysregulated neurotransmitter systems may not respond appropriately to external stimulation and may be highly variable and desynchronized from normal periodicities.

In order to test for pathophysiology of affective disorders based upon time- and stimulus-dependent regulation of bioamine neurotransmitter systems, Siever and Davis (1985) provided six criteria that can be used to test dysregulation: 1) impairment of one or more regulatory or homeostatic mechanisms; 2) erratic pattern of basal output in the neurotransmitter system; 3) disruption in the normal periodicities of the system, including circadian rhythmicities; 4) diminished selective responsiveness of the system to external stimuli; 5) sluggish return of the system to basal activity following a perturbation; and 6) restoration of efficient regulation by pharmacological agents demonstrating clinical effectiveness.

The authors concluded that the dysregulation model meshes with what is known about the noradrenergic system in depression. Specifically, they proposed that noradrenergic neuronal firing is elevated and erratic, while the amount of norepinephrine released in response to each nerve impulse is decreased. Such a mechanism appears to be consistent with animal models of depression induced by learned helplessness, as well as with the clinical features and course of the affective disorders in humans. Furthermore, this model may be useful in reaching a developmental understanding of depression if it is applied in conjunction with temperament theory, since behavioral regulation is an underlying premise of the temperament construct.

Assessment of Current Status of Biogenic Amine Theories

A major problem in attempting to correlate blood or urinary concentrations of amine metabolites with depression stems from the fact that such metabolites may not accurately reflect the metabolism that occurs in the brain (Blombery, Koplin, Gordon, Markey, & Ebert, 1980; Hollister, Davis, & Overall, 1978). For example, the blood-brain barrier, the protective shield that exists between the blood and the extracellular fluids of the brain and prevents passage of various substances, inhibits the escape of serotonin. Moreover, serotonin metabolism is very sensitive to dietary tryptophan (van Praag & de Haan, 1980). Similar problems apply to norepinephrine metabolism (Baldessarini, 1975). Therefore, excretion rates of amines and their metabolites might loosely reflect the central and peripheral metabolism (Wilk & Watson, 1973); however, it remains difficult to assess the relation of the metabolic turnover rate to the functional state of the synapse (Kelley & Stinus, 1984). (See Table 9.1.)

This problem has been particularly evident in the area of urinary metabolites. MHPG (3-methyl-4-hydroxyphenalglycol), for example, is the major metabolite of brain norepinephrine (Deleon–Jones, Maas, Deikirmenjian, & Sanchez, 1975; Maas, Dekirmenjian, & Fawcett, 1971). However, the exact fraction of urinary MHPG deriving from brain norepinephrine remains a matter of speculation (Schatzberg et al., 1981).

MHPG levels may, in fact, be useful in predicting the subject's responsiveness to various drugs. High MHPG levels can imply responsiveness to agents that have strong effects against serotonin uptake (clomipromine or amitriptyline). Low levels of MHPG may predict responsiveness to drugs that effect norepinephrine uptake into neurons (desipramine, maprotiline, or imipramine) (Baldessarini, 1983; Depue & Evans, 1981; Goodwin, Cowdry, & Webster, 1978). MHPG measurement in infants and children has been found to correlate with results seen in adults, although age-related norms for urinary MHPG in children are needed in order to gain further refinements in the use of this technique for detecting and classifying depression (Tennes et al., 1977).

TABLE 9.1. Behavior and affective regulation mediated by hormones.

Hormone	Behavior
Serotonin[a]	Anorexia, dejected mood, sleep disturbances, reward system[b]
	Sedation, underarousal, depression[c]
	Sleep/wake cycles, central temperature, aggressive behavior[d]
	Crying[e]
	Behavioral states, sensory pathways[f,g,h,i,j]
	Anxiety, sleep disturbances[k]
	Suicide[l,m]
Catecholamines	Drive-inducing reward functions[n]
	Sedation, underarousal, depression[c]
	Protest behavior[o]
Norepinephrine[a]	Anorexia, dejected mood, sleep disturbances, reward system[b]
	Sedation, underarousal, depression[c]
Dopamine[a]	Anorexia, dejected mood, sleep disturbances, reward system[b]
	Sedation, underarousal, depression[c]
Cortisol[p]	Crying [e],[q]
	Rigid coping styles[r]
	Depression[s],[t]

Note. Unless otherwise noted, these authors correlated one or more hormones and/or neurotransmitters with behavioral regulation.
[a]Davis (1970).
[b]Depue and Evans (1981).
[c]Baldessarini (1983).
[d]Iversen (1982).
[e]Tennes and Carter (1977).
[f]Trulson and Jacobs (1979).
[h]Reader et al. (1979).
[i]Jouvet (1969).
[j]Bloom et al. (1972).
[k]Kelley and Stinus (1984).
[l]Lloyd et al. (1974).
[m]Murphy et al. (1978).
[n]Crow (1973).
[o]Breese et al. (1973).
[p]Azmitia (1978).
[q]Anders et al. (1970).
[r]Knight et al. (1979).
[s]Carroll (1972).
[t]Sachar et al. (1971, 1973, 1980).

Cortisol Response to Stress

The evidence is very strong that the production or secretion rate of cortisol over a 24-hour period is elevated in most, if not all, depressive patients (Gibbons, 1964; Sachar, 1975; Sachar, Fratz, Altmann, & Sassin, 1973; Sachar, Hellman et al., 1973). Levels of plasma free cortisol (PFC) in depressed patients are higher than those of control psychiatric inpatients (Carroll, Curtiss, & Mendels, 1976).

The hypersecretion of cortisol is thought to reflect malfunction of the limbic system (Carroll 1972; Carroll, Martin, & Davies, 1968; Sachar, Fratz et al., 1973; Sachar, Hellman et al., 1973) in addition to the patient's subjective distress (Carroll, 1972, 1976). The relation between stress and cortisol release is complex and not completely understood, but can be roughly summarized as follows: through the ascending reticular activating system, which receives input from a number of areas including the musculature, viscera, and cortex, stress triggers the limbic system and, perhaps, in particular, the amygdala. The limbic system activates the hypothalamus, which releases a corticotropin-releasing factor (CRF), which then stimulates secretion of corticotropin or adrenocorticotropic hormone (ACTH) from the anterior pituitary. ACTH transported through the blood causes cortisol to be secreted from the adrenal cortex, and as cortisol concentrations rise in the blood, some effect of cortisol feeds back to the limbic system (perhaps the hippocampus), which in turn inhibits hypothalamic neuroendocrine cells from releasing further CRF (Depue & Evans, 1981; Ganong, 1979; Guyton, 1971; Mason, 1968a, 1968b, 1968c, 1968d, 1968e).

A failure of the feedback-inhibitory influence on ACTH-cortisol release, (that is, the disinhibition of the HPA axis) is an important neuroendocrine lesion in depression (Carroll et al., 1976; Depue & Evans, 1981). It is important to realize that the responsivity of the organism to stress often varies in phase with the 24-hour circadian rhythm (Charney et al., 1981; Puig-Antich, Chambers, Halpern, Hallon, & Sachar, 1979). In the normal adult, very little cortisol is secreted during the evening and early morning hours. Levels peak at late morning and remain high until early evening. In addition to circadian fluctuations, stressful stimuli, such as the trauma of surgery, may completely override both circadian control and negative feedback mechanisms (Tennes & Mason, 1982).

A study by Knight et al. (1979) examined the impact on children caused by the anticipation of elective surgery in relation to cortisol levels. The investigation involved 19 boys and six girls between the ages of seven and 11 who had been admitted to a pediatric ward for elective surgery. The impact of stress was measured at three different points in time.

At Time I, when the child had just been told to come back for surgery in two weeks, an extensive interview was conducted to gauge the child's coping ability and determine types of defense used (employing the defense effectiveness scale). The children were instructed to collect urine samples during two 24-hour periods over the next weekend. These samples were later used to estimate cortisol production rates.

Time II was the day following admission to the hospital. During this time, when the hospital and preparation for surgery had become a concrete reality for the child, urine samples were collected for a 24-hour period. The child was interviewed a second time by a clinician blind to the results of the earlier interview.

Time III occurred on the day following surgery when the child was still in the hospital. No urine samples were taken.

The results for Time I showed no correlation between cortisol production rates and scores for defense effectiveness gleaned from the interview. The cortisol production rate ranged from 8.43 to 27.93 mg/g of creatinine per 24 hours, yielding a mean of 14.32. Comparison was made with a control group of children hospitalized for medical evaluation for which mean cortisol production was found to be 15.01 mg/g of creatinine per 24 hours, using the three-metabolite method.

Between Time I and Time II, cortisol production rates and defense effectiveness scores changed significantly. The Time II cortisol production rate ranged from 9.46 to 25.59 mg/g of creatinine per 24 hours, with a mean of 16.03. Knight et al. (1979) found that elevated cortisol levels correlated negatively with defense efficacy. When denial and displacement were used to defend against the stress of hospitalization, children had higher cortisol levels than when they used intellectualization or a mixed pattern of response.

Unfortunately, there is relatively little information about these relationships in infancy or childhood (Tennes et al., 1977; Tennes & Mason, 1982). In a preliminary report, Puig-Antich et al. (1979) noted that approximately 50% of adult endogenous or vital depressives hypersecrete cortisol. These researchers subsequently measured plasma cortisol every 20 minutes for 10–24 hours in four pre-pubertal children meeting the Research Diagnostic Criteria for major depressive disorder, endogenous subtype. Results were in line with those found for adults. Two of the four prepubertal subjects were observed to hypersecrete cortisol during illness. Cortisol returned to normal levels after clinical recovery. While these were preliminary data using a small number of patients, Puig-Antich et al. (1979) indicated that their findings support the idea that major depressive disorders in children and adults may be fundamentally the same illness occurring during different stages of development.

Experimental results have upheld a strong relationship between elevated emotion and elevated cortisol early in life. Tennes and Carter (1973) explored the relationship between plasma cortisol levels and behavioral states in 40 full-term infants on the third day of life. The behavioral states of the infants were assessed during the 30 minutes prior to routine blood sampling for phenylketonuria. There were no relationships detected between levels of cortisol and sex, birth weight, recency of circumcision, or Apgar scores. However, behavioral state was found to be related to cortisol secretion. Low cortisol levels were associated with the sleep state, while periods of fussiness and/or crying were accompanied by elevated plasma cortisol concentrations.

Anders et al. (1970) studied the relationship between behavior state and plasma cortisol response in four infants, taking blood samples on 20 occasions between the first and 15th week of their lives. Marked rises in plasma cortisol occurred after 20 minutes of crying, while levels remained relatively low and constant in quiescent periods. From the results of this experiment with a limited number of subjects, it appears that measurement of plasma cortisol is potentially as useful in infancy as it has proved to be in the adult.

Tennes and Carter (1973) also studied the cortisol levels of three infants in their sample longitudinally during the first three months of life. Data did not support a relationship of sustained increase in plasma cortisol in response to the rise in chronic fussiness/irritability frequently found in normal infants in the second month of life. However, the authors observed that the lack of this relationship may suggest that the increase in irritability during the first three months of life was a reflection of variations in physiological reactivity, which is a primary component of temperament.

Dexamethasone Suppression Test (DST)

The dexamethasone suppression test (DST) was developed as another attempt to isolate a biological marker of depression—one that does not require the measurement of hormone metabolites in the blood. Although the limbic system cannot yet be studied through direct, invasive means in humans, neuroendocrine function tests can be used to acquire inferential knowledge about the system (Carroll, 1983). The DST is one such test. When hypersecretion of cortisol is identified in patients with severe depression, the DST is used in these patients to determine whether dexamethasone would have any inhibitory effect on cortisol output (Carroll, 1984). The test involves oral administration of dexamethasone late in the evening before the patient goes to sleep. The following day, blood samples for plasma cortisol are drawn on two separate occasions. An elevated plasma cortisol concentration in either blood sample indicates a positive response. Endocrinologically, a positive response may be interpreted as signaling a disinhibitory defect of the hypothalamic-pituitary-adrenal axis (Carroll, 1984). That is, despite artificial administration of an agent known to suppress cortisol levels, the patient is unable to activate the mechanism responsible for achieving endocrine equilibrium.

As the test is applied in clinical studies under increasingly realistic field conditions, evidence is mounting that the diagnostic value of the DST is limited but useful, with an average sensitivity of around 50% (Asnis et al., 1981; Baldessarini, 1983; Fang, Tricou, Robertson, & Meltzer, 1981; Poznanski, Carroll, Banegas, Cook, & Gross, 1982). By "sensitivity" is meant the rate of positive tests among those suspected of being depressed ("true" positive rate). "Specificity" is defined as the rate of negative tests in a control population ('true' negative rate) (Baldessarini, 1983). In recent studies, sensitivity has ranged from 22% to 75% and specificity from 85% to 100%.

In children, the biological markers for depression have been investigated much less extensively than in adults (Geller, Rogol, & Knitter, 1983). The DST has proven 90% specific for depressed adults and moderately sensitive (30–60%), but the specificity of the test may be even better in children because nonsuppression of cortisol has been associated with a number of conditions not commonly observed in childhood, including anorexia nervosa, bulimia, and opiate addiction (Klee & Garfinkel, 1984).

Petty, Asarnow, Carlson, and Lesser (1985) administered the dexamethasone suppression test (DST) to 30 children; seven with major depression, six with dysthymia, and 17 with various other, nonaffective disorders. The children, who had been psychiatrically hospitalized and ranged in age from five to 12 years, either met the *DSM–III* criteria for major depressive disorder or dysthymic disorder, or clearly did not meet the criteria for either disorder.

The study found similar rates of nonsuppression were displayed by the major depressives (6 of 7, 86%), the dysthymic group (5 of 6, 83%), and a subgroup of the controls who were diagnosed as "definitely not depressed" (5 of 6, 83%). The test showed a sensitivity for major depression (87%), but had a low specificity (53%) (Petty et al., 1985).

Thus, a limited but significant number of trials have found that the DST can be useful in detecting depression in children (Branyon, 1983; Geller et al., 1983; Klee & Garfinkel, 1984; Weller, Weller, Fristad, & Preskorn, 1984). Poznanski et al. (1982) concluded from their use of the test in 18 dysphoric children, ages 6–12 years, that endogenous depression is not rare and is biochemically similar to the disorder in the adult. This conclusion supports the validity of using *DSM–III* diagnostic criteria, which apply the same symptomatology to both adults and children, for detecting depressive disorders during childhood.

Growth Hormone

Analysis of growth hormone (GH) response provides another means of examining the operation of the hypothalamic-pituitary-adrenal axis. Normal patients generally demonstrate increased GH secretion under conditions of insulin-induced hypoglycemia. Unipolar depressives, however, have been shown in many studies to have inadequate GH responses to hypoglycemia (Carroll, 1972; Depue & Evans, 1981; Sachar et al., 1971; Sachar, Fratz et al., 1973). An interesting implication of this relates to the maternal deprivation-failure-to-thrive syndrome in children, which may be similar to the anaclitic depression syndrome described in young children. (See "Case Report" of this chapter.) Neglected children sometimes not only fail to grow, but demonstrate an abnormal response to insulin-induced hypoglycemia (Powell, Brasel, & Blizzard, 1967a, 1967b). This parallel between unipolar depressives and children suffering from maternal deprivation may be helpful in elucidating the proposed proclivity for depression in children separated from their parents (Depue & Evans, 1981).

Several researchers (Money, 1977; Powell et al., 1967a, 1967b) have documented a direct cause and effect relationship between emotional abuse and subsequent physiological disturbances, manifested by deficiency of growth. The growth disorder, often referred to as psychosocial dwarfism or nonorganic failure to thrive, has a typical onset of prior to 8 months of age. Most prominent is the infant's failure to gain in length. Indeed, the disorder has been recognized to the extent of earning a classification in DSM–III (American Psychiatric Association, 1980).

With regard to the etiology of psychosocial dwarfism, Green, Campbell, and David (1984) have noted that the condition may be attributed to deprivation or lack of some necessary positive element between mother and child. That is, the condition may be characterized as an attachment disturbance.

In relation to this discussion of the neuroendocrine correlates of depression, it is significant that Powell et al. (1967a, 1967b) reported specific absence of growth hormone (GH) release in emotionally abused or deprived children and, additionally, found rapid recovery of this hormonal disturbance upon changing the child's environment. In an attempt to capture the elements of growth hormone deficiency and the high degree of spontaneous recovery when the child was removed from the depriving environment, Money (1977) labeled the syndrome "reversible hyposomatotropism."

Calling the syndrome "deprivation dwarfism," Patton and Gardner (1975) commented that the growth retardation observed in infants and children from disordered environmental situations has classically been traced to specific hormonal or metabolic disorders. The authors note that the more the social environment in which the child is reared deviates from an adaptational environment, the greater the danger of developing maladaptive patterns of physiological and endocrinological manifestations. These maladaptive patterns would be mediated through the impact of abnormal environmental stimuli on the neocortex, which controls the secretion of releasing and inhibiting factors by the hypothalamus, and consequently exerts an adverse influence on the production of tropic hormones by the pituitary gland. Specific hormonal abnormalities that have been reported in children and infants with psychosocial dwarfism include abnormally low ACTH reserve and below normal values for fasting GH levels. Growth hormone levels after stimulation (usually insulin–provoked hypoglycemia) are also low in approximately one half of the cases reported. Finally defective somatomedin production has also been reported by a number of researchers (D'Ercole, Underwood, & VanWyk, 1977; Tanner, 1973; Saenger et al., 1977; Van den Brande et al., 1975). Thus, it is postulated that growth hormone stimulates somatomedin accumulation (Gilman, Goodman, & Gilman, 1980).

Cortisol-Serotonin Interaction

The relation of cortisol to stress and the increased levels of cortisol in depressed patients has been discussed. Also discussed is the potential value of using chronic cortisol levels to assess a given individual's reactivity to stress—an important component of temperament—and perhaps even to predict the particular strategy that an individual will adopt when exposed to stress (aggressive versus withdrawn). In relation to these elements, and to the permissive amine and dysregulation hypotheses, it is important to realize that serotonin is a major regulator of neuroendocrine rhythms, especially cortisol secretion (Heniger, Charney, & Sternberg, 1984).

Meltzer, Perline, and Tricov (1984) administered 200 mg of oral 5-hydroxytryptophan, the precursor of serotonin, to 25 patients with major depression, six schizoaffective depressed patients, and 16 bipolar manic patients. They found that serum cortisol levels were significantly higher after administration of the precursor in depressed patients than in controls. In addition, the increase in cortisol was positively correlated with Hamilton ratings of depressed mood, helplessness, and worthlessness as well as with the Schedule of Affective Disorders and Schizophrenia Change. A predicted positive correlation was also found between suicidal acts and the 5-hydroxytryptophan-induced increase in cortisol. In fact, the largest cortisol response observed occurred in a depressed patient who later committed suicide.

The authors conclude that their data confirm the significance of the reported relationship among low cerebrospinal fluid levels of 5-hydroxyindoleacetic acid (the major metabolite of serotonin), increased activity of the hypothalamic-pituitary-adrenal axis, and the more violent suicide attempts seen in depressed and nondepressed patients.

In another study, Meltzer, Lowy, Robertson, Goodnick, and Perline (1984) tested the effects of antidepressant drugs in the eight unipolar and seven bipolar depressed patients and the seven manic patients included in their first study. After a three- to five-week period of treatment with lithium carbonate or a MAO inhibitor, the mean increase in cortisol induced by 200 mg of 5-hydroxytryptophan was augmented. Treatment with tricyclics and second generation antidepressants reduced the mean cortisol response in patients with major depression.

Tricyclics and second-generation antidepressants apparently normalized the cortisol response to serotonin, indicating that such treatments enhance serotonergic action, leading to a down-regulation of serotonin receptors. The fact that lithium carbonate enhanced cortisol response provides evidence that long-term lithium treatment improves serotonergic function as well. These data support the idea of a permissive role of a decreased serotonin concentration in depression. The enhanced cortisol response to 5-hydroxytryptophan in this study was likely the result of supersensitivity of serotonin receptors, a condition that may have been secondary to an abnormality in presynaptic function. This abnormality could be a chronic condition in patients with affective disorders (Meltzer, Lowy, et al., 1984).

These studies illustrate the fact that evidence is growing to support the value of the amine and dysregulation hypotheses and that data are accumulating that validate the idea that downward changes in serotonin levels can operate as a "predisposer" to vulnerability for depression, mediating the individual's reactivity to stress.

Developmental Psychoendocrinology: Therapeutic Implications for Definition and Treatment of Depression

Avoidance and Learned Helplessness

One useful way to explore the role of biogenic amines in depression lies in an examination of avoidance to aversive stimuli (e.g., avert gaze, turn away) and learned helplessness, two stress-related phenomena. In neonates, active avoidance of the mother or caregiver presents a theoretical problem. Although attachment theory is based on the premise that an infant has an inherent need to maintain proximity to an attachment figure, this drive is mediated by other drives in both the infant and the caregiver. The result is that the infant and caregiver do not attempt to maintain constant physical contact, but the infant alternates exploratory behavior with contact-seeking behavior. Upon being reunited with their caregivers following a long or even relatively short separation, some infants commonly will avert their gaze and, if picked up, will signal an inclination to be put down immediately. Such examples of active avoidance of the caregiver are not attributable to exploratory behavior on the part of the infant and do not seem to fit in with an attachment model of behavior.

Gaze aversion and similar behaviors (physical avoidance, apparent lack of recognition of the mother, etc.) recently have been viewed as possibly being part of a strategy to maintain proximity when the infant is separated from or rejected by the mother. Main and Weston (1982) have hypothesized that, similar to locomotion and crying, avoidance functions as a means of bridging gaps in the attachment bond. In this paradigm, avoidance is compellingly seen as a way of maintaining behavioral organization.

Behavioral disorganization can result when the infant is placed in a conflict situation regarding the attachment bond. This occurs, in theoretical terms, when an infant is simultaneously subjected to threats from the mother while being denied physical contact. The infant is thus placed in an irresolvable conflict, since any threat from the environment generates an urge to withdraw from the source of the threat and to seek out the caregiver. Approach, therefore, is not possible when it is most needed. This dilemma causes increased activation of the attachment behavior system, but approach is still not possible, and this leads to even greater levels of irresolvable conflict. In short, Main and Weston describe the development of a positive feedback loop.

It is not difficult to speculate how this positive feedback system might eventuate in a depressive state (Main, Kaplan, & Cassidy, 1985). The loop cannot be broken as long as the attention of the infant is focused on the attachment figure. The only solution lies in a shift in attention, and, in making the avoidance response, this is precisely what the infant does. In effect, the infant is acting on his or her own behalf to preserve his or her behavioral organization and thus to maintain control and to continue to exert flexibility in his or her interactions with the environment (Main & Weston, 1982).

This explanation implies that the infant is a highly sophisticated organism, capable of finding the only solution that might preserve his or her psychological well-being. In light of the data showing early functioning of the hypothalamic-pituitary-adrenal axis, such sophisticated analysis on the part of the infant does not seem unreasonable. However, the next step clearly is to determine what happens when even the avoidance response is not possible (i.e., does depression result when the infant is given no chance to break the positive feedback loop described above?).

The Learned Helplessness Paradigm presents another model within which to study the interrelationship of biogenic amines and depression. The theory states that following the experience of traumatic, uncontrollable events, major emotional, cognitive, and motivational deficits color the psychological experience of the individual (Abramson, Seligman, & Teasdale, 1978).

If animals are subjected to inescapable shock and later given the opportunity to escape the aversive stimulus by learning a simple task, they seem unable or unwilling to do so. Their behavior suggests that they have "learned to be helpless" (Anisman, 1975; Overmeir & Seligman, 1967; Seligman, 1975). Interestingly, the degree of inability to later learn to avoid the aversive situation appears directly related to the lack of control that the animal has over the shock during its initial exposure (Seligman & Maier, 1967). Therefore, it appears that even a relatively minor volitional action, such as averting the eyes or rejecting the caregiver, will have some value in keeping the infant from experiencing the full force of behavioral disorganization. The symptoms of learned helplessness parallel those of depression: 1) low initiation of voluntary response, 2) negative cognitive set, 3) time course, 4) low aggression, 5) loss of appetite, 6) physiological changes (in norepinephrine for example) (Seligman, 1975). In animals, the Learned Helplessness Paradigm has been studied in detail and has been associated with variations in several neurotransmitters, primarily norepinephrine (NE). Exposure to inescapable shock has been reported to increase MHPG production, to decrease brain NE, and to increase the turnover of NE (Weiss, Glazer, & Podhorecky, 1974; Weiss, Stone, & Harrell, 1970). Seligman has suggested that a susceptibility to a belief that maintains a learned helplessness response is the critical underlying factor for depression. However, it may be that such a belief is secondary to a primary cause—namely, a set of stressors that have begun a pattern of neuroendocrine dysregulation.

In an experiment to measure the effects of stress-induced depression on brain norepinephrine levels, Weiss, Glazer, Pohorecky, Bailey, and Schneider (1979) ran a simultaneous series on three rats. An "avoidance-escape" animal was able to avoid shocks to its tail by performing a specific response before the shock came. A second, "yoked" animal received the same shocks as the avoidance-escape animal, but no response that it made could control the delivery of shocks. Finally, a third animal, the control animal, was included in each experiment with an identical setup, but received no shocks. This last animal served as a baseline for comparison with the other animals.

Weiss et al. (1979) found that the avoidance-escape animals showed higher levels of NE in the brain than did the nonshock control animals. The yoked animals showed roughly similar NE levels to control when few shocks were given and lower levels when many shocks were given. This latter result is consistent with earlier studies of brain NE levels associated with the application of a severe stressor (Weiss et al., 1970, 1974). The variations in brain NE levels were somewhat localized. The avoidance-escape animals showed no NE depletion in the hypothalamus and an elevation of NE levels in the brain stem and cortex. The yoked animals, on the other hand, displayed much NE depletion in the hypothalamus and less depletion in the brain stem and cortex (Weiss et al., 1979).

Using dogs as subjects, Overmeir and Seligman (1967) found that stressful inescapable shock produces a behavioral deficit or inability to cope. Specifically, the study showed that when the subjects received strong, inescapable shocks, they were thereafter unable to learn a shuttle avoidance-escape response. Weiss et al. (1979) have suggested that the behavioral findings of Overmeir and Seligman might follow from the neurochemical differences in rate of amine synthesis and release for yoked and avoidance-escape subjects as found in their own experiments (Weiss et al., 1970, 1979).

Another series of experiments tested the behavioral deficit due to a cold swim (Glazer, Weiss, Pohorecky, & Miller, 1975; Weiss & Glazer, 1975; Weiss, Glazer, Pohorecky, Brick, & Miller, 1975). Using five groups of animals, two were subjected to cold swims of 3.5 minute and 6.5 minute duration, respectively; two received equivalent treatment except the water was warm, and the last group was not put in water and served as the control group. Thirty minutes after the swim, all groups were tested for avoidance-escape responses in a shuttle box. The groups subjected to cold swims were found to have significantly impaired ability to respond in the avoidance-escape test. The stress, as the experiment showed, reduced central noradrenergic activity. This result would seem to reinforce the possibility that avoidance-escape deficits are mediated by reduction in central noradrenergic activity (Weiss et al., 1979).

It is likely that inescapable shock depletes brain NE levels by causing a rate of NE release so high that a regulated synthesis process cannot be maintained by the organism. NE levels remain low, because the released NE is metabolized by the enzyme MAO (presumably intraneurally after reuptake) (Weiss et al., 1979). In order to prevent NE depletion, Weiss et al. (1979) gave subjects a dose of MAO inhibitor. Animals given the drug before exposure to inescapable shock subsequently performed the avoidance-escape task as well as did the nonshock control subjects. The inhibitor thus eliminated the behavioral deficit due to inescapable shock, which lends strength to the suggestion that the behavioral deficit was, indeed, a result of neurochemical changes, primarily norepinephrine depletion, as suggested in Weiss et al. (1979).

To some extent, these results can be generalized to humans. Van der Kolk, Greenberger, Boyd, & Krystal (1985) have hypothesized that the behavioral consequences of unavoidable shock in animals are paralleled by those seen in patients who have been exposed to massive psychic trauma, specifically patients who are diagnosed according to the *DSM–III* criteria as having post-traumatic stress disorder (PTSD).

In brief, these investigators provide evidence arguing that the overall behavioral constriction manifested in lack of motivation and diminished occupational performance seen in PTSD patients is associated with NE depletion secondary to unavoidable trauma, the same effect that is seen in animals subjected to trauma during the learned helplessness facsimile. They further postulate that the hyperreactivity observed in these patients can be attributed to a "chronic adrenergic hypersensitivity following transient catecholamine depletion from acute trauma" (Van der Kolk et al., 1985, p. 317). (See Tables 9.2 and 9.3.) Whether or not the effects of behavioral disorganization in the infant are sufficiently traumatizing to allow a parallel to be drawn between this phenomenon and inescapable shock is unknown. However, the study of avoidance in the infant in relation to neurotransmitters certainly seems warranted as a potential means to detect and treat a highly probable pathway to depression.

In another study (Reus, Peeke, & Miner, 1985), researchers were able to correlate positive responses on the dexamethasone suppression test in depressed patients with impaired ability to distinguish between familiar and novel stimuli. The very defects highlighted in the study are similar to the defects observed in subjects exposed to a learned helplessness sit-

TABLE 9.2. Hormones related to separation reactions.

Hormone	Reference
Norepinephrine	Kalin & Carnes (1984); McKinney (1977)
Dopamine	Kalin & Carnes (1984); McKinney (1977)
Cortisol	Kalin & Carnes (1984); Gunnar et al. (1981); Levine et al. (1978); Vogt & Levine (1980);

Note. Unless otherwise noted, studies found relationship of neurotransmitters/hormones and separation experiences in nonhuman primates.

TABLE 9.3. Examples of hormonal dysregulation in depression.

Hormone	Reference
All Hormones	Carroll (1981); Dörner (1983)[a]
Serotonin	Åsberg et al. (1976)[b]; Åsberg, Thoren, & Traskman (1976); Birkmayer & Riederer (1975); Depue & Evans (1981)[c] Goodwin & Bunney (1973); Kelley & Stinus (1984); van Praag & de Haan (1980)
Cortisol	Baldessarini, (1983); Carroll (1978); Carroll et al. (1975, 1981); Fang et al. (1981); Ferguson et al. (1964); Gibbons & Fahy (1966); Puig-Antich et al. (1979, 1984); Prange et al. (1977); Sachar (1976); Sachar et al. (1970, 1971, 1973, 1980)
Norepinephrine	Bond et al. (1972)[i]; Bunney et al. (1971, 1972)[e]; Depue & Evans (1981)[f]; Goodwin & Bunney (1973)[g]; Lingjaerde (1983); Maas et al. (1971); Schildkraut (1970)
Dopamine	Bunney et al. (1971, 1972)[e]; Garver & Davis (1979); Sjöström & Roos (1972)
Growth hormone	Puig-Antich et al. (1981, 1984); Sachar et al. (1980)
Acetylcholine	Janowski et al. (1972, 1974)
MHPG	Baldessarini (1983)[j]; Bond et al. (1972)[d]; Bunney et al. (1972)[j]; Maas et al. (1968, 1971, 1973); Schatzberg et al. (1982); Schildkraut (1978)[j]

[a]Dysregulation of hormones due either to genetic flaw or environment may lead to permanent, stable effects.
[b]Dysregulation of serotonin characterized distinct subgroup of depressives.
[c]Concluded serotonin underlies regulation of sleep patterns and affective behaviors.
[d]Increase of noradrenaline in mania and decrease in depression.
[e]Norepinephrine and dopamine increased prior to "switch process" from depression to mania.
[f] NE underlies regulatory function for anorexia, dejected mood, sleep disturbances, and reward system.
[g]NE levels generally decreased by stress.
[h]Fall in urinary MHPG in depression and return to normal levels in recovery and/or mania.
[i]Fall in urinary MHPG in depression and higher than normal levels in mania.
[j]Urinary MHPG indicated three subgroups of unipolar depressives.

uation. It is not, at this juncture, possible to comment on whether the cognitive and affective deficits manifested by learned helplessness subjects are caused by an endocrine dysfunction, whether the experience of learned helplessness precipitates a defect in the hypothalamic-pituitary-adrenal axis, or whether both phenomena exist concurrently as part of a larger etiological framework for depressive pathology. Nevertheless, it is clear from all of the above mentioned studies that neuroendocrinological defects, whether they are in the form of norepinephrine depletion or excess levels of cortisol, are frequently present in patients with clinical learned helplessness.

Feasibility of Neurochemical Diagnostic Criteria

The possibility for developing neurochemical diagnostic criteria for depression in the infant certainly seems to exist. Except for relatively few brain stem nuclei, monoamine neurons comprise some of the earliest forming neuronal populations within the brain (Lauder, 1983). Considerable evidence also indicates that the hypothalamic-pituitary-adrenal axis is functionally reactive to the environment at or shortly after the time of birth (Anders et al., 1970; Anders & Zeanah, 1984; Gunnar et al., 1985; Gunnar, Fisch, & Malone, 1984; 1985; Meyer-Bahlberg, 1984; Talbert, 1975).

Furthermore, *in vitro* studies indicate that even during fetal life the hypothalamic-pituitary-adrenal axis can respond to stress-induced ACTH release and can secrete steroid precursors of sex hormones (Yanaihara & Arai, 1981). During delivery, the anterior pituitary of the fetus secretes increasing amounts of ACTH as delivery progresses. Arai, Yanaihara, and Okinaga (1976) postulate that the fetal adrenal axis is active during the delivery process and during the change from intrauterine to extrauterine life. Other studies indicate that during fetal life, the chromaffin tissue of the adrenal glands responds to the stress of hypoxia by releasing catecholamines, especially norepinephrine, into the fetal circulation. This causes alpha-receptor stimulation and peripheral vasoconstriction, resulting in increased perfusion of the fetal heart and brain and, necessarily, a decreased perfusion of the other, less vital fetal organs (Behrman, Lees, Peterson, DeLannoy, & Seeds, 1970; Campbell, Dawes, Fishman, & Hyman, 1967; Cohn et al., 1974; Goodwin, 1976; Meschia, 1978; Phillippe, 1983; Sheldon, Peeters, Jones, Makowski, & Meschina, 1979).

Greenberg and Gardener (1960) examined the ability of neonates to respond to insulin-induced hypoglycemia. In a group of seven male infants in the first week of life, the application of 0.3 U/k of regular insulin intramuscularly, resulted not only in a more than 20 mg/dl reduction of blood glucose, but in a rise of urinary epinephrine excretion, from 0.086 to 0.66 ng/kg/min. These results are consistent with the catecholamine responses to hypoglycemia in human adults (Christenson, Alberti, & Brandsborg, 1975; Phillippe, 1983).

Another significant finding is that elevations in serum cortisol have been correlated with behavioral distress or crying in the neonate (Anders et al., 1970; Tennes & Carter, 1973). The correspondence between adrenocortical activity and crying implies that factors that reduce crying might also reduce the degree of hormonal stress response in infants.

To test the above hypothesis, Gunnar et al. (1984) performed circumcisions on 18 healthy male newborns, two to five days old. Half were randomly assigned to a group that was encouraged to suck on a pacifier during the procedure, while the other half served as no-pacifier controls. Blood samples for cortisol were taken immediately before circumcision and 30 minutes later. Behavioral observations were made for 30 minutes before, during, and after circumcision. The experimental group showed a reduction in crying of about 40% induced by the pacifier. However, serum levels of cortisol after the procedure did not differ between groups. Members of both groups showed marked elevations in serum cortisol 30 minutes after the beginning of circumcision. Cortisol levels prior to the procedure did not differ between groups.

These findings strongly favor the contention that measures of adreno-cortical activity can be used to detect variations in response to stressful events in neonates. In fact, in this experiment, such measures provided information regarding the infant's response to stress, which was not de-tectable by behavioral means. Thus, observation of both behavioral and adrenocortical responses appears to be a valuable way of examining stress and coping mechanisms in the neonate (Gunnar et al., 1984).

Circumcision, performed without anesthesia, provides a valuable aver-sive experience for studying stress in neonates. Gunnar et al. (1985) sought to determine the time course of circulating cortisol following circumcision and also investigated whether behavioral changes paralleled the adreno-cortical time course in a predictable fashion. Eighty healthy newborns, age two to three days old were observed for 30 minutes prior to heel stick blood sampling to determine baseline cortisol levels. Circumcision without anesthesia was then performed and the infants were assigned to one of four treatment groups wherein blood sampling was performed 30, 90, 120, and 240 minutes after the start of circumcision. The behavioral state of each infant was observed during the procedure and for 30 minutes fol-lowing. Behaviorally, the newborns responded to the combined circum-cision and blood sampling with short-lived but intense distress. There was a marked increase in cortisol production in response to the stress, but this increase normalized by 150–250 minutes following the procedure.

This study and others of its kind illustrate the remarkable coping capacity of the newborn. Not only is the healthy neonate capable of undergoing minor surgery, but only a few minutes following surgery, the infant is able to feed and interact normally with the mother (Gunnar et al., 1985).

Attachment

The great value of being able to intervene therapeutically at an early de-velopmental stage is illustrated dramatically in the nature and dynamics of infant attachment. Attachment behavior is regarded as a class of be-havior that is as socially important as the behaviors of mating and parenting (Bowlby, 1969). The parent provides regulation of the infant's behavioral, neurochemical, autonomic, and hormonal functions through various as-pects of the relationship including nutrition, affection, sensory stimulation, and rhythmic responsiveness (Anders & Zeanah, 1984; Papousek & Pa-pousek, 1984).

Secure attachment to the caregiver has been shown to be positively related to self-esteem, curiosity, exploration, independence, coping with novelty and failure, and peer competence (Arend, Gove, & Sroufe, 1979; Lewis, Feiring, McGuffog, & Jaskir, 1984; Londerville & Main, 1981; Matas, Arend, & Sroufe, 1978; Waters, Whippman, & Sroufe, 1979). Sep-aration from the caregiver results in a profound grief reaction characterized by many negative shifts in physiological function. In fact, stable attachment bonds are vitally important for adequate neurobiological development in the infant and in all social animals (Bakwin, 1949; Kalin & Carnes, 1984; Spitz & Wolf, 1946). Among the biological alterations noted to occur upon a traumatic separation are negative changes in sleep patterns, immune function, monoamine systems, heart rate, body temperature, and endocrine function (Kalin & Carnes, 1984).

During the first year of life, the ontogeny of behavioral systems is slow and development varies greatly from child to child (Rothbart & Derryberry, 1981). But, by the beginning of the second year, the attachment bond is strong in most infants, and they will react with great distress to separation from the caregiver (Bowlby, 1969).

The results of a study by Matas et al. (1978) illustrate the developmental importance of the quality of attachment. The relationship between quality of attachment in infancy—the organization of attachment behavior—and quality of play and problem solving at two years of age was examined in 48 infants. Infants who were judged to be securely attached at 18 months were observed to be more cooperative, persistent, and enthusiastic than those infants who were more insecurely attached. Thus, secure attachment apparently enhances the individual's later ability to cope with the environment. Infants and children separated from their parents and placed in a nonsupportive environment often show severe psychological manifestations of stress (Bowlby, 1960; Spitz & Wolf, 1946; Spitz & Wolf, 1949). Bowlby describes the syndrome that follows separation as characterized by a sequential pattern of responses. In the first, or protest phase, the child is acutely distressed. The despair phase follows in a matter of days, and the infant becomes increasingly withdrawn and inactive (Bowlby, 1960). In *DSM–III* (American Psychiatric Association, 1980), the disruption of attachment bonds is associated with the development of infant reactive attachment disorder, separation anxiety disorder, bereavement, and major depressive disorder.

Aspects of the reaction to separation from the caregiver provide an excellent paradigm for depression and depressive-like phenomena in infants. Psychoendocrine correlates in one year old infants separated from their mothers for one hour have been reported to be in line with the results seen in highly emotional versus more reserved adults. That is, infants who exhibited marked distress upon departure of the mother secreted increased amounts of cortisol, just as do adults when they are confronted with psychological stress (Bliss et al., 1956; Tennes & Mason, 1982).

The researchers reported a "modest" but nevertheless consistent linear association between levels of cortisol excretion and the infant's manifest anxiety. It was discovered, therefore, that infants who displayed the most distress and who remained in an agitated state throughout the period of maternal absence excreted the highest levels of cortisol. Infants who protested their caregivers' departure briefly and displayed little manifest anxiety excreted cortisol in significantly lower levels. Finally, a third type of infant response was observed. These infants were initially distressed at the caregivers' departure, but subsequently became withdrawn and in-active, retreating from social contact. Measurements revealed significantly lower levels of cortisol in this group than in either the mildly distressed or agitated infants. The researchers hypothesized that such infants might subsequently mature into adults who used defense mechanisms effectively to maintain low levels of corticosteroids.

The investigators tied their findings to a report by Ainsworth (1979) in which the latter researcher found that infants of one year who were responsive to caregiver reunion after separation (as manifested by high pleasure at the caregiver return) had high levels of cortisol. Infants who evinced an "ambivalent" response at caregiver return excreted moderate cortisol levels. Lastly, a group of infants who avoided the caregiver on return (analogous to the infants in the Tennes and Mason study who with-drew from social contact) were the lowest excretors of cortisol.

These findings raise several questions. Perhaps the most seminal issues remain the extent to which caregiver interaction affects the infant's hor-monal response pattern and the degree to which the infant's constitu-tionally determined capacity (temperament) to regulate his or her endocrine system impacts on the relationship with the caregiver. Although these questions have yet to be answered, the data from Tennes and Mason (1982) and Ainsworth (1979) indicate that the association between attachment behaviors and endocrine function in infants merits further attention.

The hypothesis that the nonemotive infants may have been serotonin deprived and therefore vulnerable to stress receives support from the fact that the antidepressant imipramine, which selectively blocks serotonin reuptake, has been found to significantly improve despair responses in infant rhesus monkeys (Kalin & Carnes, 1984). Moreover, neuroendocrine abnormalities of the hypothalamic-pituitary-adrenal axis have also been identified in these infant primates. Thus, it was found that four days after peer separation, some juvenile rhesus monkeys failed to suppress plasma cortisol concentrations normally after dexamethasone administration. Significantly, 4 of the 11 monkeys in the study had originally tested as being dexamethasone suppressors while they had been housed with their peers. Following separation, these 4 monkeys manifested a nonsuppressor response on the DST. This finding is highly pertinent in that it suggests that a stress-related external event may precipitate an abnormal neu-roendocrinological response. If such a finding can be analogized to human infants, some light may be shed on one of the vital issues raised in this chapter. That is, the Kalin and Carnes data suggest that separation or a severance of the attachment bond may trigger or cause a defect in the neuroendocrine regulation.

The large number of opiate receptor binding sites in the limbic system and the fact that endogenous opioids are released during stressful situations clearly illustrate the importance of these substances with regard to de-pressive states (Akil, Madden, Patrick & Barchas, 1976; Amir & Amit,

1978; Csontos et al., 1979). Willer et al. (1979) have proposed a mechanism for the release of opiates that in some ways resembles the one governing secretion of cortisol. This proposal maintains that under normal conditions, the opiate-containing neurons are tonically inactive. In this paradigm, opiates are released only under stressful, novel, or aversive conditions.

Herman and Panksepp (1978) studied the effects of morphine and naloxone on separation distress and approach attachment and found that distress at separation was alleviated by morphine and potentiated by naloxone. They concluded that their data supported the idea that an endorphin-based process similar to addiction may underlie the maintenance of social attachments, implying that separation distress may reflect a condition of endogenous opiate withdrawal. Avoidance has been associated with endorphin levels in rats (Bugnon, Block, Lenys, & Fellmann, 1970).

The value of studying attachment is clear. An interruption of this bond gives rise to a defined behavioral syndrome that has been associated with a number of neuroendocrine correlates, including elevated levels of cortisol and diminished levels of endogenous opioids. Additionally, an increased level of serotonin apparently reduces the despair response, at least in infant rhesus monkeys (Kalin & Carnes, 1984). Further study of the interplay as well as the separate actions of serotonin, cortisol, and the endogenous opiates will undoubtedly prove rewarding and may advance most rapidly if observed in connection with the attachment bond. At the most optimistic level, study of the interplay between the dynamics of attachment bonding and developmental endocrinology may eventually provide a means of diagnosing vulnerability to stress that, if corrected in infancy, might interrupt the formation of a depressive disorder.

Conclusion

Of the factors whose interaction can result in depression (genetic predisposition, reactivity to stress, compromised developmental milestones, and psychosocial and physiological stressors) reactivity to stress is perhaps among the most important to the study of developmental endocrinology, both in terms of producing depression and because it has neurochemical correlates that can be measured. Neurochemically, the reaction to stress can be measured by many means, primarily the production of cortisol, norepinephrine, serotonin, and dopamine.

The construct of temperament, as outlined by Rothbart and Derryberry (1981, 1982) is useful in uncovering the developmental correlates of reactivity. Their theory is based on hierarchical levels of control—the same principle of organization seen in neurochemical functioning—and has reactivity as a central component. A merging of this temperament model with what is known about the neuroendocrine correlates of depression would seem to present an ideal strategy to employ in the attempt to define the developmental underpinnings of the depressive state.

At this time, unfortunately, few temperament measurement instruments have proved sufficiently sophisticated to show long-term predictive validity from early infant measurements. To date, the attachment model has proved more fruitful in this regard. The phenomena of attachment and the depressive-like syndrome that follows its premature interruption may prove to be among the most useful infant behaviors for investigators of depression.

This approach is experimentally sound as well, since there is now little doubt that the infant's limbic system is active from birth and capable of responding adequately to trauma shortly, if not immediately, thereafter. The value of studying the elements of attachment in conjunction with psychoendocrine measures is illustrated by the emergence of data implicating serotonin as central to the dynamics of this bond. There is a strong consensus that serotonin depression exists and that subnormal levels of serotonin may predispose an individual to depression. It is also known that serotonin plays an early role as a modulator in neonatal inhibitory maturation and that it is a primary regulator of cortisol. Thus, serotonin is not only crucially involved in the ontogeny of temperament, but adequate production of this indoleamine hypothetically causes proper secretion of cortisol in response to environmental stress. This in turn allows for adequate coping behavior, thus reducing the risk of the development of a depressive condition.

The fact that affective states are improved in infant rhesus monkeys in the presence of an excess of serotonin is significant. Furthermore, the data showing that secure attachment enhances the infant's later ability to cope, thus lowering the likelihood of later depression, are very interesting in light of serotonin's observed role as a protection against depression. It seems clear that studies of the dynamics of the attachment bond and the behaviors that result from its premature severance are proving invaluable for the task of unraveling the early neurochemical correlates of depression.

Within the context of the attachment model, the elements of temperament can be used as parameters to quantify early behavioral correlates of depression that may then be linked to maturational endocrine events. This multifactorial approach may provide the means not only of preventing many primary forms of depression, but of eliminating the later formation of the inimical positive feedback dynamic in which depressive feelings or traumatic life events produce depressive behavior, which ultimately generates a more profound sense of depression.

CHAPTER 10

Clinical Paradigm

The preceding chapters propose a new perspective for analyzing infant behavioral disorganization, particularly aberrant behavior suggestive of depression and depressive-like phenomena. Developmental psychopathology provides a convenient framework within which to view the nuances of chronological change occurring during infancy. Using the developmental model, a diagnostic approach is offered, from which prospective predictions about infant behavioral abnormalities can be derived. Moreover, as is noted, applying the developmental model also permits researchers to unravel retrospectively the etiologies of a depression manifesting in childhood that may have its roots in the experiences of early infancy.

The specific variables of development that are most useful for tracing the evolution of, or predicting, depression, include *temperament, attachment, self, object-representation,* and *empathy.* Each of these early developmental milestones, discussed through documented data, is correlated with specific behavioral manifestations. These behaviors are analyzed both in terms of normal displays and as deviant manifestations raising challenges to be resolved before the infant-caregiver dyad can progress to a more mature phase of development.

Pathogenic origins of deviant behavior are further explored by focusing on face-to-face interaction studies, studies of learned helplessness in children and infants, and patterns of infant neuroendocrinological mechanisms. Implicit in these latter discussions is the notion of an essential bifurcation of development. That is, normal developmental patterns are discussed and are juxtaposed against configurations indicative of abnormality or psychopathology. Armed with this composite spectrum of infant and early childhood behavioral manifestations, it is now appropriate to apply the developmental model specifically to the area of childhood and infant depression.

Models of Childhood Depression

The concept that depression in infancy and childhood exists as a discrete clinical entity is still in the early stages of clarification. In studying this phenomenon, the investigator is initially confronted with the perplexity of articulating a specific operational definition for depression arising in those early age groups.

Over the past thirty years there have been remarkable changes in attitude and approach to the question of infant and childhood depression. Four primary schools of thought can be identified in the effort to establish an operational model for the study of depressive-like phenomena occurring in infancy and childhood. The theoretical foundations of these four schools run the gamut from total rejection of the notion that children can experience depression in childhood to the espousal of childhood depression as a disorder comparable to that found in adults. In addition, when grappling with the concept of adult depression, researchers have had to account for the developmental factor—making the formulation of a precise definition even more problematic.

The Developmental Symptomatology Argument

The first clearly delineated explanation of childhood depression adopted the view that depression, as a syndrome analogous to that existing in adults, does not occur in childhood (Rie, 1966; Rochlin, 1959). It is somewhat surprising that Spitz and Wolf's (1946) findings of widespread institutionalized infants a decade earlier were minimized, at best, by this school of thought. At most, according to this school of thought, symptomatology resembling depressive-like phenomena, as defined based on adult criteria, was perceived as a manifestation of a specific developmental stage, rather than as a particular indication of pathology. Indeed, the theoretical formulations of psychoanalysts such as Mahler (Mahler, Pine & Bergman, 1975) posit a naturally occuring depressive period in early life.

This argument, referred to as the Developmental Psychoanalytic Theory, was buttressed by findings from an epidemiological study conducted by Lapouse in 1966. Examining 482 randomly selected children, ranging in age from six to 12 years, the researcher reported that various forms of behavior commonly classified under the rubric of depression were markedly widespread. Lapouse was skeptical about this high prevalence of symptomatic behavior and suggested that these behavioral manifestations might, in actuality, be indicative of normal developmental phenomena, rather than of psychiatric disorder.

Despite the superficial appeal of Lapouse's argument, two major problems are inherent in the developmental symptomatology approach. First, the, "symptomatology" is so loosely defined that the risk of overinclusive diagnosis is presented. More important is the fact that merely because symptoms are transient and recede over time does *not* mean that they are clinically insignificant. Indeed, one of the major premises of the developmental psychopathology approach advocated in the preceding chapters is that the mechanisms of development occur over a chronological period. A behavioral manifestation associated with an early phase of development may recede as another type of behavioral organization rises to prominence. But the disappearance of one "symptom" does not mean that the underlying conflict has been resolved. Rather, the conflict may merely be submerged and overshadowed by developmental achievement in other areas. Thus, as discussed in Chapter 8, the ability to moderate discrepancies and derive pleasure from perceived contingencies may not obliterate an experience of disrupted contingency that occurred earlier, nor is the negative affect associated with the non-contingent experience or extreme discrepancies necessarily erased from evocative memory. The developmental symptomatology approach, therefore, has failed to account for the potential repercussive effect of depressive-like phenomena.

The "Depressive Equivalents" Argument

The second approach for defining childhood depressive-like phenomena conceived of depression as an entity unto itself and posited that the overt manifestations of this syndrome were *not* identical to the adult model (Cytryn & McKnew, 1974; Glaser, 1968; Renshaw, 1974; Toolan, 1962). According to this school, children were assigned a diagnosis of depression because of a wide variety of behavioral problems, even if no clear dysphoria or mood changes were apparent. Among the behaviors encompassed by this approach and included as indicative of childhood depression were aggression, hyperactivity, enuresis, sleeping and eating disturbances, and miscellaneous somatic complaints, all thought to be signals of an underlying yet "unseen" depressive disorder. Clusters of these symptoms were labeled *masked depressions* or *depressive equivalents*.

Several problems arose in establishing the validity of the depressive equivalents argument. For example, the various classifications used relied, at times, on contradictory diagnostic criteria. Often the criteria necessary for distinguishing a child whose aggression "masked" genuine depression from one whose aggression was symptomatic of another psychiatric disorder were not articulated, or if the criteria were voiced, they were not reliable enough for use in validation studies (Cytryn & McKnew, 1974). Hence, when the masked depression or depressive equivalency theory was used to formulate a diagnosis, childhood depression on occasion appeared as a ubiquitous phenomenon.

Nevertheless, the depressive equivalent school had the advantage of according childhood depression legitimacy in its own right, as a clinical entity distinct from adult depression. Criticism, however, may be leveled at the model for several reasons. First, no cohesive theoretical formulations are offered to explain the depressive equivalent symptomatology. It is not sufficient to observe that because eating and sleeping disorders coupled with aggression are considered part of a syndrome of depression in adults, similar symptom patterns in children are indicative of depression. The depressive equivalent or "masked" depression school, in other words, neglects to reveal what lies behind the "mask." Moreover, the depressive equivalent model ignores the factor of development in analyzing childhood depression. As argued earlier, only by using a developmental model that traces the appearance of normal behavioral manifestations through an organized chronological sequence can a researcher pinpoint deviations of development and their corresponding etiologies.

The Epidemiological Approach

The epidemiological approach, the third major school of thought on childhood depression, accepts the concept that depression exists as a distinct clinical entity during childhood (Albert & Beck, 1975; Arajarvi & Huttunen, 1972; Kashani, Barbero, & Bolander, 1981; Ling, Oftedal, & Weinberg, 1970; McConville, Boag, & Purohit, 1973; Poznanski & Zrull, 1970; Weinberg, Rutman, Sullivan, Penick, & Dietz, 1973). Problems with this approach have centered on the methodology pursued. This approach relies predominantly on epidemiological studies which may offer an uneven portrait of the syndrome of childhood depression, both in terms of diagnosis and prevalence. A prime reason for the inconsistent results gleaned from these epidemiological studies has been the use of subjective, non-standardized criteria for the diagnosis of depression.

Compounding the problem of an inexact operational definition is the fact that some epidemiological studies focus on "major" depression and do not consider "minor" depressive-like phenomena. Other difficulties arise due to the age differences and heterogencity of the population sampled, e.g., outpatients, children in residential nurseries, medical mixed with general populations, etc. With such a wide variety in the sample, disparities are almost inevitable. Finally, the epidemiological model seeks to isolate a single factor that provides a necessary and sufficient explanation for childhood depression. This concentration on a unifactorial approach has been supplanted in psychiatric research by multifactorial models of causation. It should be stressed that one of the key advantages of the developmental approach advocated in the preceding chapters is its ability to encompass a full spectrum of data derived from such diverse areas as neuroendocrinology, research in maternal–infant interaction, and traditional psychiatric theory. Thus, the epidemiological approach, which stresses a more parochial view, is ultimately incapable of explaining and integrating the broad spectrum of data now available on infant behavior.

Despite the drawbacks of the model, it should be noted that methodology borrowed from the epidemiological model has often proved helpful in contributing to an organized theory of infant and childhood depression. For example, the New York Longitudinal Study (Chess & Thomas, 1985) utilized research methods to isolate the impact of temperament on subsequent pathology in infancy and childhood.

Adult Model Approach: *DSM–III*

Finally, the fourth school of thought addressing the issue of childhood depression is the model most prevalently used today. Labeled the Adult Model approach, this school theorizes that childhood depression is fully analogous to adult depression and can be studied in the same way through a multifactorial approach. As an investigative strategy, this school starts with the known, an understanding of depression in adulthood. The hypothesis of the Adult Model is that if it is possible to delineate and measure depressive syndromes in adults, it is possible to do the same with children.

In 1973, the pioneers of this approach, W.A. Weinberg and associates, modified and adapted the Feighner Adult Diagnostic Criteria (Feighner et al., 1972) for use with children. Using these criteria they diagnosed childhood depression in 42 of 72 children, six to 12 years of age, who were referred to an educational diagnostic center. Investigators for the development of *DSM–III* recognized Weinberg et al.'s achievement in this area and formulated one unified set of criteria to be used for both adults and children. *DSM–III*, as it was developed by the American Psychiatric Association in 1980, employs a multifactorial approach and is currently the instrument used to diagnose depression in childhood. For example, in articulating features of major depressive episodes, the *DSM–III* notes that such episodes may begin at any age including infancy, and that age of onset is fairly evenly distributed throughout adult life.

In addition, some of the phenomenological and developmental experiences of the child can be effectively integrated into diagnosis and treatment by utilizing Axis IV (psychosocial stressors) and Axis V (level of adaptive functioning) of *DSM–III*. This synthesis allows the clinician to differentiate the way in which developmental adaptation takes place in the face of challenge (e.g., psychosocial stressor) and helps to qualify expected (i.e., congruent) or unexpected (i.e., incongruent) emotional responses during a specific developmental epoch within the life of the child. For example, how does the stranger anxiety phenomenon (congruent at eight months) influence the experience and manifestations of infant depression? How does the "low keyed" behavior of the rapprochement subphase of the separation-individuation model (congruent at 15 months) color the expression of a full depressive episode? By utilizing all the elements of the diagnostic criteria articulated in *DSM–III*, pathological and nonpathological manifestations of the child may be clearly delineated.

DSM–III may also serve as a useful tool for diagnosing infant and childhood depression inferentially, by focusing on populations with a clinically depressed caregiver. In 1979, Phillips demonstrated the dynamic relationship between disabilities and/or depression in parents (*DSM–III* diagnosed) and subsequent manifestations of depression in their children. The predominant response to caregiver depression was passive or active depression (also fulfilling *DSM–III* criteria), and the child's response to caregiver disability was outwardly directed aggression or passivity along with withdrawal.

Nevertheless, although the specific criteria for childhood depression offered by *DSM–III* provides the clinician with a convenient model for diagnosis, by fusing the criteria of adult and childhood symptomatology, *DSM–III* fails to give sufficient emphasis to the developmental framework. As pointed out in Chapter 1, and as Bemporad and Rathbun (1982) have noted, the developmental framework is crucial to articulating accurate criteria of childhood depression, because it considers how the child's abilities and limitations, at each developmental stage, impose their characteristic stamp on affect, dysphoria, and symptom complexes. *DSM–III*'s advocacy of adult models applied to child psychiatry has been challenged for allegedly not taking into account the effect of developmental changes on symptoms throughout childhood and early adolescence. Although there is empirical evidence that the symptoms and features of childhood depression are similar to those of adult depression, a widely held consensus also exists that infantile experiences are likely to influence the individual's predisposition to depressive–like symptomatology at a later age (Katz, 1979). The implications of the face-to-face interaction, neuroendocrinological, and learned helplessness studies of the past decade suggest that *DSM–III* criteria for depression in children may be incomplete

Although *DSM–III* states that there may be features associated with depression that are age specific, these are not yet part of the diagnostic criteria (Cantwell, 1983a,1983b). It is not difficult to understand why *DSM–III* has had difficulty explicitly designing age-specific criteria. Even depressive affect, for example, one of the major features associated with depressive symptomatology, can be diagnostically problematic when dealing with infants and children who either cannot yet verbalize their feelings or who may be in the throes of normal developmental transition.

Part of the problem of identifying the cause of age-related symptomatology may be attributed to the shortage of studies describing changes in the nature of self-understanding during development (Brim, 1976). In addition, psychological research on the development of self-concept has been largely limited to assessing self-esteem in children (Damon & Hart, 1982). Hypothetically, self-esteem can be quantified along a scale of feelings from positive to negative, and theorists have attempted to do so because of the presumed impact of self-esteem on the social relations and general mental viability of children. However, this approach has not met with a great deal of success. Studies correlating self-esteem to interpersonal relations, achievement, and other factors have not yielded compelling results (Wylie, 1979).

A more concrete example of the elusive nature of the age-specific features in depression is revealed in Cantwell's (1983b) summary of Puig-Antich's extensive work with biological markers for depression. Cantwell (1983a, 1983b, 1983c) noted that approximately 50% of melancholic subtype adults with major depressive disorder display hypersecretion of cortisol during the acute phase of their illness. However, when children and adults with major depressive disorder of the melancholic subtype are compared, only about half as many children as adults are found to hypersecrete cortisol. As Cantwell notes, the reason for this finding may be that cortisol production is a developmental phenomenon linked to chronological age. In addition, levels of cortisol production may be temperamentally determined, meaning that certain children are individually predisposed to produce higher levels of the hormone than other children. These considerations illustrate the difficulty in accurately defining age-specific features associated with depression in children, and they help to explain why the DSM–III formulation may not offer a comprehensive listing of the diagnostic criteria for depression in children.

For purposes of validity, then, any studies attempting to prove or disprove the relationships between infant behavioral manifestations and adult symptomatology must do so within a framework that takes into consideration the heterogeneous nature of the depressive condition. It is also necessary to quantify the degree to which depressive symptomatology in the adult is related to the original developmental process, although applying a developmental framework may itself raise new problems in arriving at precise diagnostic criteria for infant and childhood depression.

These factors led Kovacs and Paulauskas (1984) to propose that novel conceptual strategies may be needed in order to discern the dynamics of developmental psychopathology. In their sample of 80 school age depressed children (eight to 13 years), the authors found the less developmentally mature children suffered the most chronic depressions and, during major depressive episodes, required more time to recover than the more developmentally mature children.

A study of depression in female children by Garber (1984) yielded more predictable results. In this trial with 137 girls between the ages of seven and 13, Garber found an increase in the frequency of depressive symptoms with increasing age. Nevertheless, the researcher noted that within the developmental context, there are a number of possible explanations for these findings, including hormonal changes associated with puberty, genetic factors, frequency of environmental stressors, and the possible presence of the cognitive set associated with learned helplessness.

As another example of the complexity involved in developmental research, Freeman, Poznanski, Grossman, Buschbaum, and Banegas (1985) recently reported on six children between six and 12 years of age who were diagnosed as both psychotic and depressed. Evaluation of the study subjects was comprised of semistructured parent and child interviews, the Schedule for Affective Disorders and Schizophrenia for School Aged Children (K-SADS), and the Children's Depression Rating Scale—Revised (CDRS-R). Dexamethasone suppression tests were given to five of the six children; of these four showed positive results. The six children with psychotic features met *DSM–III* and Research Diagnostic Criteria (RDC) for depression. Longitudinally, the children were given repeat CDRS-R at two weeks, six months, one year, and two years, as well as repeated K-SADS after one and two years. The six children with psychotic features (hallucinations and/or delusions) comprised nearly one fifth (18.2%) of the depressed sample. The authors concluded that since this group has only recently been described and longitudinal studies are limited, it is not yet feasible to arrive at an appropriate diagnostic classification for psychotic depressed children. However, this study may represent an example of how *DSM–III* criteria, coupled with alternative techniques that embody a developmental approach, may yield data on previously unrecognized forms of child and infant depression.

In summary, the *DSM–III* model, which utilizes the same diagnostic criteria for both adult and childhood depression, has permitted researchers to identify specific types of depressive disorders in children. The short-comings of the *DSM–III* model become glaringly apparent, however, when the developmental psychopathology model is applied. Tracing development through the evolution of various chronological milestones—such as temperament, attachment, self-object representation, and empathy—facilitates the recognition of aberrant behavioral manifestations that are distinct to children and infants. In addition, integrating neuroendocrinological data into the developmental model alerts researchers to an underlying layer of biochemical events that may correlate with overt affective manifestations. The flexibility of the developmental paradigm also enables application of such theories as Learned Helplessness to infant and childhood behavior. Thus, the eclecticism inherent in the Developmental Psychopathology Paradigm ultimately allows the researcher to incorporate a broad spectrum of behavioral data into a coherent framework that permits correlations between adult and childhood psychopathology, but that, at the same time, acknowledges the unique experiences of the infant and the young child.

Case Report

George was an infant placed in a residential nursery at eight days of age. He immediately seized the attention of the caregivers because he was fussier than the other newborns, cried for attention, seemed to want to be cuddled, and often emitted what was described as an "angry cry" if he was denied contact. These traits were stable, enduring throughout the time George was in the nursery. Additionally, by four months of age, George exhibited a pronounced long-lasting social smile.

At eight months of age, George displayed the classic signs of stranger anxiety. This was considered atypical, since nursery children generally do not have the experience of forming a single caregiver bond, the prerequisite for developing later anxiety manifestations in the presence of a stranger. Moreover, one month later, at nine months of age, George displayed symptomatology of anaclitic depression, characterized by weeping, withdrawal, apathy, weight loss, sleep disturbance, and overall decline in developmental functioning.

This episode of depression was noteworthy in several respects. First, although George did not have a preexisting bond with a single mother surrogate, he did experience a multiplicity of concerned caregivers. Significantly, a quantitative reduction in caregiving behavior was directly correlated with the onset of depression. In addition, subsequent increase in caregiving behavior directed toward George facilitated his recovery from the depressive interlude. Finally, this initial anaclitic episode lasted for seven and one half months, when George was between nine and 17 months of age. Following his "recovery," George made quick strides in development. When adopted at 20 months, he was depicted as a curious, attractive, and sociable infant.

Nevertheless, during his preschool years, George experienced three major depressive episodes, each associated with separation from a primary maternal figure. Each episode began with agitated behavior and was followed by depressive symptomatology and subsequent apathy. Equally pertinent, each depression was punctuated with an outbreak of severe atopic dermatitis.

During his first adoption at 20 months, George adjusted well to his new home. His new mother, however, was hospitalized for a hysterectomy when George was 25 months old, and became clinically depressed following the operation. Eventually, finding that she could no longer "cope" with her adopted son, she relinquished George to the nursery when he was a little over two years old.

Upon return to the nursery, George exhibited signs of depression. He was found to have food allergies and a serious atopic dermatitis covering his entire body. In the winter of that year, he suffered severe bouts of measles, mumps, and chicken pox. However, a nursery caregiver took special interest in him, devoting much attention and time to the infant. The pair were often observed playing together. George recovered physically, and within a period of six months after the nurse had begun to care for him, he was once again an alert and sociable infant.

When he was three and one half, George was again adopted. His initial adjustment was difficult. At first he engaged in much rebellious or protest-like behavior. There were several incidents of fecal smearing and provocative disobedience toward his adoptive mother. After several weeks his behavior changed markedly, however. Now the child was observed staring off into space for long periods. He sat alone in the basement, rocking repetitively and twisting his fingers in writhing movements. Eventually these "down in the dumps" manifestations receded and George resumed an outgoing personality. But his dermatitis recurred intermittently, and he would occasionally cling to his mother. After several months, this second adoption was disrupted when George's mother accepted a full-time job. The pattern of rebelliousness followed by reclusive staring periods that had surfaced during the beginning of this adoption returned with increased intensity. Again George was returned to the nursery.

With this return, however, George re-established a relationship with the special caregiver he had known earlier. While he exhibited marked depressive symptomatology and his allergies had returned, these disturbances receded within a short time. George's caregiver was especially encouraging and supportive of him during this period, and she gradually recognized that much of the child's psychopathology and physical symptomatology occurred during her separation from him.

Throughout his childhood George remained in the orphanage and displayed signs of good adjustment. Disturbing symptoms periodically returned, though, when a situation threatening separation from his caregiver was presented. For example, George developed a transient school phobia and clung to his caregiver. Atopic dermatitis flared when he was sent to the orphanage's summer camp and removed from his caregiver during this period.

George entered therapy when he was seven and one half years old. The treatment, consisting primarily of psychoanalysis, explored issues of early object loss. At age 10, George was adopted yet again. This time, the adoption seemed to stick. Upon follow-up assessment of George and his new parents two and one half years later, George was evaluated as an energetic, well-adjusted child. Although a reflective, withdrawn side to his personality was revealed when George expressed hesitancy and denial in discussing his previous life in the orphanage and his earlier therapy, his peer relationships were good and he was reported as doing extremely well in school (Harmon, Wagonfeld, & Emde, 1982).

Maternal Deprivation

Among the variables that recur repeatedly in discussions of infant and childhood depression is maternal deprivation. It is one of the contentions of this book that maternal deprivation, whether as a consequence of a literal separation because of caregiver absence or as a result of inadequate caregiver responsiveness due to conditions such as maternal depression, significantly correlates with the outcome of infant behavioral organization. Neuroendocrinological changes, a product of stress, may resemble the hormonal fluctuations encountered in adult depressives. Indeed, as discussed previously, maternal behavior interacts with temperament dimensions, establishes the type of attachment bond formed within the dyad, transmits empathy to the infant, and is a guiding factor in the development of the infant's emerging sense of self and object representation. Moreover, maternal behaviors displayed during face-to-face encounters and during exposure of the infant to discrepancy and contingency relationships may lay the groundwork for normal adjustment or for the debilitating path to learned helplessness

Tronick, Rick, and Cohn (1982), for example, in their face-to-face studies comparing infant response during periods of normal maternal facial interaction with infant manifestations during periods of simulated depression, discerned two distinctive patterns of cycling. During periods of normal interaction, the researchers reported that infants tended to display a more flexible pattern of response, encompassing brief positive, monitoring, and play expressions. In contrast, when infants were subjected to simulated maternal depression, their overall patterning of behaviors was more rigid, with cycling occurring almost exclusively among negative states. Thus, overt depressed expressions dominated, along with gaze aversion and expressions typical of protest. Significantly, Tronick et al. noted that the infants tend to become absorbed in the cycle of negative affective states and that this absorption signifies some form of taxing the infant's regulatory capabilities.

Given this data, it is clear that during exposure to a discrete episode of maternal depression, albeit simulated in the clinical setting, the ability of infants to extricate themselves from the impact of negative affect is impaired. Depressive-like phenomena, in this case, are manifested as a form of affective impairment. However, since Tronick et al. emphasized particularly that infants in this condition have difficulty emerging from the cycle of negative affect, it may be suggested that, in some instances, the negative affect may have more lingering effects, and in some cases may transform into an enduring negative mood. That is, for infants of clinically depressed caregivers, the continual, sustained experience of negative affect may provoke an enduring negative mood in their infants. Moreover, in cases of maternal deprivation, where separation from the caregiver is prolonged rather than discrete, an initial negative affect experienced by the infant may have generalized into a perpetual state of depression, characterized by negative mood. In the latter cases, the negative mood has transferred across tasks and situations. This hypothesis is given further credence by the work of Lester, Hoffman, and Brazelton (1985), who confirm the existence of specific social rhythms, implicitly organized within a temporal structure, during infant-caregiver interaction. As a consequence of this temporal structure, the researchers inferred that the infant develops expectancies about future interaction which are introduced into each subsequent encounter. Spelke (1979) has also identified the phenomena of temporal synchrony. If, then, infants do develop temporal patterns, along with concomitant expectancies, it is not unusual that they may transfer these expectancies across situations, particularly if later situations are similar to earlier ones. The phenomenon of depression in infants who have experienced maternal deprivation, then, may represent one example of the manner in which what began as a negative affect is generalized into a mood pervasive enough to warrant the label of overt depression.

Prior to discussing the specific impact of maternal deprivation on infant behaviors indicative of depressive–like phenomena, it is worth noting that other infant-caregiver situations may also be particularly suited to precipitating a response suggestive of incipient depression. By employing a developmental framework, designed to trace infant maturation through the milestones of temperament, attachment, self and object representation, future investigations should focus on *populations at risk,* in which infant or child abuse, sexual abuse, or neglect has occurred. In addition, studies which probe the effects of long-term separation of caregiver and infant due to hospitalization, trials involving handicapped infants and children, and investigations of developmental phenomena in the offspring of emotionally ill parents, may provide further evidence to substantiate the genesis of depression. Thus, the following discussion highlights the impact of maternal separation on infant psychopathology as merely one scenario to which the developmental approach can be applied in a clinical setting, in order to discern the mechanisms triggering the onset of infant depressive disorders.

Broadly defined, maternal deprivation is an event or set of circumstances that result in lack of appropriate sensory, perceptual, reciprocal, and/or consistent interaction with the caregiver. Contact with the caregiver may be inadequate in quantity, intensity, and variability, or may not be based on contingent responsiveness. At the extreme end of the deprivation spectrum are those instances in which children have little or no contact with a human caregiver. Most of these examples are from the 19th century and involve so-called "feral children," who had been abandoned and left to live in the wild. Accounts of these children are of particular interest because, although the deprivation is quite extreme—indeed, complete— reports of such cases suggest that once returned to civilization these children did not appear to have exhibited any symptoms of depression. One might surmise from this observation that it is only through contact with caregivers that clinical depression emerges. However, these accounts may also suggest that in the absence of affective development, full-fledged depression does not occur (Squires, 1927; Zingg, 1940).

In contrast to these long-term cases of deprivation are studies in which temporary separation from caregivers (on the occasion of a birth of a sibling, family discord, or mother's inability to care properly for the child) serve to illustrate the first effects of maternal deprivation and to demonstrate how this phenomenon is related to the initial signs of depression. Unfortunately, scant prospective documentation of the consequences of deprivation exists. Instead, investigators generally work retrospectively with a depressed child to determine elements contributing to the illness, and whether or not deprivation was present at some early time. Another problem in the literature on maternal deprivation is the omission of descriptions of affective manifestations among maternally deprived infants and children. One explanation may be that many deprived children display little affect, but such a condition may well correspond to the detachment phase (Bowlby, Ainsworth, Boston, & Rosenbluth, 1965) following deprivation. As an example, a child who appears detached six months after being separated from the caregiver may have displayed more blatant signs of depression four months earlier. Thus, the long-term study of the maternally deprived child is highly desirable, with the understanding that not all children respond to maternal deprivation on a precise timetable.

Another problem in assessing the impact of maternal deprivation has been the difficulty of defining the concept. For example, Krieger & Liotta (1979) describe maternal deprivation as a syndrome "characterized by growth failure, developmental retardation and affective abnormalities which develop in an adverse environment and improve after removal from it" (p. 142). Koluchova (1979) defined the phenomenon of maternal deprivation as "a state which occurs when a child is not given an opportunity to meet one or more basic psychological wants" (p. 163), with normal mother-infant interaction comprising one of these wants.

As early as 1965, Bowlby, Ainsworth, Boston and Rosenbluth pointed out the difficulties in achieving a definition of maternal deprivation by noting the multi-factorial nature of the experience of such children and highlighting the fact that isolating the variable of maternal deprivation poses problems. These researchers commented:

. . . a group of children for whom a separation experience in early childhood was the *only* adverse factor in their histories, hardly exists; almost always there is a medical or social reason for separation, and this frequently in itself is emotionally disturbing. . . . The best that can be done is to study a group of children whose experiences associated with separation are reasonably well known and to compare the characteristics of such a group with those found in other groups. (p. 212, emphasis added)

Nevertheless, most researchers studying the effects of maternal deprivation agree about reported responses of children who have been maternally deprived. The developmental alterations frequently associated with maternal deprivation include environmental retardation (Powell, Brasel, & Blizzard, 1967a). Maternal deprivation has also been described as one facet of the role of early maternal care in personality development (Rutter, 1972, 1979; Yarrow, 1961, 1964), as well as in the precipitation of depressive disorders. Yarrow (1961) contributed to the definition of maternal deprivation by outlining four potential preconditions in which the phenomenon can occur: "institutionalization, separation from a mother or mother substitute, multiple mothering [and] . . . distortions in the quality of mothering" (pp. 459–460). Thus, to reach an adequate, all-inclusive model of maternal deprivation and its effects, it is important to keep in mind the wide spectrum of situations that it covers and what each of these situations has in common.

The feral child studies, previously mentioned, reflect the view that severe isolation from a caregiver figure bears directly on the extent of developmental impairment. Reports of such children indicate prominent manifestations of mental, emotional, and physical retardation attributed to maternal deprivation, as well as reports of speech impairment. Additionally, such children were reported to display minimal capacity for sadness or joy. The feral children who did make significant progress in learning and language skills after their discovery appeared to have had some early contact with a caregiver. Later work on deprived children supports the idea that degree or severity of deprivation has a direct bearing on developmental level. On this topic, Spitz and Wolf (1946) wrote: ". . . clinical pictures vary in severity from temporary developmental arrest to inhibition of already acquired functions . . . and in extreme cases result in irreversible progressive personality distortion" (p. 321).

Once maternal deprivation has been basically clarified, a contrast between the portrait of the maternally deprived child and the clinically depressed child is appropriate. Under the diagnostic criteria outlined in *DSM–III*, depressed children and infants display loss of interest or pleasure in usual activities, along with dysphoric mood. Mood change is accompanied by behavioral alterations, including significant increase or decrease in appetite with corresponding fluctuations in weight, sleep abnormalities, reduced energy, diminished ability to think or concentrate, feelings of worthlessness, self-reproach, or inappropriate guilt. Recurrent thoughts of death and attempts at or suicidal ideation complete the picture.

Goldfarb's (1943) long-term observations of the effects of maternal deprivation as a result of institutionalization, have revealed some of the overlap between deprivation and depressive symptomatology. His appraisal of the institutionalized child is, to a certain degree, a description of a depressed child. He described a personality that is "meager and undifferentiated . . . passive or apathetic," with a "qualitative and quantitative deficiency in the general inhibitory process" (p. 127). Manifestations include hyperactivity, restlessness, and inability to concentrate.

Provence and Ritvo's (1961) study of deprived children revealed a similar picture; their study group displayed "little evidence of enjoyment and none of the experimental zest of the normal baby. . ." (p. 197). Similarly, Krieger and Liotta (1979) found deprived infants to be "generally withdrawn and apathetic" (p. 145).

To explore the interrelationships between maternal deprivation and childhood depression further, it is helpful to take into consideration five points. The first is that each entity may be manifested at mild or severe extremes, as well as at intermediate levels. Second, varying degrees of deprivation and depression may appear in conjunction with one another, creating several clinical pictures of the deprived/depressed child. For example, severe depression may be found in the child whose deprivation is severe. Third, the situation is further complicated by the difficulty of determining whether a child is truly displaying symptoms of long–term depression or whether he or she is being examined during the "despair" phase that may comprise a "natural" part of the evolution of deprivation, i.e., protest, despair, detachment, withdrawal (Bowlby et al., 1965). In such cases, the symptoms of despair may well be considered identical to the clinical picture of a *DSM–III* depressed child. Fourth, it is therefore essential that the clinician understand how the two entities are related, and thoroughly analyze the stage of separation that a deprived child is experiencing. Finally, the clinician should bear in mind that these conditions may be present to the exclusion of each other.

For the purposes of this analysis, maternal deprivation is hypothesized to be a crucial etiological variable in the genesis of childhood and infant depression. With respect to the causal link between maternal deprivation and clinical depression, Spitz and Wolf's (1946) work is highly persuasive. In their discussion of anaclitic depression among institutionalized children, they cite the grief reaction displayed by infants over six months of age upon separation from their parents, and draw parallels between many of these behavioral responses and the behavioral manifestations seen among depressed adults. The symptomatology associated with this study population included listlessness, passivity, loss of appetite, apathy, weight loss, sleep disorders, crying, affectlessness, and withdrawal.

For these children, it appeared that maternal deprivation acted as a central event precipitating depression. By definition, psychoanalytic use of the term *anaclitic* refers to the infant's love for his or her mother, and the infant's original dependence on her for care. The Spitz and Wolf study involved 133 infants in a nursery. They reported that it is during the second half of the first year that such infants initially appear cognizant of their loss, an event characterized by affect distress, notably crying. The crying phase was followed by withdrawal. By the end of one year, all children who remained maternally deprived displayed alteration in development. Spitz and Wolf wrote that maternal deprivation was considered "an etiologically significant factor" in these cases (p. 319). They further identified a syndrome among these infants including: apprehension, sadness, and weepiness, and characterized as well by lack of contact, rejection of the environment and withdrawal, retardation of development, retardation of reaction to stimuli, slowness of movement, dejection, stupor, loss of appetite, refusal to eat, and weight loss. Perhaps most telling, Spitz and Wolf noted a "physiognomic expression" which "in an adult would be described as depression" (p. 316). Significantly, Spitz and Wolf also wrote that "[t]he factor which appears to be of decisive etiological significance in our cases is the loss of the love object" (p. 320). While Spitz and Wolf explain these feelings in traditional psychoanalytic terms, the data can be construed from a developmental perspective as well.

Thus, in analyzing whether the deprivation symptomatology cited by Spitz and Wolf is indicative of infant depression, it is important to keep in mind the full spectrum of variables that provoke the syndrome. For example, the developmental perspective accords great weight to individual constitutional variation (i.e., temperament), which may make some infants more susceptible to experiencing the negative impact of maternal deprivation. The formation of an attachment bond, and its concomitant empathic exchange, is also generally lacking in these infants. The developmental model requires the coalescence of these milestone behaviors if normal self-object representation is to occur. Thus, maternal deprivation implies a deviation from the normal achievement of every significant developmental milestone discussed previously.

Deutsch (1959), perhaps unwittingly at the time, published a classic case in 1919, subsequently translated and republished in 1959, that helps make the connection between caregiver deprivation and childhood depression more acute. The case involved the separation between a two year old boy and a nurse who served as his surrogate mother. The nurse, whose name was Paula, abruptly left the little boy, Rudi, when he was two years old, without saying goodbye or expressing any formal farewell. At bedtime Rudi called for his biological mother, permitting her to undress him and put him to bed without protesting Paula's absence. Though not normally prone to sleep disturbances, Rudi awoke one or two hours later weeping loudly. He again called for his mother, insisting that she stay with him through the entire night, during which he did not sleep. Every few minutes he sought reassurance, asking, "Mummy, are you still there?" This was unusual in that before the departure of his nurse Rudi's behavior had been to ward off his mother in favor of Paula. Toward morning he slept for a short time. After awakening, he refused to take any food, showing a facial expression of extreme despair each time food was offered. His mother finally succeeded in feeding him a small portion, after which the boy, who had been fully toilet trained, wet himself and soiled his pants. This behavior remained the same through the nights that followed, and on the third day the mother faced the situation by asking Rudi "Where is Paula?" He replied with great indifference. By the fifth day he began to sleep normally, and no longer wet or soiled himself. At the ninth day, Rudi returned to his former sociable self. Eventually, he came to have great affection for his new nurse, and his sleeping, eating, and toilet habits were again normal. Deutsch concluded that even though Little Rudi overcame his first bitter disappointment in nine days, there was no way to determine how this first great accomplishment would influence the future of his psychic functions, the vicissitudes of his life, and his further strivings. According to the developmental psychopathology model, although Rudi recovered from this early deprivation experience, the aftermath of the separation may emerge at a later day in the form of depressive symptomatology.

Clinical Studies of Maternal Separation

A series of clinical studies exploring the ramifications of early infant and childhood separation from caregivers further elucidates the connections between maternal deprivation and depressive symptomatology. As noted earlier, maternal deprivation can assume a variety of forms. For the purposes of most clinical studies, brief maternal separations, due either to an episode of hospitalization occurring in infancy or to the removal of the child from the mother as a consequence of attending school, have proven to be the most feasible types of situations to explore. In this analysis, brief maternal separation is considered as a paradigm for studying the effects of maternal deprivation. In addition, the studies discussed below involve infants and children of various types, permitting convenient comparison of separation phenomena occurring from early infancy through early childhood. Thus, this series of studies facilitates the viewing of deprivation experience from a developmental perspective.

The results of the studies indicate that, more often than not, one isolated incident does not result in prolonged displays of depressive symptomatology. Thus, while depressive-like phenomena generally erupt immediately following the separation experience, such phenomena seem to disappear or recede if the caregiver relationship is resumed. This book posits two hypotheses for such an inhibitory process. First, despite the fact that studies have found that depressive-like manifestations retreat if the caregiver relationship is reinstated, the symptomatology may in fact not actually disappear, but instead may go into remission. That is, the repercussions or sequelae of the separation incident may be in eclipse, but this does not necessarily mean that the underlying sense of loss provoking the symptomatology has been resolved. Indeed, the Developmental Psychopathology Model argues that while the effects of one experience may be overshadowed by development in another area, subsequent problems rooted in earlier experience can surface at a later developmental period. Second, the Learned Helplessness Paradigm indicates that either repeated bouts of separation or sufficient separation experiences in an infant temperamentally and/or neuroendocrinologically predisposed to experiencing depressive-like phenomena may eventually culminate in depression. In other words, it is the cumulative effect of several separation episodes that may ultimately erode the infant's resistance and make him or her vulnerable to depression. As an example, when viewed in this context, the "avoidant" and "resistant" responses during the Strange Situation (Ainsworth, 1969) may gain a new interpretive gloss. Such responses may represent the final outcome of several previous separation experiences and, in these instances, the infant may be viewed as manifesting ambivalence toward the caregiver due to these earlier separation experiences.

Spitz and Wolf were among the first researchers to use modern empirical methods to document the impact of maternal deprivation on the very young. Faithful to the theoretical principals of psychoanalysis, they called the syndrome they observed, anaclitic depression. Other psychoanalysts, while departing more from orthodox views, also noted the impact of separation from the mother. Children who are separated from their mothers often exhibit an initial period of protest, followed by a behavioral reaction described by one researcher as "despair" (Bowlby, 1961). Beginning with these findings, one research team (Reite, Short, Seller, & Pauley, 1981) explored the mother-infant bond in pigtailed monkeys. Normal interaction between the infant monkeys and their mothers was observed and at a mean age of 19 weeks, infants were surgically implanted with multichannel biotelemetry systems, enabling recording of EKG, body temperature, eye movement, muscle activity, and EEGs. After a three to five day period of baseline recording, mothers were separated from infants. Mothers were placed in isolated cages while infants remained in social groups. After 10 days of separation, the mothers were returned to the social groups; physiological and behavioral monitoring continued for another four days, during the "reunion period."

Results showed that the infants vigorously protested separation from the mother, with much cooing and screeching. Activity recordings displayed a marked increase immediately after separation with rest periods decreasing markedly. In contrast, immediately following reunion, infant activity scores were low and rest scores increased. On the second day of separation, the researchers commented on the slouched posture and the saddened facial expressions of the infants. Heart rate immediately following separation increased and was agitated. The researchers also found that while these overall physiological trends were apparent in the entire group of infant monkeys, infants were also found to vary individually with respect to behavioral measures, implying constitutional differences. The researchers concluded that the data demonstrate that separation may be accompanied by a complex series of physiological changes that underscore the importance of attachment bonds and suggest a general impairment of autonomic homeostatic regulatory processes.

Researchers seeking to understand how separation affects infants and children have been locked in debate over whether there is a critical period, generally thought to occur immediately after birth, in which a unique bond is formed, and which, if disrupted, can have enduring consequences on the attachment behavior of the child. Klaus and Kennell (1976) have emphasized the importance of such a period in early development. In a study exploring the effect of minimal maternal-infant contact and prolonged separation following birth, Rode, Chang, Fisch, and Sroufe (1981) found that attachment patterns are not the product of a single episode in any infant's life, but rather, coalesce over time. Additionally, evidence was found for the resilience of infants in forming attachment patterns. The researchers examined a sample of 24 infants (20 premature and 4 seriously ill, full term infants) who had experienced prolonged separation due to hospitalization following birth. Infant attachment relationships with their caregivers at approximately 12 months of age were assessed by means of the Ainsworth Strange Situation. According to this categorization, 17 of the infants were categorized as securely attached, 3 of the infants were labeled anxious avoidant, and 4 of the infants displayed an anxious resistant response. Such figures are comparable to those found among infants who are not separated at birth. Moreover, secure versus insecure infants could not be differentiated on Bayley developmental scores, by birth weight, gestational age, days of neonatal intensive-care hospitalization, or parental visiting patterns.

The researchers concluded that attachment patterns are the norm despite physical separation of caregiver and infant at birth. Nevertheless, it should be pointed out that these infants were visited by parents frequently during hospitalization and that the family situations in these cases were "stable." The researchers posited that attachment is an evolving process, occurring during the first year of life, that takes time to reach full fruition. In addition, they emphasized the apparent "resiliency" of attachment relationships. Comments in the area of resiliency suggest, once again, that it may be repeated bouts of separation that result in infant and childhood depressive-like phenomena, rather than a single, isolated episode. Moreover, the flexibility or resiliency of these infants in reestablishing attachment bonds does not mean that the experience of separation has been fully resolved. Rather, an inhibitory process (alluded to earlier) may be at work, so that the earlier separation experience may be merely overshadowed by later developmental trends.

Field (1977) focused on the effects of separation using experimental manipulation of maternal-infant face-to-face interactions in three and one half month old infants. Interactive sequences were videotaped in 12 infants who had been separated from parents due to prematurity and respiratory distress syndrome at birth. These infants had also received low Brazelton interaction scores. A second group of 12 nonseparated, post-term, post-mature infants receiving low Brazelton scores was also studied, as was a third group of healthy, term infants. Field particularly examined infant display of gazing activity and maternal efforts at imitating infant behavior. Among the findings of the study was an absence of interaction differences between postmature and premature infants, suggesting that separation contributed less to later interaction disturbances than it did to the deficits tapped by the Brazelton Neonatal Scale shortly after birth.

The study involved maternal manipulations of attention-getting and imitation behavior. Despite these manipulations, an absence of differences between risk and nonrisk groups in the amounts of maternal activity and infant gaze during imitation was found. Unlike the imitation interactions, however, the spontaneous interactions of the normal and high-risk dyads were dramatically different. Significantly, mothers of normal infants were less active, and normal infants engaged in substantially more gazing behavior than infants in the other groups.

Field noted that the fact that the high-risk dyads at least matched the postmature pairs on interaction behaviors, despite the early separation that they had experienced, suggests some form of compensatory experience for their separation. Compensation may, for example, have taken the form of very sensitive nurse-neonate interaction during extended hospitalization. Field concluded that the lack of difference between the postmature and high-risk dyads does not suggest that early separation had no effect on later infant-mother interaction. Instead, the separation effect appears to be of lesser import than the infant's interaction style at birth (as demonstrated through the Brazelton score) and the continuity of style, as well as maternal behavior during later interactions.

Another study conducted by Field (Field, Vega-Lahr, & Jagadish, 1984) explored the aftermath of separation in the context of nursery school entrances among infants and toddlers. Play behaviors and sleep patterns of 11 infants (15 months) and 20 toddlers (24 months) were observed during the first and fourth week of the month preceding and following their entrance into new nursery classes. Activity level was monitored during free-play sessions, sleep-state changes were recorded, and parents answered questionnaires on behavioral, sleep, eating, toileting, and illness changes. Comparison observations during the week immediately before and after entrance to new nursery classes revealed greater amounts of fussing, verbal interaction, physical contact (aggressive and affectionate), wandering, and fantasy play behavior among both groups. In addition, during this period, latency to sleep was longer and crying was more frequent preparatory to sleep. In contrast to toddlers, infants were less agitated prior to entrance, but more agitated during the first week in their new class.

According to Field, the fact that toddlers manifested behavior changes *prior* to separation while infants did not manifest increased negative affect and sleep disturbance until *after* the separation experience suggests that at some time late in infancy, the necessary cognitive development has occurred for the experience of an anticipatory reaction to separation stress. Field's phrase, "anticipatory reaction to separation stress," is crucial to this discussion. Implicitly, the phrase suggests that once evocative memory is present, the experience of a separation, along with its affective correlates, is retained. This experience can be retriggered with the onset of appropriate cues. Thus, the resilience reported earlier in infants who experienced separation and were later reunited with caregivers was just that. The symptomatology of separation distress reminiscent of depression may superficially vanish, but the experience itself is retained in memory. Moreover, as discussed in Chapter 7, evocative memory may develop earlier than previously supposed.

Field, Gewirtz, et al. (1984) further explored the theme of school separation in an examination of leavetaking and reunion behaviors among infants, toddlers, and preschoolers who were dropped off and picked up at their nursery school each day. The study focused on a developmental comparison of behaviors evinced by the three groups, including infants (mean age nine months), toddlers (mean age 24 months), and preschoolers (mean age 48 months). Toddlers most frequently showed distress behaviors during parental departure. Children dropped off by mothers versus fathers showed more attention-getting behavior and crying. During the second semester of observation, parents and children spent less time relating to each other during leavetaking. Children protested departures less frequently and parents left the classroom more quickly.

During the first semester, toddlers were most distressed by leavetaking, even though they had experienced daily leavetaking since early infancy. But while distress behaviors of the toddlers significantly diminished, the infants showed increasing amounts of clinging and hovering across the two semesters. According to the investigators, these data suggest that proximity-maintaining behaviors may be more influenced by developmental age than by amount of experience with leavetaking. Also, implicit is the fact that repeated experiences of separation may have a cumulative effect up to a specific developmental stage.

In a related study involving the separation stress of young children (mean age, 55 months) transferring to new schools, Field, Vega-Lahr, and Jagadish (1984) documented observations made two weeks prior to separation from classmates. Comparing children who were leaving for a new school versus children who were staying in the same school environment, Field reported in the former an increase in fantasy play, physical contact, negative statements and affect, fussiness, activity level, tonic heart rate, and alterations in eating and sleeping patterns. Once again, Field commented on the "anticipatory" reactions to separation of the departing children, and noted that these clusters of behaviors were similar to manifestations observed in young children separated from their mothers during hospitalization for birth of another child.

Each of these studies reveals a particular clinical response manifested by the infant during an episode of maternal separation. These responses, as noted, are indicative of depression or depressive-like phenomena. Nevertheless, infant response during these trials should not be viewed in isolation. While the manifestation of overt behavior is obvious to the researcher, it is crucial to realize that on a more complex level, the infant's well-endowed psychological and physiological equipment is being subjected to stress and, thus, the response may be viewed as one method of coping with a newly experienced discrepant situation. In short, as previous chapters have discussed, the response of the infant to maternal separation is actually the final outcome of a myriad of factors, including infant temperament and biochemical predisposition, maternal attachment, and empathic patterns, infant capacity for determining locus of control, and previous experiences with discrepancy and contingency.

Conclusion

The preceding sections detail much of the relevant data currently available in the area of infant and childhood depression. Clearly, the early paradigms of depressive-like phenomena among these young age groups provided inadequate and ultimately unsatisfying theories for explaining behavioral disorganization in infants and children. The diagnostic criteria offered by *DSM–III* certainly posit a more coherent perspective for analyzing childhood depression. Indeed, at the very least, *DSM–III* recognizes the phenomenon of depression among young age groups as a distinct clinical entity. But as has been emphasized, by grafting an identical symptomatology onto both the adult and childhood manifestations of depression, the *DSM–III* analysis gives short shrift to the fundamental developmental processes implicit during the infancy and childhood years.

If, then, *DSM–III* represents an under-inclusive theoretical framework, the researcher is left to uncover new variables, to devise further instrumentation, and to integrate innovative data from a broad range of fields. Studies documenting the effect of caregiver deprivation on infant behavioral manifestations, for example, have provided more profound insights into the types of responses infants and young children display under these circumstances. The case history of Little Rudi (Deutsch, 1959) referred to earlier suggested that young children undergo a distinctive sequence of behaviors in coping with the effects of deprivation. Deutsch further indicated that the effects of caregiver deprivation may be more devastating than would appear; although overt signs of behavioral disorganization eventually receded, she noted that the ultimate repercussions of exposure to deprivation were unclear. Thus, Deutsch inadvertently hinted that it is only through a developmental perspective that permits long-term chronological charting that researchers can discern the etiologies of subsequent pathology.

The clinical studies discussed next used brief maternal separation episodes as representative of deprivation exposure in miniature. At first glance, these investigations appear to indicate that maternal separation does result in behavior disorganization, some of which resembles depression, but that the symptomatology remits upon reunion with the caregiver. Upon closer scrutiny, however, the data hint that such experiences may exert a more lingering carry-over effect that reappears when the infant or young child is placed in a situation similar enough to evoke stress. Field, for example, speaks of the phenomenon of anticipatory distress.

The case report discussed at the beginning of this chapter may represent one instance in which repeated bouts of separation resulted in an enduring symptomatology resembling depression. Although George (Harmon, Wagonfeld, & Emde 1982) displayed a remarkable resiliency between his depressive episodes, with each repeated separation challenge his symptomatology resumed. The case is notable as well because the interplay among developmental milestones, outlined in the first portion of this book, is clear. As described, George was a decidedly "fussy" infant whose behavior manifestations within the first month of life signaled that he was an infant with a "difficult" temperament. The history of multiple caregivers, coupled with several adoptive mothers, created an unstable environment for the development of attachment and empathic behavior. Within such a troubled environment, it might be predicted that self-object representation, while progressing through its usual chronological sequence, would ultimately emerge in a disorganized fashion. Moreover, the infant's atopic dermatitis, whose outbreaks coincided with separation experiences, indicate that an underlying sensitivity in neuroendocrinological function may be activated in times of distress.

Applying the Learned Helplessness Paradigm to this case, one might argue that the repeated experiences of caregiver separation represented reinforced non-contingencies or extreme discrepancies to which George responded with distress. It is notable that after the rejection of his first adopted home, George's symptomatology was manifested in more aggressive types of behavioral disorganization; only with the second rejection did the symptomatology—excessive staring, sitting alone in the basement, twisting fingers—indicate a more profound pathology, clearly reminiscent of traditional depressive disorder. One explanation for this may be that George was "protesting" (to borrow Bowlby's terminology) the negative affect brought on by the non-contingent experience. But upon experiencing a replica of the initial rejection, George's motivation had been undermined, and he evinced the affective and cognitive deficits associated with Learned Helplessness depression. Moreover, by the time of his second adoption, George was developmentally in possession of a differentiated sense of self and the potential for negative self-attribution was increased.

By using the Developmental Model, this case elucidates more coherently how early maternal separation can ultimately result in depressive symptomatology. The paradigms outlined previously suggest possible scenarios for how such depression may emerge. Nevertheless, the final paradox is that despite early exposure to often devastating circumstances, infants generally do "recover" sufficiently to progress through childhood and adulthood before symptomatology resurfaces. It is the challenge of developmental psychopathology to ensure that this recovery is indeed genuine, and that the early roots of infant depression are fully eradicated.

One manner in which developmental psychopathology may meet the challenge of clarifying the etiology and operational criteria of infant depression, is to correlate the types of depressive-like phenomena encountered in the studies discussed above, with instances of more enduring depression documented in infants and children who have, for example, experienced prolonged maternal separation. Furthermore, articulating a connection between infant depressive-like phenomena and well-established subtypes of depression known to occur in children and adults (for example, major affective and dysthymic disorders), remains an ambitious task for the future.

Although much work is yet to be done in order to clarify the parameters of infant depression, the developmental model focusing on key milestones of achievement offers researchers an appropriate blueprint with which to interpret data. From this model, an articulation of the ultimate theory of infant depression may be accomplished.

References

Abramson, L. (1977). *Universal versus personal helplessness: an experimental test of the reformulated theory of learned helplessness and depression.* Unpublished dissertation, University of Pennsylvania.

Abramson, L., & Sackeim, H. A. (1977). A paradox in depression: Uncontrollability and self–blame. *Psychological Bulletin, 84*, 838–851.

Abramson, L. Y., Seligman, M. E. P., & Teasdale, J. D. (1978). Learned helplessness in humans: Critique and reformulation. *Journal of Abnormal Psychology, 87*, 49–74.

Achor R. W. P., Hanson, N. O., & Gifford, R. W., Jr. (1955). Hypertension treated with rauwolfia serpentina (whole root) and with reserpine: Controlled study disclosing occasional severe depression. *Journal of the American Medical Association, 159*, 841–845.

Adams, R. J., & Maurer, D. (1984). Detection of contrast by a newborn and 2–month–old infant. *Infant Behavior and Development., 7*, 415–422.

Ahrens, R. (1954). Beitrag zur Entwicklung des physiognomie und mimikerkennens. *Zeitschrift für experimentelle unde angewandte Psychologie, 2*, 412–454.

Ainsworth, M. D. S. (1969). Object relations, dependency and attachment: A theoretical review of the infant–mother relationship. *Child Development, 40*, 969–1025.

Ainsworth, M. D. S. (1972). Attachment and dependency: A comparison. In J. Gerwirtz (Ed.), *Attachment and dependency* (pp. 97–137). Washington, DC: Winston.

Ainsworth, M. D. S. (1973). The development of infant–mother attachment. In B.M. Caldwell & H.N. Ricciuti (Eds.), *Review of child development research* (pp. 1–94). Chicago: University of Chicago Press.

Ainsworth, M. D. S. (1979, April). *Attachment: Retrospect and prospect.* Presidential address at the meeting of the Society for Research in Child Development, San Francisco.

Ainsworth, M. D. S., & Bell, S. M. (1979). Attachment, exploration, and separation: Illustrated by the behavior of one–year–olds in a Strange Situation. *Child Development, 41*, 49–67.

Ainsworth, M. D. S., Bell, S. M., & Stayton, D. J. (1971). Individual differences in strange–situation behavior in 1–year–olds. In H.R. Schaffer (Ed.), *The origins of human social relations* (pp. 17–57). London/New York: Academic Press.

Ainsworth, M. D. S., Blehar, M. C., Waters, E., & Wall, S. (1978). *Patterns of attachment: A psychological study of the Strange Situation.* Hillsdale, NJ: Erlbaum.

Ainsworth, M. D. S., & Wittig, B. A. (1969). Attachment and exploration behavior of one–year–olds in a strange–situation. In B.M. Foss (Ed.), *Determinants of infant behavior: Vol. 4.* (pp. 113–136). London: Methuen.

Akil, H. J., Madden, J., Patrick, R. L., & Barchas, J. D. (1976). Stress induced increase in endogenous opiate peptides: Concurrent analgesia and its partial reversal by naloxone. In H.W. Kosterlitz (Ed.), *Opiates and endogenous opiate peptides* (pp. 63–70). Amsterdam: North Holland.

Akiskal, H. S., & McKinney, W. T. (1975). Overview of recent research in depression: Integration of ten conceptual models into a comprehensive clinical frame. *Archives of General Psychiatry, 32,* 285–303.

Albert N., & Beck, A. T. (1975). Incidence of depression in early adolescence: A preliminary study. *Journal of Youth and Adolescence, 4,* 301–307.

Alloy, L. B., & Abramson, L. Y. (1979). Judgment of contingency in depressed and nondepressed students: Sadder but wiser? *Journal of Experimental Psychology [General], 108,* 441–485.

Alloy, L. B., Abramson, L. Y., & Viscusi, D. (1981). Induced mood and the illusion of control. *Journal of Personality and Social Psychology, 41,* 1129–1140.

Allport, G. W. (1937). *Personality: a psychosocial interpretation.* New York: Holt.

Als, H. (1985). Reciprocity and autonomy: Parenting a blind infant. *Zero to Three, 5,* 8–10.

Altman, N., Sachar, E. J., Gruen, P. H., Halpern, J. S., & Eto, S. (1975). Reduced plasma LH concentration in post–menopausal depressed women. *Psychosomatic Medicine, 37,* 274–276.

American Psychiatric Association. (1980). *Diagnostic and statistical manual of mental disorders [DSM–III]* (3rd ed.). Washington, DC: Author.

Ames, R. E. (1975). A methodology of inquiry for self–concept. *Educational Theory, 21,* 322–344.

Amir, S., & Amit, Z. (1978). Endogenous opiod ligands may mediate stress– induced changes in the affective properties of pain related behavior in rats. *Life Sciences, 23,* 1143–1152.

Amsterdam, B. K. (1972). Mirror self–image reactions before age two. *Developmental Psychobiology, 5,* 297–305.

Amsterdam, B. K., & Levitt, M. (1980). Consciousness of self and painful self–consciousness. *Psychoanalytic Study of the Child, 35,* 67–83.

Anders, T.F., Sachar, E.J., Kream, J., Rolfwang, H.P., & Hellman, L. (1970). Behavioral state and plasma cortisol response in the human newborn. *Pediatrics, 46,* 532–537.

Anders, T. F., & Zeanah, C. H. (1984). Early infant development from a biological point of view. In J.D. Call, E. Galenson, & R.L. Tyson (Eds.), *Frontiers of infant psychiatry: Vol. 2.* (pp. 55–69). New York: Basic Books.

Anisman, H. (1975). Time–dependent variations in aversively motivated behaviors: Non–associative effects of cholinergic and catecholaminergic activity. *Psychological Review, 82,* 359–385.

Antell, S.E., & Keating, D.P. (1983). Perception of numerical invariance in neonates. *Child Development, 54*, 695–701.

Anthony, E. J. (1983). An overview of the effects of maternal depression on the infant and child. In H. L. Morrison (Ed.), *Children of depressed parents: Risk, identification, and intervention* (pp. 1–16). New York: Grune & Stratton.

Antonucci, T. C., & Levitt, M.J. (1984). Early prediction of attachment security: A multivariate approach. *Infant Behavior and Development, 7*, 1–18.

Arai, K., Yanaihara, T., & Okinaga, S. (1976). Adrenocorticotropic hormone in human fetal blood at delivery. *American Journal of Obstetrics and Gynecology, 125*, 1136.

Arajarvi, T., & Huttunen, M. (1972). Encopresis and enuresis as symptoms of depression. In A. L. Annell (Ed.), *Depressive states in childhood and adolescence* (pp. 212–217). Stockholm: Almquist & Wiksell.

Arend, R., Gove, F., & Sroufe, L.A. (1979). Continuity of individual adaptation from infancy to kindergarten: A reductive study of ego resilience and curiousity in pre–schoolers. *Child Development, 50*, 950–959.

Argyle, M., & Kendon, A. (1967). The experimental analysis of social performance. *Advances in Experimental Social Psychology, 3*, 55–99.

Arimura, A., Saito, T., Bowers, C. Y., & Shally, A. V. (1967). Pituitary– adrenal activation in rats with hereditary hypothalamic diabetes insipidus. *Acta Endocrinologica, 54*, 155–165.

Åsberg, M., Thoren, P., & Traskman, M. (1976). Serotonin depression—a biochemical subgroup within the affect disorders? *Science, 191*, 478–480.

Åsberg, M., Thoren, P., Traskman, L., Berllsson, L., & Ringberger, V. (1976). 5–HIAA in the cerebrospinal fluids: A biological suicide predictor? *Archives of General Psychiatry, 33*, 1193–1197.

Asnis, G. M., Sachar, E. J., Halbreich, U., Nathan, R. S., Ostrow, L., & Halpern, F.S. (1981). Cortisol secretion and dexamethasone response in depression. *American Journal of Psychiatry, 138*, 1218–1221.

Azmitia, E. C. (1978). The serotonin–producing neurons of the midbrain median and dorsal raphe nuclei. In L. L. Iversen, S. D. Iverson & S. H. Snyder (Eds.). *Handbook of Psychopharmacology: Vol. 9*. (pp. 233–314). New York: Plenum Press.

Bakwin, H. (1949). Emotional deprivation in infants. *Journal of Pediatrics, 35*, 512–521.

Baldessarini, R. J. (1975). The basis for amine hypotheses in affective disorders. *Archives of General Psychiatry, 32*, 1087–1093.

Baldessarini, R.J. (1983). *Biomedical aspects of depression and its treatment* (pp. 22–160). Washington, DC: American Psychiatric Press.

Bandura, A. (1977). Self–efficacy: Toward a unifying theory of behavioral change. *Psychological Review, 84*, 191–215.

Barnett, M. A., King, L. M., & Howard, J. A. (1979). Inducing affect about self or other: Effects of generosity in children. *Developmental Psychology, 15*, 164–167.

Barrera, M. E., & Maurer, D. (1981). Discrimination of strangers by the three–month–old. *Child Development, 52*, 558–563.

Beck, A. T. (1967). *Depression: clinical, experimental and theoretical aspects.* New York: Harper & Row.

Beck, A. F., Ward, C. H., Mendelson, M., Mock, J., & Erlbaum, J. (1969). An inventory for measuring depression. *Archives of General Psychiatry, 9*, 295–302.

Behrman, R. E., Lees, M. H., Peterson, E. N., DeLannoy, C. W., & Seeds, A. E. (1970). Distribution of the circulation in the normal and asphyxiated fetal primate. *American Journal of Gynecology, 108*, 956.

Bell, R. Q. (1968). Adaptation of small wristwatches for mechanical recording of activities in infants and children. *Journal of Experimental Child Psychology, 6*, 302–305.

Bell, R. Q., Weller, G. M., & Waldrop, M. F. (1971). Newborn and preschooler: Organization of behavior and relations between periods. *Monographs of the Society for Research in Child Development, 36*(1–2, Serial No. 142).

Bell, S. M. (1970). The development of the concept of object as related to infant–mother attachment. *Child Development, 11*, 291–311.

Belsky, J. Garduque, L., & Hrncir, E. (1984). Assessing Performance, competence, and executive capacity in infant play: Relations to home environment and security of attachment. *Developmental Psychology, 20*, 406–417.

Bemesderfer, S., & Cohler, B. J. (1983). Depressive reactions during separation period: Individuation and self among children of psychotic depressed mothers. In H. L. Morrison (Ed.), *Children of depressed parents: risk, identification, and intervention* (pp. 159–188). New York: Grune & Stratton.

Bemporad, D. B., & Rathbun, J.M. (1982). Childhood depression from a developmental perspective. In L. Grinspoon (Ed.), *Psychiatry 82: The American Association annual review* (pp. 272–281). Washington, DC: American Psychiatric Press.

Berntson, G. G., & Micco, D. J. (1976). Organization of brainstem behavioral systems. *Brain Research Bulletin, 1*, 471–483.

Bertenthal, B. I., & Fischer, K. W. (1978). Development of self–recognition in the infant. *Developmental Psychology, 14*, 44–50.

Bibring, E. (1953). The mechanism of depression. In P. Greenacre (Ed.), *Affective disorders: Psychoanalytic contribution to their study* (pp. 13–48). New York: International Universities Press.

Biederman, J., & Jellinek, M.S. (1984). Current Concepts of Psychopharmacology in children. *New England Journal of Medicine, 310*, 968–972.

Birkmayer, W., & Riederer, P. (1975). Biochemical post–mortem findings in depressed patients. *Journal of Neural Transmission, 37*, 95.

Birns, B. (1965). Individual differences in neonates' responses to stimulation. *Child Development, 36*, 249–256.

Birns, B., Barten, S., & Bridger, W. (1969). Individual differences in temperamental characteristics of infants. *Transactions of the New York Academy of Science, 31*, 1071–1081.

Blanchard, M., & Main, M. (1979). Avoidance of the attachment figure and social–emotional adjustment in day–care infants. *Developmental Psychology, 15*, 445–446.

Blass, E. M., Ganchrow, J. R., & Steiner, J. E. (1984). Classical conditioning in newborn humans 2–48 hours of age. *Infant Behavior and Development, 7*, 223–235.

Blehar, M. C., Lieberman, A. F., & Ainsworth, M. D. S. (1977). Early face–to–face interaction and its relationship to later infant–mother attachment. *Child Development, 48*, 182–194.

Bliss, E. L., Migeon, C. H., Branch, C. H., & Samuels, L. T. (1956). Reaction of the adrenal cortex to emotional stress. *Psychosomatic Medicine, 18*, 56–76.

Blombery, P. A., Koplin, I. J., Gordon, E. K., Markey, S. P., & Ebert, M. H. (1980). Conversion of MHPG to vanillymandelic acid. *Archives of General Psychiatry, 37*, 1095–1098.

Bloom, F. E., Hoffer, B. J., Siggins, G. R., Barker, J. L., & Nicoll, R. A. (1972). Effects of serotonin on central neurons: Microiontophoretic administration. *Federation Proceedings, 31*, 97–106.

Bond, P. A., Jenner, F. A., & Sampson, G. A. (1972). Daily variations of the urine content of 3–methoxy–4–hydroxyphenylglycol in two manic depressive patients. *Psychological Medicine*, 81–85.

Borton, R. W. (1979). *The perception of causality in infants.* Unpublished doctoral dissertation, University of Washington.

Bower, T. G. R. (1972). Object perception in infants. *Perception, 1*, 15–20.

Bower, T. G. R., Broughton, J., & Moore, M. K. (1971). Development of the object concept as manifested in changes in the tracking behavior of infants between 7 and 20 weeks of age. *Journal of Experimental Child Psychology, 11*, 182–193.

Bower, T. G. R., & Patterson, J. G. (1973). The separation of place, movement, and object in the world. *Journal of Experimental Child Psychology, 15*, 161–168.

Bowlby, J. (1958). The nature of the child's tie to its mother. *International Journal of Psychoanalysis, 39*, 350–373.

Bowlby, J. (1960). Grief and mourning in infancy and early childhood. *Psychoanalytic Study of the Child, 15*, 9–52.

Bowlby, J. (1961). Childhood mourning and its implications for psychiatry. *American Journal of Psychiatry, 118*, 481–498.

Bowlby, J. (1969). *Attachment and Loss: Vol. I. Attachment.* New York: Basic Books.

Bowlby, J. (1973). *Attachment and Loss: Vol. II. Separation Anxiety and Anger.* London: Hogarth.

Bowlby, J. (1980). *Attachment and Loss: Vol. III. Loss.* New York: Basic Books.

Bowlby, J. (1982). *Attachment and Loss: Vol. I. Attachment* (2nd Ed.) New York: Basic Books.

Bowlby, J., Ainsworth, M. D., Boston, M., & Rosenbluth, D. (1965). Effects of mother–child separation. *British Journal of Medical Psychology, 29*, 211–247.

Branyon, D. W. (1983). Dexamethason suppression test in children (Letter to the editor). *American Journal of Psychiatry, 140*, 1385.

Brazelton, T. B. (1973). *Neonatal Behavioral Assessment Scale.* Philadelphia: J. B. Lippincott.

Brazelton, T. B., Koslowski, B., & Main, M. (1974). The origins of reciprocity: The early mother–infant interaction. In M. Lewis & L. A. Rosenblum (Eds.), *The effect of the infant on its caregiver* (pp. 49–76). New York: John Wiley.

Breese, G. R., Smith, R. D., Mueller, R. A., Howard, J. L., Prange, A. J., & Lipton, M. A. (1973). Indication of adrenal catecholamine synthesizing enzymes following mother–infant separation. *Nature/New Biology, 246*, 94–96.

Bremner, J. G. (1978a). Egocentric versus allocentric spatial coding in nine–month–old infants: Factors influencing the choice of code. *Developmental Psychology, 14*, 346–355.

Bremner, J. G. (1978b). Spatial errors made by infants: Inadequate spatial clues or evidence of egocentrism? *British Journal of Psychology, 690*, 77–84.

Bretherton, I., & Ainsworth, M. D. S. (1974). Responses of one–year–olds to a stranger in a Strange–situation. In M. Lewis & L. Rosenblum (Eds.), *The origins of behavior, Vol. 2, Fear* (pp. 33–78). New York: John Wiley.

Bridges, L. J., Grolnick, W. S., Frodi, A., & Connell, J.P. (1984). Determinants and correlates of mastery motivation and attachment across the second year: A structural modeling approach. *Infant Behavior and Development, 7*, (Special ICIS Issue), Abstract No. 48.

Brim, O. G., Jr. (1976). Life–span development of the theory of oneself: implications for child development. *Advances in Child Development and Behavior, 11*, 241–251.

Brodie, H. K. H., Murphy, D. L., Goodwin F. K., & Bunney, W. E. (1971). Catecholamines and mania: The effect of alpha–methyl–para–tyrosine on manic behavior and catecholamine metabolism. *Clinical Pharmacology and Therapeutics, 12*, 218–224.

Bronson, G. W. (1982). Structure, status and characteristics of the nervous system at birth. In P. Stratton (Ed.), *Psychobiology of the Human Newborn* (pp. 99–118). New York: John Wiley.

Broughton, J. (1978). Development of concepts of self, mind, reality and knowledge. *New Directions for Child Development, 1*, 75–100.

Brown, W. A., & Mueller, B. (1979). Alleviation of manic symptoms with catecholamine agonists. *American Journal of Psychiatry, 136*, 230–231.

Bugnon, C., Bloch, B., Lenys, D., & Fellmann, D. (1970). Etude cytoimmunologique chez le foetus humain et chez l'homme adulte de neurones hypothalamiques susceptibles d'elaborer divers peptides de type endorphines, ACTH, LPH et MSH a partir d'un precurseur commun. *Journal de Physiologie (Paris), 75*, 67–87.

Bunney, W. E., Brodie, K. K. H., Murphy, D. L., & Goodwin, F. K. (1971). Studies of alphamethyl–*para*–tyrosine, L–DOPA, and tryptophan in depression and mania. *American Journal of Psychiatry, 127*, 872–881.

Bunney, W. E., & Davis, J. M. (1965). Norepinephrine in depressive reactions. *Archives of General Psychiatry, 13*, 483–494.

Bunney, W. E., Murphy, D. L., Goodwin, F. K., & Borge, G. F. (1972). The "Switch Process" in manic-depressive illness. *Archives of General Psychiatry, 27*, 295–302.

Buss, A. H., & Plomin, R. (1975). *A Temperament Theory of Personality.* New York: John Wiley.

Buss, A. H., Plomin, R., & Willerman, L. (1973). The inheritance of temperaments. *Journal of Personality, 41*, 513–524.

Buss, D. M., Block, J. H., & Block, J. (1980). Preschool activity level: Personality correlates and developmental implications. *Child Development, 51*, 401–408.

Butterworth, G. (1977). Object disappearance and error in Piaget's Stage IV task. *Journal of Experimental Child Psychology, 23*, 391–401.

Butterworth, G., & Jarret, N. (1981). The geometry of pre–verbal conversation. *Bulletin of the British Psychological Society, 34*, 217.

Campbell, A. G. M., Dawes, G. S., Fishman, A. P., & Hyman, A. I. (1967). Regional redistribution of blood flow in the mature fetal lamb. *Circulation Research, 21*, 229.

Campos, J. J., Barrett, K., Lamb, M. E., Goldsmith, M. E., & Stenberg, C. (1983). Socioemotional development. In M.M. Haith & J.J. Campos (Eds.), *Handbook of child psychology: Vol. 2. Infancy and developmental psychobiology* (pp. 783– 916). New York: John Wiley.

Campos J. J., Hiatt, S., Ramsay, D., Henderson, C,. & Svejda, M. (1978). The emergence of fear of heights. In M. Lewis & L. Rosenblum (Eds.), *The development of affect*. New York: Plenum.

Cannon, W.B., & de la Paz, D. (1911). Emotional secretion of the adrenal secretion. *American Journal of Physiology, 27,* 64–70.

Cantwell, D. P. (1983a). Assessment of childhood depression: An overview. In D. P. Cantwell & G. A. Carlson (Eds.), *Affective disorders in childhood and adolescence: An update* (pp. 3–18). New York: SP Medical and Scientific Books.

Cantwell, D. P. (1983b). Overview of etiologic factors. In D. P. Cantwell & G. A. Carlson (Eds.), *Affective disorders in childhood and adolescence: An update* (pp. 206–219). New York: SP Medical and Scientific Books.

Cantwell, D. P. (1983c). Childhood depression: Issues regarding natural history. In D. P. Cantwell and G. A. Carlson (Eds.), *Affective disorders in childhood and adolescence: An update* (pp. 266–278). New York: SP Medical and Scientific Books.

Caplovitz, K., Morgan, G., & Mardashi, S. (1982). Mastery motivation in infancy: What does persistance index? *Program and proceedings of the developmental psychobiology research group second biennial retreat, 2,* (Summary) Estes Park, CO.

Cardinali, D. P. (1983). Molecular mechanism of neuroendocrine integration in the central nervous system: An approach through the study of the pineal gland and its innervating sympathetic pathway. *Psychoneuroendocrinology, 8,* 3–30.

Carey, W. B., Fox, M., & McDevitt, S. C. (1977). Temperament as a factor in early school adjustment. *Pediatrics, 60,* 621–624.

Carey, W. B., & McDevitt, S. C. (1978). Stability and change in individual temperament diagnoses from infancy to early childhood. *Journal of the American Academy of Child Psychiatry, 17,* 331–337.

Carlsson, A., Lindvist, M., & Magnusson, T. (1957). 3,4–Dihydroxyphenylalanine and 5–hydroxytryptophan as reserpine antagonists. *Nature, 180,* 1200.

Caron, A. J., Caron, R. F., Caldwell, R. C., & Weiss, S. (1973). Infant perception of the structural properties of the face. *Developmental Psychology, 9,* 385–399.

Carroll, B. J. (1972). The hypothalmic pituitary adrenal axis in depression. In B. Davies, B. J. Carroll, & R. M. Mowbray (Eds.), *Depressive illness: Some research studies* (pp. 143–159). Springfield, IL: Charles C. Thomas.

Carroll. B. J. (1976). Limbic system pituitary adrenal cortex regulation in depression and schizophrenia. *Psychosomatic Medicine, 38,* 106–121.

Carroll, B. J. (1978). Neuroendocrine function in psychiatric disorders. In M. A. Lipton, A. DiMascio, & K. F. Killman (Eds.), *Psychopharmacology: A generation of progress* (pp. 487–497). New York: Raven Press.

Carroll, B. J. (1981). Implications of biological research for the diagnosis of depression. In J. Mendlewicz (Ed.), *New advances in the diagnosis and treatment of depressive illness* (pp. 85–107). Amsterdam: J. Elsevier.

Carroll B. J. (1983). Biologic markers and treatment response. *Journal of Clinical Psychiatry, 44,* 30–40.

Carroll. B. J. (1984). Dexamethasone suppression test for depression. In E. Usdin et al. (Eds.), *Frontiers in biochemical and pharmacological research in depression* (pp. 179–188). New York: Raven Press.

Carroll. B. J., Curtiss, G. C., & Mendels, J. (1976). Neuroendocrine regulation in depression: II. Discrimination of depressed from nondepressed patients. *Archives of General Psychiatry, 33*, 1051–1057.

Carroll, B. J., Health, B., & Jarrett, D. B. (1975). Corticosteroids in brain tissue. *Endocrinology, 97*, 290–300.

Carroll. B. J., Martin, F. I. R., & Davies, B. (1968). Resistance to suppression by dexamethasone of plasma 11–OHCS level in severe depressive illnesses. *British Medical Journal, 3*, 285–287.

Cattell, R. B. (1965). *The scientific analysis of personality.* Baltimore: Penguin Books.

Chance, M. R. A. (1962). An interpretation of some agonistic postures: The role of "cut–off" acts and postures. *Symposia of the Zoological Society of London, 8,* 71–89.

Charney, D. S., Menkes, D. B., & Heniger, G. R. (1981). Receptor sensitivity and the mechanism of action of antidepressant treatment. *Archives of General Psychiatry, 38*, 1160–1180.

Chess, S., & Thomas, A. (1984). Origins and evolution of behavior disorders: *From infancy to early adult life.* New York: Brumer/Mazel.

Chess, S., & Thomas, A. (1985). Temperamental differences: A critical concept in child health care. *Pediatric Nursing, 11*, 167–171.

Chess, S., Thomas, A., & Hassibi, M. (1983). Depression in childhood and adolescence: A prospective study of six cases. *Journal of Nervous and Mental Disease, 171*, 411–420.

Christenson, N. J., Alberti, K. G., & Brandsborg, O. (1975). Plasma catechoalmines and blood substrate concentrations, studies in insulin induced hypoglycemia after adrenaline infusions. *European Journal of Clinical Investigation, 5*, 415.

Cicchetti, D. (1984). The emergence of developmental psychopathology. *Child Development, 55*, 1–7.

Clarke–Stewart, K.A. (1973). Interactions between mothers and their young children: Characteristics and consequences. *Monographs of the Society for Research in Child Development, 38*, 5–6.

Clifton, R. K, & Graham, F. K. (1968). Stability of individual differences in heart rate activity during the newborn period. *Psychophysiology, 5*, 37–50.

Cobliner, W. G. (1965). Some maternal attitudes toward conception. *Mental Hygiene, 49*, 550–557.

Cohen, L. B., DeLoache, J. S., & Pearl, R. (1977). An examination of interference effects in infants' memory for faces. *Child Development, 48*, 88–96.

Cohen, L. B., DeLoache, J. S., & Strauss, M. S. (1979). Infant visual perception. In J.D. Osofsky (Ed.), *Handbook of infant development* (pp. 393–438). New York: John Wiley.

Cohen, L. B., Dibble, E., & Grawe, J. M. (1977). Fathers' and mothers' perceptions of children's personality. *Archives of General Psychiatry, 34*, 480–487.

Cohn, J. F., & Tronick, E. Z. (1983). Three–month–old infants's reaction to simulated maternal depression. *Child Development, 54*, 185–193.

Connell, D. (1976). *Individual differences in attachment related to habituation to a redundant stimulus.* Unpublished doctoral dissertation, Syracuse University.

Coopersmith, S. (1959). A method for determining types of self–esteem. *Journal of Abnormal Sociology and Psychology, 59,* 87–94.

Coppen, A. (1967). The biochemistry of affective disorders. *British Journal of Psychiatry, 113,* 1237–1264.

Corman, H. H., & Escalona, S. K. (1969). Stages of sensorimotor development; A replication study. *Merrill–Palmer Quarterly, 15,* 351–361.

Costa, E., Fratta, W., Hong, J. S., Maroni, F., & Yang, H.–Y. T. (1978). Interactions between enkephalinergic and other neuronal systems. *Advances in Biochemical Psychopharmacology, 18,* 217–226.

Crittenden, P. M. (1983). The effect of mandatory protective daycare on mutual attachment in maltreating mother–infant dyads. *Child Abuse and Neglect, 7,* 297–300.

Crow, T. J. (1973). Catecholamine–containing neurons and electrical self–stimulation: A theoretical interpretation and some psychiatric implications. *Psychological Medicine, 3,* 66–73.

Csontos, K., Rust, M., Hollt, V., Mahr, W., Kromer, W., & Teschemacher, H.J. (1979). Elevated plasma B–endorphin levels in pregnant women and their neonates. *Life Sciences, 25,* 835–844.

Cytryn, L., & McKnew, T. (1974). Factors influencing the changing clinical expression of the depressive process in children. *American Journal of Psychiatry, 131,* 879–881.

Damon, W., & Hart, D. (1982). The development of self–understanding from infancy through adolescence. *Child Development, 53,* 841–864.

Darwin, C. (1877). A biographical sketch of an infant. *Mind, 2,* 285–294.

Davis, H., IV. (1979). The self-schema and subjective organization of personal information in depression. *Cognitive Theraputic Research, 3,* 415–425.

Davis, H., IV, & Unruh, W. R. (1981). The development of the self–schema in adult depression. *Journal of Abnormal Psychology, 90,* 125–133.

Davis, J. M. (1970). Theories of biological etiology of affective disorders. *International Review of Neurobiology, 12,* 145–175.

Davis, J. M., & Rovee–Collier, C. K. (1983). Alleviated forgetting of a learned contingency in 8–week–old infant. *Developmental Psychology, 19,* 353–365.

Dayton, G. O., Jones, M. H., Aiu, P., Rowson, R. A., Steele, B., & Rose, M. (1964). Developmental study of coordinated eye movements in the human infant: 1. Visual acuity in the newborn human: A study based on induced optokinetic nystagmus recorded by electrooculography. *Archives of Opthalmology, 71,* 865–870.

Decarie, T. G. (1965). *Intelligence and affectivity in early childhood: An experimental study of Jean Piaget's object concept and object relations* (E. P. Brandt & L. W. Brandt, Trans.). New York: International Universities Press.

Decarie, T. G. (1978). Affect development and cognition in a Piagetian context. In M. Lewis & L.A. Rosenblum (Eds.), *The Development of affect* (pp. 183–204). New York: Plenum.

Decarie, T. G. & Simineau, K. (1979). Cognition and perception in the object concept. *Canadian Journal of Psychology, 33,* 396–407.

DeCasper, A. J., & Carstens, A. A. (1981). Contingencies of stimulation: Effects on learning and emotion in neonates. *Infant Behavior and Development, 4*, 19–35.

Deleon–Jones, F., Maas, J.W., Dekirmenjian, H., & Sanchez, J. (1975). Diagnostic subgroups of affective disorders and their urinary excretion of catecholamine metabolites. *American Journal of Psychiatry, 132*, 1141–1148.

Depue, R. A., & Evans, R. (1981). The psychobiology of depressive disorders: From pathophysiology to predisposition. In B. A. Maher & W. B. Maher (Eds.), *Progress in experimental personality research* (pp. 1–114). New York: Academic Press.

D'Ercole, A. J., Underwood, L. E., & Van Wyk, J. J. (1977). Serum somatomedin–C in hypopituitarism and in other disorders of growth. *Journal of Pediatrics, 90*, 375–381.

Derryberry, D. & Rothbart, M. K. (1984). Emotion, attention and temperament. In C. E. Izard, J. Kagan, & R. B. Zajonc (Eds.), *Emotions, cognition and behavior* (pp. 132–166). Cambridge, England: Cambridge University Press.

Deutsch, H. (1959). A two–year–old boy's first love comes to grief. (M. Sommerfeld, Trans.). In L. Jessner & E. Pavenstedt (Eds.), *Dynamic Psychopathology of Childhood* (pp. 1–5). New York: Grune & Stratton. (Original work published 1919.)

Diamond, S. (1957). *Personality and Temperament.* New York: Harper.

Diener, C. I., & Dweck, C. S. (1980). An analysis of learned helplessness: II. The processing of success. *Journal of Personality and Social Psychology, 39*, 940–952.

Dixon, J. C. (1957). Development of self–recognition. *Journal of General Psychology, 91*, 251–256.

Dodd, B. (1979). Lip reading in infants: Attention to speech presented in– and out–of–synchrony. *Cognitive Psychology, 11*, 478–484.

Donovan, W. L. (1981). Maternal learned helplessness and physiologic response of infant crying. *Journal of Personality and Social Psychology, 40*, 919–926.

Dörner, G. (1983). Hormone–dependent brain development. *Psychoneuroendocrinology, 8*, 205–212.

Drillien, C. M. (1964). *The growth and development of the prematurely born infant.* Baltimore: Williams & Wilkins.

Dunst, C. J., & Lingerfelt, T. (1985). Maternal ratings of temperament and operant learning in two to three month old infants. *Child Development, 56*, 555–563.

Dweck, C. S. (1975). The role of expectations and attributions in the alleviation of learned helplessness. *Journal of Personality and Social Psychology, 31*, 674–685.

Dweck, C. S., & Bush, E. S. (1976). Sex differences in learned helplessness: I. Differential debilitation with peer and adult evaluators. *Developmental Psychology, 12*, 147–156.

Dweck, C. S., Davidson, W., Nelson, S., & Enna, B. (1978). Sex differences in learned helplessness: II. The contingencies of evaluative feedback in the classroom, and III. Experimental analysis. *Developmental Psychology, 14*, 268–276.

Dweck, C. S., Goetz, T. E., & Strauss, N. L. (1980). Sex differences in learned helplessness: IV. An experimental and naturalistic study of failure generalization and its mediators. *Journal of Personality and Social Psychology, 38*, 441–452.

Dweck, C.S., & Reppucci, N.D. (1973). Learned helplessness and reinforcement responsibility in children. *Journal of Personality and Social Psychology 25*, 109–116.

Earls, F. (1982). Application of DSM–III in an epidemiological study of preschool children. *American Journal of Psychiatry, 139*, 242–243.

Ehrensing, R. H., Kastin, A. J., Schalch, D. S., Friesen, H. G., Vergas, J. R., & Schally, A. V. (1974). Affective state and thyrotropin and prolactin responses after repeated injections of TRH in depressed patients. *American Journal of Psychiatry, 131*, 714–718.

Ekman, P., Friesen, W. V., & Ellsworth, P. (1972). *Emotion in the human face.* New York: Pergamon Press.

Emde, R. N. (1983). The prerepresentational self and its affective core. *Psychoanalytic Study of the Child, 38*, 165–192.

Emde, R. N. (1984). The affective self: Continuities and transformations from infancy. In J. D. Call, E. Galenson, & R. L. Tyson (Eds.). *Frontiers in child development: Vol. 2.* (pp. 38–54). New York: Basic Books.

Escalona, S. K. (1963). Patterns of infantile experience and the developmental process. *Psychoanalytic Study of the Child, 18*, 197–244.

Ettigi, P. G., & Brown, G. M. (1977). Psychoneurondocrinology of affective disorder: An overview. *American Journal of Psychiatry, 134*, 493–501.

Exline, R. V. (1982). Gaze behavior in infants and children: A tool for the study of emotions? In C. E. Izard (Ed.), *Measuring emotions in infants and children* (pp. 164–177). Cambridge, England: Cambridge University Press.

Exline, R. V., Gray, D., & Schuette, D. (1965). Visual behavior as affected by interview content and sex of respondent. *Journal of Personality and Social Psychology, 1*, 201–209.

Fagan, J. F. (1972). Infants' recognition memory for faces. *Journal of Experimental Child Psychology, 14*, 453–476.

Fagan, J. F. (1976). Infants' recognition of invariant features of faces. *Child Development, 47*, 627–638.

Fagen, J. W. (1980). Stimulus preference, reinforcer effectiveness, and relational responding in young infants. *Child Development, 51*, 372–378.

Fagen, J. W., Morrongiello, B. A., Rovee–Collier, C., & Gekowski, M. J. (1984). Expectancies and memory retrieval in three–month–old infants. *Child Development, 55*, 936–943.

Fagen, J. W., & Ohr, P. S. (1985). Temperament and crying in response to the violation of a learned expectancy in early infancy. *Infant Behavioral Development, 8*, 157–166.

Fang, V. S., Tricou, B. J., Robertson, A., & Meltzer, H. Y. (1981). Plasma ACTH and cortisol levels in depressed patients: Relation to dexamethasone suppression test. *Life Sciences, 29*, 931–938.

Fantz, R. L. (1963). Pattern vision in newborn infants. *Science, 140*, 296–297.

Fantz, R. L. (1965). Visual perception from birth as shown by pattern selectivity. *Annals of the New York Academy of Science, 118*, 793–814.

Fantz, R. L. (1973). Pattern vision in newborn infants. In L. J. Stone, H. T. Smith, & L. B. Murphy (Eds.), *The Compent Infant.* New York: Basic Books.

Fantz, R. L., & Miranda, S. B. (1975). Newborn infant attention to form of contour. *Child Development, 46*, 224–228.

Fast, I. (1976). Some relationships of infantile self–boundary development to depression. *International Journal of Psychoanalysis, 48*, 259–266.

Faucett, R. L., Litin, E. M., & Achor, R. W. P. (1957). Neuropharmacologic action of rauwolfia compounds and its psychodynamic implications. *Archives of Neurolical Psychiatry, 77*, 513–518.

Feighner, J. P., Robins, E., Guze, S. B., Woodruff, R. A., Winokur, G., & Munoz, R. (1972). Diagnostic criteria for use in psychiatric research. *Archives of General Psychiatry, 26*, 57–63.

Ferguson, H. C., Bartram, A. C., Fowlie, H. C., Cathro, D. M., Birchall, K., & Mitchell, F. L. (1964). A preliminary investigation of steroid excretion in depressed patients before and after electroconvulsive therapy. *Acta Endocrinologica, 47*, 58–68.

Feshbach, N. D., & Roe, K. (1968). Empathy in six– and seven–year–olds. *Child Development, 39*, 133–145.

Field, T. M. (1977). Effects of early separation, interactive deficits, and experimental manipulations on infant–mother face–to–face interaction. *Child Development, 48*, 763–771.

Field, T. M. (1977). Face–to–face interactions between normal and high risk infants and their mothers. *Dissertations Abstracts International, 37*, 4675–4676.

Field, T. M. (1979). Visual and cardiac responses to animate and inanimate faces by young term and preterm infants. *Child Development, 50*, 188 194.

Field, T. M. (1981). Infant gaze aversion and heart rate during face–to–face interactions. *Infant Behavior and Development, 4*, 307–315.

Field, T. M. (1982). Affective displays of high–risk infants during early interaction. In T. Field & A. Fogel (Eds.), *Emotion and Early Interactions* (pp. 101–125). Hillsdale, NJ: Erlbaum.

Field, T. M. (1984a). Early interactions between infants and their postpartum depressed mothers. *Infant Behavior and Development, 7*, 517–522.

Field, T. M. (1984b). Perinatal risk factors for infant depression. In J.D. Call, E. Galenson, & R.L. Tyson (Eds.) *Frontiers in psychiatry: Vol. 2.* (pp. 152 159). New York: Basic Books.

Field, T. M., Cohen, D., Garcia, R., & Greenberg, R. (1984). Mother–stranger discrimination by the newborn. *Infant Behavior and Development, 7*, 19–25.

Field, T. M., Gewirtz, J. L., Cohen, D., Garcia, R., Greenberg, R., & Collins, K. (1984). Leave-takings and reunions of infants, toddlers, pre-schoolers, and their parents. *Child Development, 55*, 628–635.

Field, T. M., Vega–Lahr, N., & Jagadish, S. (1984). Separation stress of nursery school infants and toddlers graduating to new classes. *Infant Behavior and Development, 7*(3), 277–284.

Field, T. M., Woodson, R., & Greenberg, R. (1982). Discrimination and imitation of facial expression by neonates. *Science, 219*, 179–181.

Finkelstein, N. W., & Ramey, C. T. (1977). Learning to control the environment in infancy. *Child Development, 48*, 806–819.

Finlay, D., & Ivinskis, A. (1984). Cardiac and visual responses to moving stimuli presented either successively or simultaneously to the central and peripheral visual fields in 4–month–old infants. *Developmental Psychology, 20*, 29–36.

Flagle, J. R. (1982). *The effects of occupational therapy intervention on task performance in Down's Syndrome children.* Unpublished master's thesis. Colorado State University.

Fogel, A., Diamond, G. R., Langhorst, B. H., & Demos, V. V. (1982). Affective and cognitive aspects of the two–month–old's participation in face–to–face interaction with its mother. In E. Tronick (Ed.), *Social Interchchange in infancy: Affect, cognition, and communication* (pp. 37–57). Baltimore: University Park Press.

Fontaine, R. (1984). Imitative skills between birth and six months. *Infant Behavior and Development, 7,* 323–333.

Fraiberg, S. (1969). Libidinal object constancy and mental representation. *Psychoanalytic Study of the Child, 25,* 9–47.

Fraiberg, S. (1982). Pathological defenses in infancy. *Psychoanalytic Quarterly, 51,* 612–635.

Freeman, L. N., Poznanski, E. O., Grossman, J. A., Buschbaum, Y. Y., & Banegas, M. D. (1985). Psychotic and depressed children: A new entity. *Journal of the American Academy of Child Psychiatry, 24,* 95–102.

Freis, E. D. (1954). Mental depression in hypertensive patients treated for long periods with large doses of reserpine. *New England Journal of Medicine, 251,* 1006–1008.

Freud, A. (1965). *Normality and Pathology in Childhood.* New York: International Universities Press.

Fries, M. E. (1937). Factors in character development, neuroses, psychoses, and delinquency. *American Journal of Orthopsychiatry, 7,* 142–181.

Fries, M. E. (1941a). Mental hygiene in pregnancy, delivery, and the puerperium. *Mental Hygiene, 25,* 221–236.

Fries, M. E. (1941b). National and international difficulties—a suggested national program for alleviation. *American Journal of Orthopsychiatry, 11,* 562–535.

Fries, M. E. (1944). Psychosomatic relationships between mother and infant. *Psychosomatic Medicine, 6,* 159–162.

Fries, M. E., & Lewi, B. (1938). Interrelated factors in development: A study of pregnancy, labor, delivery, lying–in period, and childhood. *American Journal of Orthopsychiatry, 8,* 726– 752.

Fries, M. E., & Woolf, P. J. (1953). Some hypotheses on the role of the congenital activity type in personality development. *Psychoanalytic Study of the Child, 8,* 48–62.

Frodi, A., & Thompson, R. (1985). Infant's affective responses in the Strange Situation: Effects of prematurity and of quality of attachment. *Child Development, 5,* 1280–1290.

Gaensbauer, T. J. (1982). Regulation of emotional expression in infants from two contrasting caretaker environments. *Journal of the American Academy of Child Psychiatry, 21,* 163–171.

Gaensbauer, T. J., Harmon, R. J., Cytryn, L., & McKnew, D. (1984). Social and affective development in infants with a manic–depressive parent. *American Journal of Psychiatry, 141,* 223–229.

Gaensbauer, T. J., Harmon, R. J., & Mrazek, D. (1980). Affective behavior patterns in abused and/or neglected infants. In N. Frude (Ed.), *Psychological approaches to prevention of child abuse.* London, Batesford Academic and Educational Ltd..

Ganong, W. F. (1963). The central nervous system and the synthesis and release of adrenocorticotropic hormone. In A.V. Ivalbandov (Ed.), *Advances in neuroendocrinology* (pp. 99–149). Urbana, IL: University of Illinois Press.

Ganong, W. F. (1977). Neurotransmitters involved in ACTH secretion: Catecholamines. *Annals of the New York Academy of Science, 297*, 509–517.

Ganong, W. F. (1979). *Review of Medical Physiology* (9th Ed). Los Altos, CA: Lange Medical Publications.

Garber, J. (1984). The developmental progression of depression in female children. *New Directions for Child Development, 26*, 29–58.

Garmezy, N., Masten, A. S., & Tellegen, A. (1984). The study of stress and competence in children: A building block for developmental psychopathology. *Child Development, 55*, 97–111.

Garver, D. L., & Davis, J. M. (1979). Biogenic amine hypotheses of affective disorders. *Life Sciences, 5*, 383–394.

Garver, D. L., Hirschowitz, J., Fleishmann, R., & Djuric, P. E. (1984). Lithium response and psychoses: A double blind, placebo–controlled study. *Psychiatry Research, 12*, 57–68.

Gekoski, M. J., & Fagen, J. W. (1984). Noncontingent stimulation, stimulus familiarization, and subsequent learning in young infants. *Child Development, 55*, 2226–2233.

Geller, B., Rogol A. D., & Knitter, E. F. (1983). Preliminary data on the dexamethasone suppression test in children with major depressive disorder. *American Journal of Psychiatry, 140*, 620–622.

George, C., & Main, M. (1979). Social interactions of young abused children: Approach, avoidance and aggression. *Child Development, 50*, 306–318

Gershon, E. S., Dunner, D. L., & Goodwin, F. K. (1971). Toward a biology of affective disorders. *Archives of General Psychiatry, 25*, 1–15.

Gesell, A., & Ames, L. (1937). Early evidence of individuality in the human infant. *Scientific Monthly, 45*, 217–225.

Gewirtz, J. L. (1961). A learning analysis of the effects of normal stimulation, privation and deprivation on the acquisition of social motivation and attachment. In B. Foss (Ed.), *Determinants of infant behavior: Vol. 1.* (pp. 213–290). New York: John Wiley.

Gibbons, J. L. (1964). Cortisol secretion rate in depressive illness. *Archives of General Psychiatry, 10*, 572–575.

Gibbons, J. L. & Fahy, T. J. (1966). *Neuroendocrinology, 1*, 358–363.

Gibson, E. J. (1969). *Principles of perceptual learning and development.* New York: Appleton–Century–Crofts.

Gilman, A. G., Goodman, L., & Gilman, A. (1980). *Goodman and Gilman's the pharmacological basis of therapeutics* (6th Ed.). New York: Macmillan.

Ginsburg, H., & Opper, S. (1978) *Piaget's theory of intellectual development.* Englewood Cliffs, NJ: Prentice Hall.

Glaser, K. (1968). Masked depression in children and adolescents. *Annual Progress in Child Psychiatry and Child Development, 1*, 345–355.

Glazer, H. L., Weiss, J. M., Pohorecky, L. A., & Miller, N. E. (1975). Monoamines as mediators of avoidance–escape behavior. *Psychosomatic Medicine, 37*, 535–543.

Goldberg, S. (1977). Social competence in infancy: A model of parent–infant interaction. *Merrill–Palmer Quarterly, 23*, 163–177.

Goldfarb, W. (1943). The effects of early institutional care on adolescent person-ailty. *Journal of Education, 12*, 106–129.

Goldsmith, H. H. (1983). Genetic influences on personality from infancy to adult-hood. *Child Development, 54*, 331–355.

Goldsmith, H. H., & Campos, J. J. (1982). Toward a theory of infant temperament. In R. N. Emde & R. J. Harmon (Eds.) *The development of attachment and affiliative systems* (pp. 161–193). New York: Plenum.

Goldsmith, H. H., & Gottesman, I. I. (1981). Origins of variations in behavioral style: A longitudinal study of temperament in young twins. *Child Development, 52*, 91–103.

Goodman, C. S., & Gilman, A. (1970). *The pharmacological basis of therapeutics* (4th Ed., p. 1628). New York: Macmillan.

Goodwin, F. K. (1976). Discussion remarks. In E. Usdin, D. A. Hamburg, & Y. D. Barchas (Eds.), *Neuroregulators and psychiatric disorders* (p. 192). New York: Oxford University Press.

Goodwin, F. K., & Bunney, W. E. (1973). A psychobiological approach to affective illness. *Psychiatric Annals, 3*, 19–51.

Goodwin, F. K., Cowdry, R. W., & Webster, M. H. (1978). Predictors of drug response in the affective disorders: Toward an integrated approach. In M. A. Lipton, A. Dimacscice, & K. F. Killam (Eds.), *Psychopharmacology: a gen-eration of progress* (pp. 1277–1288). New York: Raven Press.

Graham, F. K. (1979). Distinguishing among orienting, defense and startle re-sponses. In M. D. Kimmel, E. H. Van Olst, & J. F. Orlebeke (Eds.), *The ori-enting reflex in humans* (pp. 137–167). New York: Erlbaum.

Gratch, G. Appel, K. J., Evans, W. F., LeCompte, G. K., & Wright, N. A. (1974). Piaget's Stage IV object concept error: Evidence of forgetting or object con-ception? *Child Development, 45*, 71–77.

Green, W. H., Campbell, M., & David, R. (1984). Psychosocial dwarfism: A critical review of the evidence. *Journal of the American Academy of Psychiatry, 23*, 39–48.

Greenberg, R. E., & Field, T. (1982). Temperament ratings of handicapped infants during classroom, mother, and teacher interactions. *Journal of Pediatric Psy-chology, 7*, 387–405.

Greenberg, R. E., Gardener, E. I. (1960). The excretion of free catecholamines by newborn infants. *Journal of Clinical Endocrinology, 20*, 1207.

Greenspan, S. I. (1981). *Psychopathology and adaptation in infancy and early childhood: Principles of clinical diagnosis and preventive intervention.* New York: International Universities Press.

Guardo, C. J., & Bohan, J. B. (1971). Development of a sense of self–identidy in children. *Child Development, 42*, 1909–1921.

Guillemin, R., & Burgus, R. (1955). The hormones of the hypothalamus. *Scientific American, 227*, 24–33.

Guillemin, R., & Rosenberg, B. (1972). Humoral hypothalmic control of anterior pituitary: A study with combined tissue cultures. *Endocrinology, 55*, 599–607.

Gunnar, M. R., Fisch, R. O. Korsvik, S., & Donhoue, J. (1981). The effects of circumcision on serum cortisol and behavior. *Psychoneuroendocrinology, 6*, 269–276.

Gunnar, M. R., Fisch, R. O., & Malone, S. (1984). The effects of pacifying stimulus on behavioral and adrenocortical responses to circumcision in the newborn. *Journal of the American Academy of Child Psychiatry, 23*, 34–38.

Gunnar, M. R., Malone, S., Vance, G., & Fisch, R.O. (1985). Coping with aversive stimulation in the neonatal period: Quiet sleep and plasma cortisol levels during recovery from circumcision. *Child Development, 56*, 824–834.

Guyton, A. C. (1971). *Textbook of medical physiology* (4th Ed.). Philadelphia: W. B. Saunders.

Haith, M. M. (1979). Visual cognition in early infancy. In R. B. Kearsley & I. E. Sigel (Eds.), *Infants at risk: Assessment of cognitive functioning* (pp. 23–48). Hillsdale, NJ: Erlbaum.

Haith, M. M., Bergman, T., & Moore, M. J. (1977). Eye contact and face scanning in early infancy. *Science, 198*, 853–855.

Hammen, C., & Zupan, B.A. (1984). Self–schemas, depression, and the processing of personal information in children. *Journal of Experimental Child Psychology, 37*, 598–608.

Harmon, R. J., & Culp, A. M. (1981). The effects of premature birth on family functioning and infant development. In I. Berlin (Ed.), *Children and our future* (pp. 1–9). Albuquerque, NM: University of New Mexico Press.

Harmon, R. J., Morgan, G. A., Jacobs, T., Glicken, A. D., Culp, A.M., Busch, F., Rossnagel, N. A., and Butterfield, P. M. (1982). Comparison of risk and low–risk infant's motivation on a maternal report questionnaire and mastery tasks. *Program and Proceedings of the Developmental Psychobiology Research Group Second Biennial Retreat, 2*, 25 (Summary). Estes Park, CO.

Harmon, R. J., Wagonfeld, S., & Emde, R. N. (1982). Anaclitic depression: A follow–up from infancy to puberty with observations and psychotherapy. *Psychoanalytic Study of the Child, 37*, 67–94.

Harris, P. L. (1975). Development of search and object permanence during infancy. *Psychological Bulletin, 82*, 332–344.

Harris, P. L. (1983). Infant cognition. In P. H. Mussen (Ed.), *Infancy and developmental psychobiology: Vol. 2.* (pp. 692–782). New York: John Wiley.

Harris, P., & MacFarlane, A. (1974). The growth of the effective visual field from birth to seven weeks. *Journal of Experimental Child Psychology, 18*, 340–348.

Harter, S. (1974). Pleasure derived by children from cognitive challenge and mastery. *Child Development, 45*, 661–669.

Harter, S. (1977). The effects of social reinforcement and task difficulty level on the pleasure derived by normal and retarded children from cognitive challenge and mastery. *Journal of Experimental Child Psychology, 24*, 476–494.

Harter, S. (1978). Effectance motivation reconsidered: Toward a developmental model. *Human Development, 21*, 34–64.

Harter, S. (1982). The perceived competence scale for children. *Child Development, 53*, 87–97.

Harter, S. (1983). Developmental perspectives on the self–system. In E. M. Hetherington (Ed.), *Handbook of child psychology: Vol. 4. Socialization, personality and social development* (pp. 275–385). New York: John Wiley.

Harter, S., & Pike, R. (1984). The pictorial scale of perceived competence and social acceptance for young children. *Child Development, 55*, 1969–1982.

Hartmann, H. (1952). The mutual influences in the development of ego and id. In *Essays on ego psychology: selected problems in psychoanalytic theory* (pp. 155–182). New York: International Universities Press.

Hazen, N. L., & Durrett, M. E. (1982). Relationship of security of attachment to exploration and mapping abilities in 2–year–olds. *Developmental Psychology, 18*, 751–759.

Heard, D. H. (1978). From object relations to attachment theory: A basis for family therapy. *British Journal of Medical Psychology, 51*, 67–76.

Heckhausen, H. (1967). *The anatomy of achievement motivation.* New York: Academic Press.

Heckhausen, H. (1981). The development of achievement motivation. *Review of Child Development Research, 6*, 600–668.

Henderson, N. D. (1982). Human behavior genetics. *Annual Review of Psychology, 33*, 403–440.

Heniger, G. R., Charney, D. S., & Sternberg, D. E. (1984). Serotonergic function in depression. *Archives of General Psychiatry, 41*, 398–402.

Herman, B. H., & Panksepp, J. (1978). Effects of morphine and naloxone on separation distress and approach attachment: Evidence for opiate mediation of social affect. *Pharmacology Biochemistry & Behavior, 9*, 213–220.

Hinde, R. A. (1982). Attachment: Some conceptual and biological issues. In C. Parkes & J. Stevenson–Hinde (Eds.), *The place of attachment in human attachment* (pp. 60–76). New York: Basic Books.

Hiroto, D. S. (1974). Locus of control and learned helplessness. *Journal of Experimental Psychology, 102*, 187–193.

Hiroto, D. S., & Seligman, M. E. P. (1975). Generality of learned helplessness in man. *Journal of Personality and Social Psychology, 31*, 311–327.

Hoffer, W. (1952). The mutual influences in the development of ego and id: Earliest stages. *Psychoanalytic Study of the Child, 7*, 31–41

Hoffer, W. (1955). *Psychoanalysis: Practical and research aspects.* Baltimore: Williams & Wilkins.

Hoffman, M. L. (1975). Developmental synthesis of affect and cognition and its implications for altruistic motivation. *Developmental Psychology, 11*, 607–622.

Hoffman, M. L. (1977). Empathy, its development and prosocial implications. *Nebraska Symposium on Motivation, 25*, 169–217.

Hoffman, M. L. (1981). Is altruism part of human nature? *Journal of Personality and Social Psychology, 40*, 121–137.

Hoffman, M. L. (1982a). Development of prosocial motivation: Empathy and guilt. In N. Eisenberg (Ed.), *The development of prosocial behavior* (pp. 281–313). New York: Academic Press.

Hoffman, M. L. (1982b). The measurement of empathy. In C.E. Izard (Ed.), *Measuring emotions in infants and children* (pp. 279–296). Cambridge, England: Cambridge University Press.

Hoffman, M. L. (1983). Affective and cognitive processes in moral internalization. In E. T. Higgins, D. N. Ruble, & W. W. Hartup (Eds.), *Social cognition and social development: A sociocultural perspective* (pp. 236–274). Cambridge, England: Cambridge University Press.

Hoffman, M. L. (1984). Interaction of affect and cognition in empathy. In C. E. Izard, J. Kagan, & R. B. Zajonc (Eds.). *Emotions, Cognition and Behavior* (pp. 103–131). Cambridge, England: Cambridge University Press.

Hollister, L. E., Davis, K. L., & Overall, J. E. (1978). Excretion of MHPG in normal subject: Implications for biological classification of affective disorders. *Archives of General Psychiatry, 35*, 1410–1415.

Hubert N. C., Wachs, T. D., Peters–Martin, P., & Gandour, M. J. (1982). The study of early temperament: Measurement and conceptual issues. *Child Development, 53*, 571–600.

Hunt, J., & Uzgiris, I. C. (1964, September). *Cathexis from recognitive familiarity: An exploratory study.* Paper presented at the 1964 Convention of the American Psychological Association, Los Angeles, CA.

Iversen, L. L. (1982). Neurotransmitters and CNS Disease. *Lancet, 2,* 914–918.

Iversen, S. D., & Koob, G. F. (1977). Behavioral implications of dopaminergic neurons in mesolimbic system. *Advances in Biochemical Psychopharmacology, 16,* 209–214.

Izard, C. (1971). *The face of emotion.* New York: Appleton–Century–Crofts.

Izard, C. E. (1977). *Human emotions.* New York: Plenum Press.

Izard, C. E. (1978). On the ontogenesis of emotions and emotion–cognition relationship in infancy. In M. Lewis and L. A. Rosenblum (Eds), *The development of affect.* New York: Plenum Press.

Izard, C. E. & Buechler, S. (1981). Theoretical perspectives on emotions in developmental disabilities. In M. Lewis & L. T. Taft (Eds.). *Developmental disabilities: theory, assessment and intervention* (pp. 353–369). New York: SP Medical and Scientific Books.

Izard, C. E., Huebner, R. R., Risser, D., McGinness,G., & Dougherty, L. (1980). The young infant's ability to produce discrete emotional expressions. *Developmental Psychology, 16,* 132–140.

Janowski, D. S., El–Yousef, M. K., Davis, J. M., & Sekerke, H. J. (1972). A cholinergic adrenergic hypothesis of mania and depression. *Lancet, 2,* 632–635.

Janowski, D. S., El–Yousef, M. K., & Davis, J. M. (1974). Acetylcholine and depression. *Psychosomatic Medicine, 36,* 248–257.

Jennings, K. D., Connors, R. E., Sankaranarayan, P., & Katz, J. (1982, October). *Mastery motivation in physically handicapped and nonhandicapped preschool children.* Paper presented at the American Academy of Child Psychiatry Meeting, Washington, DC.

Jennings, K., Yarrow, L., & Martin, P. (1984). Mastery motivation and cognitive development: A longitudinal study from infancy to three and one half years. *International Journal of Behavior and Development, 7,* 441–461.

Jensen, K. (1959). Depressions in patients treated with reserpine for aterial hypertension. *Acta Psychiatrica et Neurologica Scandinavica, 34,* 195–204.

Joffe, W. G., & Sandler, J. (1965). Notes on pain, depression and individuation. *Psychoanalytic Study of the Child, 20,* 394–424.

Johnson, W. F., Emde, R. W., Pannabecker, B. J., Stenberg, C., & Davis, H. (1982). Maternal perception of infant emotion from birth through 18 months. *Infant Behavior and Development, 5,* 313–322.

Johnson, W. F., & Moeller, D. (1972). *Living with change: The semantics of coping.* New York: Harper & Row.

Jones, S. S. (1985). On the motivational bases for attachment behavior. *Developmental Psychology, 21,* 848–857.

Jouvet, M. (1969). Biogenic amines and the states of sleep. *Science, 163,* 32–41.

Kagan, J. (1971). *Change and continuity in infancy.* New York: John Wiley.

Kagan, J. (1974). Discrepancy, temperament, and infant distress. In M. Lewis & L. A. Rosenblum (Eds.), *The origins of fear* (pp. 229–248). New York: John Wiley.

Kagan, J. (1976). Emergent themes in human development. *American Scientist, 64,* 186–196.

Kagan, J. (1978). On emotion and its development: A working paper. In M. Lewis & L. A. Rosenblum (Eds.), *The development of affect* (pp. 11–41). New York: Plenum Press, 1978.

Kagan, J. (1979). Structure and process in the human infant: The ontogeny of mental representation. In M. H. Bornstein & W. Kessen (Eds.), *Psychological development from infancy: Image to intention* (pp. 159–182). Hillsdale, NJ: Erlbaum.

Kagan, J. (1980). Perspectives on continuity. In O. G. Brim & J. Kagan (Eds.), *Constancy and change in human development* (pp. 26–74). Cambridge, MA: Harvard University Press.

Kagan, J. (1981). *The second year: The emergence of self–awareness*. Cambridge, MA: Harvard University Press.

Kagan, J. (1982). Comments on the construct of difficult temperament. *Merrill Palmer Quarterly, 8*, 21–24.

Kagan, J. (1982). The emergence of self. *Journal of Child Psychology and Psychiatry and Allied Disciplines, 23*, 363–381.

Kagan, J. (1984). Continuity and change in the opening years of life. In R. N. Emde & R. J. Harmon (Eds.), *Continuities and discontinuities in development* (pp. 15–39). New York: Plenum Press.

Kagan, J., Henker, B. A., Hen–Tov, A., Levine, J., & Lewis, M. (1966). Infants' differential reactions to familiar and distorted faces. *Child Development, 37*, 519–532.

Kagan, J., & Moss, H.A. (1962). *Birth to maturity*. New York: John Wiley.

Kalin, N. H., & Carnes, M. (1984) Biological correlates of attachment bond disruption in human and nonhuman primates. *Progress in Neuropsychopharmacology and Biological Psychiatry, 8*, 459–469.

Kalmanson, B. (1982). Removing obstacles to attachment: Infant–parent psychotherapy with an adolescent mother and her baby. *Zero to Three, 3*, 10–13.

Kaplan, L.J. (1972). Object constancy in the light of Piaget's vertical decalage. *Bulletin of the Menninger Clinic, 36*, 322–334.

Karabenick, J. D., & Heller, K. A. (1976). A developmental study of effort and ability attributions. *Developmental Psychology, 12*, 559–560.

Kashani, J., Barbero, G. J., & Bolander, F. (1981). Depression in hospitalized pediatric patients. *Journal of the American Academy of Child Psychiatry, 20*, 123–134.

Kashani, J., Burk, J. P., & Reid, J. C. (1985). Depressed children of depressed parents. *Canadian Journal of Psychiatry, 30*, 265–269.

Kashani, J. H., Ray, J. S., & Carlson, G. A. (1984). Depression and depressive–like states in preschool–age children in a child development unit. *American Journal of Psychiatry, 141*, 1397–1402.

Kastin, A. J., Ehrensing, R. H., Schalch, D. S., & Anderson, M. S. (1972). Improvement in mental depression with decreased thyrotropin response after administration of thyrotropin–releasing hormome. *Lancet, 2*, 740–742.

Katz, J. (1979). Depression in the young child. In J. Nowells (Ed.), *Modern perspectives in the psychiatry of infancy* (pp. 435–449). New York: Brunner/Mazel.

Kaufman, I. C. (1977). Developmental considerations of anxiety and depression: Psychological studies in monkeys. In T. Shapiro (Ed.), *Psychoanalysis and contemporary science: An annual of integrative and interdisciplinary studies: Vol. 5.* (pp. 317–336). New York: International Universities Press.

Kaye, K., & Fogel, A. (1980). The temporal structure of face–to–face communication between mothers and infants. *Developmental Psychology, 16*, 454–464.

Keller, A., Ford, L. H., Jr., & Meacham, J. A. (1978). Dimensions of self–concept in preschool children. *Developmental Psychology, 14*, 483–489.

Kelley, A. E., & Stinus, L. (1984). Neuroanatomical and neurochemical substrates of affective behavior. In N. A. Fox & R. J. Davidson (Eds.), *The Psychobiology of Affective Development* (pp. 1–75). Hillsdale, NJ: Erlbaum.

Kendon, A. (1967). Some functions of gaze–direction in social interaction. *Acta Psychologica (Amsterdam), 26*, 22–63.

Keogh, B.K. (1982). Children's temperament and teachers' decisions. *Ciba Foundation Symposium, 89*, 269–279.

Kevill, F., & Kirkland, J. (1979). Infant crying and learned helplessness. *Journal of Biological Psychology, 21*, 3–7.

Klaus, M. H., & Kennell, J. H. (1976). *Maternal–infant bonding*. Saint Louis: C. V. Mosby.

Klee, S. H., & Garfinkel, B. D. (1984). Identification of depression in children and adolescents: the role of the dexamethasone suppression test. *Journal of the American Academy of Child Psychiatry, 23*, 410–415.

Klein, D. C., & Seligman, M. E. P. (1976). Reversal of performance deficits in learned helplessness and depression. *Journal of Abnormal Psychology, 85*, 11–26.

Klinnert, M. D., Sorce, J. F., Emde, R. N., & Svejda, M. J. (1984). Continuities and change in early emotional life: Maternal perceptions of surprise, fear and anger. In R. N. Emde & R. J. Harmon (Eds.), *Continuities and Discontinuities in development* (pp. 339–354). New York: Plenum Press.

Knight, R. B., Atkins, A., Eagle, C. J., Evans, N., Finkelstein, J. W., Fukushima, D., Katz, J., & Weiner, H. (1979). Psychological stress, ego defenses, and cortisol production in children hospitalized for elective surgery. *Psychosomatic Medicine, 41*, 40–49.

Koluchova, J. (1979). An experience of deprivation: A follow–up study. In J.G. Howells (Ed.), *Modern perspectives in the psychiatry of infancy* (pp. 163–174). New York: Brunner/Mazel.

Kopp, C. B. (1982). Antecedents of self–regulation: A developmental perspective. *Developmental Psychology, 18*, 199–214.

Kopp, C. B., Sigman, M., & Parmalee, A. H. (1974). Longitudinal study of sensorimotor development. *Developmental Psychology, 10*, 687–695.

Korner, A. F., Hutchinson, C. A., Koperski, J. A., Kraemer, H. C., & Schneider, P. A. (1981). Stability of individual differences of neonatal motor and crying patterns. *Child Development, 52*, 83–90.

Kovacs, M. (1980). Cognitive therapy in depression. *Journal of the American Academy of Psychoanalysis, 8*(1), 127–144.

Kovacs, M., & Paulauskas, S. L. (1984). Developmental stage and the expression of depressive disorders in children: An empirical analysis. *New Directions in Child Development, 26*, 59–79.

Krieger, D. T., Allen, W., Rizzo, F., & Krieger, H. P. (1971). Characterization of normal temporal pattern of plasma corticosteroid levels. *Journal of Clinical Endocrinology and Metabolism, 32*, 266–284.

Krieger, D., & Liotta, A. (1979). Pituitary hormones in brain: Where, how and why? *Science 1979, 205*, 366–372.

Kuiper, N. A., Derry, P. A., & MacDonald, M. R. (1982). Self–reference and person perception in depression: A social cognition perspective. In H. L. Mirels (Ed.), *Integration of Clinical and Social Psychology* (pp. 79–103). New York: Oxford University Press.

Kun, A. (1977). Development of the magnitude covariation and compensation schemata in ability and effort attributions of performance. *Child Development, 48*, 862–873.

LaBarbera, J. D., Izard, C. E., Vietze, P., & Parisi, S. (1976). Four– and six–month old infants' visual responses to joy, anger and neutral expressions. *Child Development, 47*, 535–538.

Lal, H., Miksic, S., & McCarten, M.A. (1978). Comparison of discrimitive stimuli produced by naloxone cyclazoane and morphine in the rat. In T.C. Colpaert & J.A. Rosencrands (Eds.), *Stimulus properties of drugs: Ten years of progress* (pp. 177–180). Amsterdam: Elsevier–North Holland.

Langer, E. J. (1975). The illusion of control. *Journal of Personality and Social Psychology, 32*, 311–328.

Langsdorf, P., Izard, C. E., Rayias, M., & Hembree, E. A. (1984). Interest expression, visual fixation, and heart rate changes in two– to eight–month old infants. *Developmental Psychology, 19*, 375–386.

Lapouse, R. (1966). The epidemiology of behavior disorders in children. *Journal of Affective Disorders of Children, 3*, 594–599.

Lauder, J. M. (1983). Hormonal and humoral influences on brain development. *Psychoneuroendocrinology, 8*, 121–155.

Lerner, J. A., Inui, T. S., Trupin, E. W., & Douglas, E. (1985). Preschool behavior can predict future psychiatric disorders. *Journal of the American Academy of Child Psychiatry, 24*, 42–48.

Lester, B. M., Hoffman, J., & Brazelton, T. B. (1985). The rhythmic structure of mother–infant interaction in term and preterm infants. *Child Development 56*, 15–27.

Levine, S., Coe, C. L., Smotherman, W. P., & Kaplan (1978). Prolonged cortisol elevation in the infant squirrel monkey after reunion with mother. *Physiology and Behavior, 20*, 7–10.

Lewis, M. (1969). Infants' responses to facial stimuli during the first year of life. *Developmental Psychology, 1*, 75–86.

Lewis, M., & Brooks, J. (1978). Self–knowledge and emotional development. In M. Lewis & L. A. Rosenblum (Eds.), *The development of affect* (pp. 205–226). New York: Plenum Press.

Lewis, M., & Brooks–Gunn, J. (1979). *Social cognition and the acquisition of self*. New York: Plenum.

Lewis, M., Brooks–Gunn, J., & Jaskir, J. (1985). Individual differences in visual self–recognition as a function of mother–infant attachment relationship. *Developmental Psychology, 21*, 1181–1187.

Lewis, M., Feiring, C., Mcguffog, C., & Jaskir, J. (1984). Predicting psychopathology in six– year–olds from early social relations. *Child Development, 55*, 123–136.

Lewis, M., & Goldberg, S. (1969). Perceptual–cognitive development in infancy: A generalized expectancy model as a function of mother–infant interaction. *Merrill–Palmer Quarterly, 15*, 81–100.

Lewis, M. & Schaeffer, S. (1979). Peer behavior and mother–infant interaction in maltreated children. In M. Lewis and L. Rosenblum (Eds.), *The uncommon child: The genesis of behavior: Vol. 3.* New York: Plenum, 1979.

Lewis, M., & Starr, M.D. (1979). Developmental continuity. In J. D. Osofsky (Ed.), *Handbook of infant development* (pp. 653–670). New York: John Wiley.

Lichtenberg, P. (1957). A definition and analysis of depression. *Archives of Neurology, 77,* 519–527.

Lidov, H. G. W., & Molliver, M. E. (1982). An immunohistochemical study of serotonin neuron development in the rat: Ascending pathways and terminal fields. *Brain Research Bulletin, 8,* 389–430.

Ling, W., Oftedal, G., & Weinberg, W. A. (1970). Depressive illness in children presenting a severe headache. *American Journal of Disease of Childhood, 120,* 122–124.

Lingjaerde, O. (1983). The biochemistry of depression. *Acta Psychiatrica Scandinavica, 302,* 36–51.

Lloyd, K. J., Farley, I. J., Deck, J. H. N., & Hornykiewicz, O. (1974). Serotonin and 5–hydroxyindoleacetic acid in discrete areas of the brainstem of suicide victims and control patients. *Advances in Biochemical Psychopharmacology, 11,* 387–397.

Londerville, S., & Main, M. (1981). Security of attachment, compliance and maternal training methods in the second year of life. *Developmental Psychology, 17,* 289–299.

Lopez, T., & Kliman, G. W. (1979). Memory, reconstruction and mourning in the analysis of a 4–year–old child: Maternal bereavement in the second year oflife. *Psychoanalytic Study of the Child, 34,* 235–271.

Maas, J. W. (1975). Biogenic amines and depression. *Archives of General Psychiatry, 32,* 1357–1361.

Maas, J. W., Dekirmenjian, H., & Fawcett, J. (1971). Catecholamine metabolism, depression and stress. *Nature (London), 230,* 330–331.

Maas, J. W., Dekirmenjian, H., & Jones, F. (1973). The identification of depressed patients who have a disorder of NE metabolism and/or disposition. *Life Sciences, 13,* 106–111.

Maas, J. W., Fawcett, J. A., & Dekirmenjian, H. (1968). 3–Methyl–4–Hydroxyphenyl–glycol (MHPG) excretion in depressive states: Pilot Study. *Archives of General Psychiatry, 19,* 129–134.

Mabry, P. D., & Campbell, B. A. (1974). Ontogeny of serotonergic inhibition of behavioral arousal in the rat. *Journal of Comparative Physiological Psychology, 86,* 193–201.

Mahler, M. (1958). Autism and symbiosis: Two extreme disturbances of identity. *International Journal of Psychoanalysis, 29,* 77–83.

Mahler, M. (1963). Thoughts about development and individuation. *Psychoanalytic Study of the Child, 18,* 307–324.

Mahler, M. (1965). On the significance of the normal separation–individuation phase: With reference to research in symbiotic child psychosis. In M. Schur (Ed.), *Drives, affects, behavior: Vol. 2.* (pp. 161–169). New York: International Universities Press.

Mahler, M. (1966). Notes on the development of basic moods; The depressive affect. In R. M. Loewenstein, L. M. Newman, M. Schur, et al. (Eds.) *Psy-*

choanalysis: A General Psychology (pp. 152–168). New York: International Universities Press.

Mahler, M. S. (1972). Rapprochment subphase of the separation–individuation process. *Psychoanalytic Quarterly, 41*, 487–506.

Mahler, M. S., & McDevitt, J. B. (1968). Observations on adaptation and defense in statu nascendi: Developmental precursors in the first two years of life. *Psychoanalytic Quarterly, 37*, 1–21.

Mahler, M. S, Pine, F., & Bergman, A. (1975). The fourth subphase: Consolidation of individuality and the beginnings of emotion object constancy. In M. S. Mahler, F. Pine, & A. Bergman (Eds.), *The psychological birth of the human infant*. New York: Basic Books.

Mahmood, T., Reveley, A. M., & Murray, R. M. (1983). Genetic studies of affective and anxiety disorders. In M. Weller (Ed.), *The scientific basis of psychiatry* (pp. 266–277). London: Bailliere Tindall.

Maier S. F., & Seligman, M. E. P. (1976). Learned Helplessness: Theory and evidence. *Journal of Experimental Psychology, 105*, 3–46.

Maier, S. F., Seligman, M. E. P., & Soloman R. L. (1969). Pavlovian fear conditioning and learned helplessness. In B.A. Campbell & R.M. Church (Eds.), *Punishment and aversive behavior* (pp. 299–342). New York: Appleton–Century Crofts.

Main, M. (1973). *Exploration, play and level of cognitive functioning as related to child–mother attachment*. Unpublished doctoral dissertation, Johns Hopkins University, Baltimore.

Main, M. (1977). Analysis of a peculiar form of reunion behavior seen in some day–care children: Its history and sequelae in children who are home reared. In R. Webb (Ed.), *Social development in childhood: Day–care programs and research* (pp. 33–78). Baltimore: Johns Hopkins University Press.

Main, M. (1981). Avoidance in the service of attachment: A working paper. In K. Immelman, G. W. Barlow, L. Petrinovich, & M. Main, (Eds.), *Behavior and development: The Bielefeld interdisciplinary project* (pp. 651–693). Cambridge, England: Cambridge University Press.

Main, M. (1983). Exploration, play and cognitive functioning related to infant–mother attachment. *Infant Behavior and Development, 6*, 167–174.

Main, M., & Goldwyn, R. (1984). Predicting rejection of her infant from Mother's representation of her own experience: Implications for the abused–abusing intergenerational cycle. *Child Abuse and Neglect, 8*, 203–217.

Main, M., Kaplan, N., & Cassidy, J. (1985). Security in infancy, childhood and adulthood: A move to the level of representation. *Monographs for the Society for Research in Child Development, 50*, 66–105.

Main, M. & Stadtman, J. (1981). Infant response to rejection of physical contact by the mother. *Journal of the American Academy of Child Psychiatry 20*, 292–307.

Main, M., Tomasini, L., & Tolan, W. (1979). Differences among mothers of infants judged to differ in security. *Developmental Psychology, 15*, 472–477.

Main, M., & Weston, D. R. (1981). The quality of the toddler's relationship to mother and to father: Related to conflict behavior and readiness to establish new relationships. *Child Development, 52*, 932–940.

Main, M., & Weston, D.R. (1982). Avoidance of the attachment figure in infancy: Descriptions and interpretations. In C. M. Parkes, & J. Stevenson–Hinde (Eds.),

The Place of Attachment in Human Behavior (pp. 31–59). New York: Basic Books.

Malatesta, C., & Haviland, J. (1982). Learning display rules: The socialization of emotion expression in infancy. *Child Development, 53*, 991–1003.

Markus, H. (1977). Self–schemata and processing information about the self. *Journal of Personality and Social Psychology, 35*, 63–78.

Mason, J. W. (1968a). A review of psychoendocrine research on the pituitary–adrenal cortical system. *Psychosomatic Medicine, 30*, 576–607.

Mason, J. W. (1968b). Overall hormonal balance as a key to endocrine organization. *Psychosomatic Medicine, 30*, 791–808.

Mason, J. W. (1968c). A review of psychoendocrine research on the pituitary thyroid system. *Psychosomatic Medicine, 30*, 666–681.

Mason, J. W. (1968d). A review of psychoendocrine research on the sympathetic adrenal medullary system. *Psychosomatic Medicine, 30*, 631–653.

Mason, J. W. (1968e). Organization of psychoendocrine mechanisms. *Psychosomatic Medicine, 30*, 631–653.

Mason, J. W. (1975). Emotion as reflected in patterns of endocrine regulation. In L. Levi (Ed.), *Emotions—Their parameters and measurements* (pp. 143–181). New York: Raven Press.

Massie, H. M. (1978). The early natural history of childhood psychosis. *Journal of the American Academy of Child Psychiatry, 17*, 29–45.

Mast, V. K., Fagen, J. W., Rovee–Collier, C. K., & Sullivan, M. V. (1980). Immediate and longterm memory for reinforcement context: The development of learned expectancies in early infancy. *Childhood Development, 51*, 700–707.

Masters, J. C. (1972). Effects of success, failure, and reward outcome upon contingent and non–contingent self–reinforcement. *Developmental Psychology, 7*, 110–118.

Masters, J. C., Barden, R. C., & Ford, M. E. (1979). Affective states, expressive behavior and learning in children. *Journal of Personality and Social Psychology, 3*, 380–390.

Masters, J. C., & Furman, W. (1976). Effects of affective states on noncontingent outcome expectancies and beliefs in internal or external control. *Developmental Psychology, 12*, 481–482.

Matas, L., Arend, R. A., & Sroufe, L. A. (1978). Continuity of adaptation in the second year: the relationship between quality of attachment and later competence. *Child Development, 49*, 547–556.

Matheny, A. P., Jr. (1980). Bayley's Infant Behavior Record: Behavioral components and twin analyses. *Child Development, 51*, 1157–1167.

Matheny, A.P., Wilson, R.S., & Nuss, S. M. (1984). Toddler temperament: Stability across settings and over ages. *Child Development, 55*, 1200–1211.

Maurer, D., & Barrera, M. (1981). Infants' perception of natural and distorted arrangements of a schematic face. *Child Development, 52*, 196–202.

Maurer, D., & Salapatek, P. (1976). Developmental changes in the scanning of faces by young infants. *Child Development, 47*, 523–527.

McCall, R. B., & Kagan, J. (1967). Stimulus–schema discrepancy and attention in the infant. *Journal of Experimental Child Psychology, 5*, 381–390.

McCall, R. B., & McGhee, P. E. (1977). The discrepancy hypothesis of attention and affect in infants. In I.C. Uzgiris & F. Weizmann (Eds.), *The Structuring of Experience* (pp. 179–210). New York: Plenum Press.

McConville, B. J., Boag, L. C., & Purohit, A. P. (1973). Three types of childhood depression. *Canadian Psychiatric Association Journal, 18*, 133–138.

McDevitt, J. B. (1975). Separation–individuation and object constancy. *Journal of the American Psychoanalytic Association, 23*, 713–742.

McDevitt, J. B. (1979). The role of internalization in the development of object relations during the separation–individuation phase. *Journal of the American Psychoanalytic Assocation, 27*, 327–343.

McDevitt, J. B., & Mahler, M. S. (1986). Object constancy, individuality, and internalization. In R. F. Lax, S. Bach, & J. A. Burland (Eds.), *Self and object constancy* (pp. 11–28). New York: The Guilford Press.

McKinney, T. D. (1977). Biobehavioral models of depression in monkeys. In I. Hanin, & E. Usdin (Eds.), *Animal models in psychiatry and neurology* (pp. 117–126). Oxford: Pergamon Press.

McKnew, D. H., Cytrn, L., Efron, M. A., Gershon, E. S., & Bunney, W. E. (1979). Offspring of parents with affective disorders. *British Journal of Psychiatry, 134*, 148–152.

Meicler, M., & Gratch, G. (1980). Do 5–month–olds show object conception in Piaget's sense? *Infant Behavior and Development, 3*, 265–282.

Melges, F. T., & Bowlby, J. (1969). Types of hopelessness in psychopathological process. *Archives of General Psychiatry, 20*, 690–699.

Meltzer, H. Y., Lowy, M., Robertson, A., Goodnick, P., & Perline, R. (1984). Effect of 5–Hydroxytryptophan on serum cortisol levels in major affective disorders: III. Effects of antidepressants and lithium carbonate. *Archives of General Psychiatry, 41*, 391–397.

Meltzer, H. Y., Perline, R. & Tricov, B. J. (1984). Effect of 5–Hydroxytryptophan on serum cortisol levels in major affective disorders: II. Relation to suicide psychosis, and depressive symptoms. *Archives of General Psychiatry, 41*, 379–387.

Meltzoff, A. N., & Moore, M. K. (1983). The origins of imitation in infancy: Paradigm, phenomena, and theories. In L. P. Lipsitt (Ed.), *Advances in Infancy: Vol. 2.* (pp. 265–301). Norwood, NJ: Ablex Publishing Company.

Mendlewicz, J., & Rainer, J. D. (1977). Adoption study supporting genetic transmission in manic–depressive illness. *Nature, 268*, 327–329.

Meschia, G. (1978). Evolution of thinking in fetal respiratory phsiology. *American Journal of Obstetrics and Gynecology*, 132–806.

Messer, D. J., & Vietze, P. M. (1984). Timing and transitions in mother–infant gaze. *Infant Behavior and Development, 7*, 167–181.

Messer, D. J., Yarrow, L. J., & Vietze, P. M. (1982, August). *Mastery in infancy and competence in early childhood.* Presented at the annual meeting of the American Psychological Association, Washington, DC.

Meyer–Bahlberg, H. F. L. (Ed.). (1984). Endocrinology and child psychiatry: Introduction. *Journal of American Academy of Child Psychiatry, 23*, 8–9.

Miller, W. R., & Seligman, M. E. P. (1973). Depression and the perception of reinforcement. *Journal of Abnormal Psychology, 82*, 62–73.

Miranda, S. B., & Fantz, R. L. (1973). Visual preferences of Down's syndrome and normal infants. *Child Development, 44*, 555–561.

Mischel, W., Ebbesen, F., & Zeiss, A. (1971). Selective attention to the self: Situational and dispositional determinants. *Journal of Personality and Social Psychology, 27*, 129–142.

Mischel, W., Ebbesen, F., & Zeiss, A. (1973). Cognitive and attentional mechanisms in the delay of gratification. *Journal of Personality and Social Psychology,* *27*, 129–142.

Money, J. (1977). The syndrome of abuse dwarfism (psychosocial dwarfism or reversible hyposomatotropism). *American Journal of Diseases of Children, 131*, 508–513.

Moore, R. Y., Halaris, A. E., & Jones, B. E. (1978). Serotonin neurons of the midbrain raphe. Ascending projections. *Journal of Comparative Neurology, 180*, 417–438.

Moore, B. S., Underwood, B., & Rosenhan, D. L. (1973). Affect and altruism. *Developmental Psychology, 8*, 99–104.

Morgan, G. A., & Harmon, R. J. (1984). Developments transitions in mastery motivation measurement and validation. In R. M. Emde & R. J. Jarmon, (Ed.), *Continuities and discontinuities in development* (pp. 263–292). New York: Plenum Press.

Morgan, G. A., Harmon, R. J., Gaiter, J. L., Jennings, K. D., Gist, N. F., & Yarrow, L.F. (1977). A method for assessing mastery motivation in one–year–old infants. In *JSAS Catalog of Selected Documents in Psychology, 7*, 68 (Ms. No. 1517, 41 pp.).

Morgan, G. A., Harmon, R. J., Malpiede, L. M., Culp, A. M., & Renner, S. (1982). *Manual for assessing mastery motivation in two–year–old children.* Unpublished manuscript, University of Colorado School of Medicine, Denver.

Morgan, G. A., Tolerton, S., Renner, J., & Harmon, R. J. (1983). *Mastery motivation tasks: Manual for one– to three–year children.* Unpublished manuscript, Colorado State University, Fort Collins.

Murphy, D. L., Campbell, I. C. & Costa, J. L. (1978). The brain serotonergic system in the affective disorders. *Progress in Neuro–Psychopharmacology, 2*, 1–31.

Nachman, P. A., & Stern, D. N. (1984). Affect retrieval: A form of recall memory in pre–linguistic infants. In J. D. Call, F. Galenson, & R. L. Tyson (Eds.), *Frontiers of infant psychiatry: Vol. 2.* (pp. 95–100). New York: Basic Books.

Nagera, H. (1966). *Early childhood disturbances, the infantile neurosis and the adulthood disturbances.* New York: International Universities Press.

Natale, M. (1978). Effect of induced elation and depression in internal– external locus of control. *Journal of Psychology, 100*, 315–321.

Nauta, W. J. H. (1979). Expanding borders of the limbic system concept. In T. Rasmussen & R. Marino (Eds.), *Functional neurosurgery* (pp. 7–23). New York: Raven Press.

Naylor, A. (1982). Results of a Mismatch. *Zero to Three, 2*, 8–11.

Nelson, C. A., & Dolgin, K. G. (1985). The generalized discrimination of facial expressions by seven–month–old infants. *Child Development, 56*, 58–61.

Nelson, C. A., Morse, P. A., & Leavitt, L. A. (1979). Recognition of facial expressions by seven– month–old infants. *Child Development, 50*, 1239–1242.

Nicholls, J. G. (1975). Causal attributions and other achievement–related cognitions: Effects of task outcomes, attainment value, and sex. *Journal of Personality and Social Psychology, 31*, 379–389.

Nicholls, J. G. (1978). The development of the concepts of effort and ability, perception of academic attainment, and the understanding that difficult tasks require more ability. *Child Development, 49*, 800–814.

Nicholls, J. G., & Miller, A. T. (1985). Differentiation of the concepts of luck and skill. *Developmental Psychology, 21*, 76–82.

Ornstein, A. (1981). Self–pathology in childhood: Developmental and clinical observations. *Psychiatric Clinics of North America, 4*, 435–453.

Oster, H. (1978). Facial expression and affect development. In M. Lewis & L. A. Rosenblum (Eds.), *The development of affect* (pp. 43–75). New York: Plenum Press.

Overmier, J. B., & Seligman, M. E. P. (1967). Effects of inescapable shock on subsequent escape and avoidance learning. *Journal of Comparative Physiological Psychology, 63*, 28–33.

Papez, J. W. (1958). Visceral brain, its component parts and their connections. *Journal of Nervous and Mental Diseases, 126*, 40–56.

Papousek, H. (1961). Conditioned head rotation reflexes in infants in the first months of life. *Acta Paediatrica, 50*, 565–576.

Papousek, H. (1967). Experimental studies of appetitional behavior in human newborns and infants. In H. W. Stevenson, E. H. Hess, & H. L. Rheingold (Eds.), *Early behavior: Comparative and developmental approaches*. New York: John Wiley.

Papousek, H. (1977). Entwicklung der Lernfähigkeit im Säglingsalter. In G. Nelson (Ed.) *Intelligenz, lernen und lernstörungen* (pp. 89–107). Berlin: Springer–Verlag.

Papousek, H. (1981). The common in the uncommon child: Comments on the child's integrative capacities and on intuitive parenting. In M. Lewis & L. A. Rosenblatt (Eds.), *The uncommon child* (pp. 317–328). New York: Plenum Press.

Papousek, H., & Papousek, M. (1975). Cognitive aspects of preverbal social interaction between human infants and adults. In M. O'Connor (Ed.), *Parent–infant interaction* (pp. 241–269). Amsterdam: Elsevier.

Papousek, H., & Papousek, M. (1977). Mothering and the cognitive head-start: Psychobiological considerations. In H. R. Schaffer (Ed.), *Studies in mother-infant interaction* (pp. 63–85). London: Academic Press.

Papousek, H., & Papousek, M. (1979). Early ontogeny of human social interaction: Its biological roots and social dimensions. In M. Von Cranach, K. Foppa, W. Lepnies, & D. Ploog (Eds.), *Human Ethology: Claims and Limits of a New Discipline* (pp. 456–490). Cambridge, England: Cambridge University Press.

Papousek, H., & Papousek, M. (1983). Interactional failures: Their origins and significance in infant psychiatry. In J. D. Call, E. Galenson, & R. L. Tyson (Eds.), *Frontiers of infant psychiatry* (pp. 31–37). New York: Basic Books.

Papousek, H., & Papousek, M. (1984). The evolution of parent–infant attachment: New psychobiological perspectives. In J. D. Call, E. Galenson & R. L. Tyson (Eds.), *Frontiers of infant psychiatry: Vol. 2.* (pp. 276–283). New York: Basic Books.

Pare, C. M. B., & Sandler, M. (1959). A clinical and biochemical study of a trial of iproniazid in the treatment of depression. *Journal of Neurology, Neurosurgery and Psychiatry, 22*, 247–251.

Parsons, J. E., & Ruble, D. N. (1977). The development of achievement–related experiences. *Child Development, 48*, 1075–1079.

Patterson, M. L. (1973). Stability of nonverbal immediacy behaviors. *Journal of Experimental Social Psychology, 9*, 97–109.

Patton, R. G., & Gardner, L. I. (1975). Deprivation dwarfism (psychosocial deprivation): Disordered family environment as cause of so–called idiopathic hypo–

pituitarism. In L. I. Gardner (Ed.), *Endocrine and genetic diseases of childhood and adolescence* (2nd Ed., pp. 85–98). Philadelphia: W. B. Saunders.

Pavlov, I. (1935). *Conditioned responses: An investigation of the psychological activity of the cerebral cortex.* London: Oxford University Press.

Pervin, L. A. (1963). The need to predict and control under conditions of threat. *Journal of Personality, 31*, 570–587.

Peters–Martin, P., & Wachs, T.D. (1984). A longitudinal study of temperament and its correlates in the first 12 months. *Infant Behavioral Development, 7*, 285–298.

Petty, L. K., Asarnow, J. R., Carlson, G. A., & Lesser, L. (1985). The dexamethasone suppression test in depressed dysthymic and nondepressed children. *American Journal of Psychiatry, 142*, 631–633.

Phillippe, M. (1983). Fetal Catecholamines. *American Journal of Obstetrics and Gynocology, 146*, 840– 855.

Philips, I. (1979). Childhood depression: Interpersonal interactions and depressive phenomena. *American Journal of Psychiatry, 136*, 511–515.

Phillips, L., & Zigler, E. (1961). Social competence: The action–thought parameter and vicariousness in normal and pathological behavior. *Journal of Personality and Social Psychology, 63*, 137–146.

Piaget, J. (1930). *The child's conception of physical causality.* London: Routledge & Kegan Paul.

Piaget, J. (1932). *The moral judgment of the child.* New York: Harcourt Brace.

Piaget, J. (1952). *The origin of intelligence in children.* New York: International Universities Press.

Piaget, J. (1954). *The construction of reality in the child.* New York: Basic Books. (Original work published in 1937).

Piaget, J. (1970). *Psychology and epistemology.* New York: Viking.

Piers, E. V. (1969a). *The Piers–Harris Children's Self Concept Scale (The way I feel about myself).* Los Angeles: Western Psychological Service.

Piers, E.V. (1969b) *Manual for The Piers–Harris Children's Self Concept Scale.* Nashville, Tenn.: Counselor Recordings and Tests.

Plomin, R. (1981). Heredity and temperament: A comparison of twin data for self–report questionnaires, parental ratings, and objectively assessed behavior. *Progress in Clinical and Biological Research, 69*, 269–278.

Plomin, R. (1983). Childhood temperament. *Advances in Clinical Child Psychology, 6*, 45–92.

Plomin, R., & Rowe, D. C. (1979). Genetic and environmental etiology of social behavior in infancy. *Developmental Psychology, 15*, 62–71.

Polak, P. R., Emde, R. N., & Spitz, R. A. (1964). The smiling response: II. Visual discrimination and the onset of depth perception. *Journal of Nervous and Mental Diseases, 139*, 407–415.

Posner, M. I., & Rothbart, M. K. (1980). The development of attentional mechanisms. *Nebraska symposium on Motivation, 1980: Cognitive Processes, 28*, 1–52.

Powell, G. F., Brasel, J. A., & Blizzard, R. M. (1967a). Emotional deprivation and growth retardation simulating idiopathic hypopituitarism: I. Clinical evaluation of the syndrome. *New England Journal of Medicine, 276*, 1271–1278.

Powell, G. F., Brasel, J. A., & Blizzard, R. M. (1967b). Emotional deprivation andgrowth retardation simulating idiopathic hypopituitarism: II. Endocrinologic evaluation of the syndrome. *New England Journal of Medicine, 276*, 1279–1283.

Poznanski, E. O., Carroll, B. J., Banegas, M. C., Cook, S. C., & Gross, J. A. (1982). The dexamethasone suppression test in prepubertal children. *American Journal of Psychiatry, 139*, 321–324.

Poznanski, E., Mokros, H. B., Grossman, J., & Freeman, L. N. (1985). Diagnostic criteria in childhood depression. *American Journal of Psychiatry, 142*, 1168–1173.

Poznanski, E., & Zrull, J.P. (1970). Childhood depression. *Archives of General Psychiatry, 23*, 8–15.

Pradhan, S. N., & Pradhan, S. (1980). Development of central neurotransmitter systems and ontogeny of behavior. In H. Parvez & S. Parvez (Eds.), *Biogenic amines in development* (pp. 641–662). New York: Elsevier/North Holland Biomedical Press.

Prange, A. J., Lipton, M. A., Nemeroff, C. B., & Wilson, I. C. (1977). The role of hormones in depression. *Life Science, 20*, 1305–1318.

Prange, A. J., Jr., Wilson, I. C., Knox, A. E., McClane, T. K., Breese, G. R., Martin, B. R., Alltop, L. B., & Lipton, M. A. (1972). Effects of thyrotropin-releasing hormone in depression. *Lancet, 2*, 999–1002.

Prange, A. J., Jr., Wilson, I. C., Knox, A. E., Alltop, L. B., & Breese, G. R. (1972). Thyroid–imipramine clinical and chemical interaction: Evidence for a receptor deficit in depression. *Journal of Psychiatric Research, 9*, 187–205.

Provence, S. A. (1980). A feeding problem. *Zero to Three, 1*, 5–9.

Provence, S. A. (1983). Case vignettes—Two depressed infants. *Zero to Three, 3*, 4–6.

Provence, S., & Ritvo, S. (1961). Effects of deprivation on institutionalized infants: Disturbances in development of relationship to inanimate objects. *Psychoanalytic Study of the Child, 16*, 189–205.

Puig–Antich, J. (1982). Major depression and conduct disorder in prepuberty. *Journal of the American Academy of Child Psychiatry, 21*, 118–128.

Puig–Antich, J., Chambers, W., Halpern, F. Hallon, C., & Sachar, E.J. (1979). Cortisol hypersecretion in prepubertal depressive illness: a preliminary report. *Psychoneuroendocrinology, 4*, 191–197.

Puig–Antich, J., Novacenko, H., Goetz, R., Corser, J., Davies, M., & Ryan, N. (1984).Cortisol and prolactin reponses to insulin–induced hypoglycemia in prepubertal major depressives during episode and after recovery. *Journal of the American Academy of Child Psychiatry, 23*, 49–57.

Puig–Antich, J., Tabrizi, M. A., Davies, M., Goetz, R., Chambers, W., Halpern, F., & Sachar, E. J. (1981). Prepubertal endogenous major depressives hyposecrete growth hormon in response to insulin–induced hypoglycemia. *Biological Psychiatry, 16*, 801–818.

Radke–Yarrow, M., Cummings, E. M., Kuczynski, L., & Chapman, M. (1985). Patterns of attachment in two– and three–year–olds in normal families and families with parental depression. *Child Development, 56*, 884–893.

Ramey, C. T., & Finkelstein, N. W. (1978). Contingent stimulation and infant competence. *Journal of Pediatric Psychology, 3*, 89–96

Ramey, C. T., & Finkelstein, N. W. (1984). Contingent stimulation and infant competence. *Journal of Pediatric Psychology, 3*, 89–96.

Ramsay D. S., & Campos, J. J. (1978). The onset of representation and entry into stage 6 of object permanence development. *Developmental Psychology, 14*, 79–86.

Randrup, A., & Braestrup, C. (1977). Uptake inhibition of biogenic amines by newer antidepressant drugs: Relevance to the dopamine hypothesis of depression. *Psychopharmacology, 53,* 309–314.

Raps, C. S., Peterson, C., Reinhard, K. E., Abramson, L. Y., & Seligman, M. E. P. (1982). Attributional style among depressed patients. *Journal of Abnormal Psychology, 91,* 102–108.

Reader, T. A., Ferron, A., Descarries, L., & Jasper, H. H. (1979). Modulatory role for biogenic amines in the cerebral cortex. *Brain Research, 160,* 217–229.

Reich, A. (1960). Pathologic forms of self–esteem regulation. *Psychoanalytic Study of the Child, 15,* 215–231.

Reite, M., Short, R., Seller, C., & Pauley, M. (1981). Attachment loss and depression. *Journal of Child Psychology and Psychiatry, 22,* 141–169.

Renshaw, D. C. (1974). Suicide and depression in children. *Journal of School Health, 44,* 487–489.

Reus, V. I., Peeke, H. V. S., & Miner, C. (1985). Habituation and cortisol dysregulation in depression. *Biological Psychiatry, 20,* 980–989.

Rholes, W. S., Blackwell, J., Jordan, C., & Walters, C. (1980). A developmental study of learned helplessness. *Developmental Psychology, 16,* 616–624.

Rie, H.E . (1966). Depression in childhood: A survey of some pertinent contributions. *Journal of the American Academy of Child Psychiatry, 5,* 653–685.

Rinsley, D. B. (1986). Object constancy, object permanence, and personality disorders. In R. F. Lax, S. Bach, & J. A. Burland (Eds.), *Self and object constancy* (pp. 193–207). New York: Guildford Press.

Robertson, J., & Bowlby, J. (1952). Responses of young children to separation from their mothers. *Courrier du Centre International de l'Enfance, 2,* 131–142.

Robson, K. S. (1967). The role of eye to eye contact in maternal–infant attachment. *Journal of Child Psychology and Psychiatry, 8,* 13–25.

Rochlin, G. (1959). The loss complex. *Journal of the American Psychoanalytic Association, 7,* 299–316.

Rode, S. S., Chang, P. N., Fisch, R. O., & Sroufe, L. A. (1981) Attachment patterns of infants separated at birth. *Developmental Psychology, 54,* 185–191.

Rosenberg, S. E. (1975). *Individual differences in infant attachment: Relationships to mother, infant and interaction system variables.* Doctoral dissertation, Bowling Green State University.

Rosenblatt, S., & Chanley, J. D. (1965). Differences in the metabolism of norepinephrine in depressions. *Archives of General Psychiatry, 13,* 495–502.

Rothbart, M. K. (1981). Measurement of temperament in infancy. *Child Development, 52,* 569–578.

Rothbart, M. K., & Derryberry, D. (1981). Development of individual differences in temperament. In M. E. Lamb & A. L. Brown (Eds.), *Advances in Developmental Psychology: Vol. 1.* (pp. 37–86). Hillsdale, NJ: Erlbaum.

Rothbart, M.K., & Derryberry, D. (1982). Theoretical issues in temperament. In M. Lewis & L. T. Taft (Eds.), *Developmental disabilities: Theory, assessment, and intervention* (pp. 383–400). New York: SP Medical and Scientific Books.

Rotter, J. B. (1966). Generalized expectancies for internal–external locus of control of reinforcement. *Psychological Monographs, 80*(1, Whole No. 609).

Rowe, D. C., & Plomin, R. (1977). Temperament in early childhood. *Journal of Personality Assessment, 41,* 150–156.

Ruble, D. C., Parsons, J. E., & Ross, J. (1976). Self–evaluative responses of children in an achievement setting. *Child Development, 47*, 990–997.

Rutter, M. (1972). Relationships between child and adult psychiatric disorders. *Acta Psychiatrica Scandanavica, 48*, 3–21.

Rutter, M. (1977). Prospective studies to investigate behavioral change. In J. S. Strauss, H. Babigian, & M. Roff (Eds.), *The origins and course of psychopathology: Methods of longitudinal research* (pp. 223–248). New York: Plenum Press.

Rutter, M. (1979). Maternal deprivation, 1972–1978: New findings, new concepts, new approaches. *Child Development, 50*, 283–305.

Rutter, M., & Garmezy, N. (1983). Developmental psychopathology. In E. M. Hetherington (Ed.), *Handbook of child psychology: Vol. 4. Socialization, personality, and sexual development* (pp. 776–911). New York: John Wiley.

Saal, D. (1975). *A study of the development of object concept in infancy varying the degree of discrepancy between the disappearing and reappearing object.* Unpublished Ph.D. dissertation, University of Houston.

Sachar, E. G. (1974). Endocrine function in affective disorders. In N. E. Kline (Ed.), *Factors in depression* (pp. 115–126). New York: Raven Press.

Sachar, E. G. (1975). Twenty–four–hour cortisol secretory patterns in depressed and manic patients. *Progress in Brain Research, 42*, 81–91.

Sachar, E. G. (1976). Neuroendocrine dysfunction in depressive illness. *Annual Review of Medicine, 27*, 389–396.

Sachar, E. G., Asnis, G., Halbreich, M., Nathan, R. S., & Halpern, F. (1980). Recent studies in the neuroendocrinology of major depressive disorders. *American Journal of Psychiatry, 139*, 942–943.

Sachar, E. G., Finkelstein, J., & Hellman, I. (1971). Growth hormone responses in depressive illness: I. Response to insulin tolerance test. *Archives of General Psychiatry, 25*, 263–269.

Sachar, E. G., Fratz, A. G., Altman, N., & Sassin, J. (1973). Growth hormone and prolactin in unipolar and bipolar depressed patients; Responses to hypoglycemia and L dopa. *Archives of General Psychiatry, 130*, 1362–1367.

Sachar, E. G., Hellman, L., Fukushima, D. K., & Gallagher, T. F. (1970). Cortisol production in depressive illness. *Archives of General Psychiatry, 23*, 289–298.

Sachar, E. G., Hellman, L., Roffwarg, H., Halpern, F., Fukushima, D., & Gallagher, T. (1973). Disrupted 24–hour patterns of cortisol secretion in psychotic depression. *Archives of General Psychiatry, 28*, 19–24.

Saenger, P., Levine, L. S., Wiedemann, E., Schwartz, E., Korth–Schutz, S., Pareira, J., Heinig, B., & New, M.I. (1977). Somatomedin and growth hormone in psychosocial dwarfism. *Padiatrie und Padologie, Supplementum (Vienna), 5*, 1–12.

Sagi, A., & Hoffman, M. L. (1976). Empathic distress in the newborn. *Developmental Psychology, 12*, 175–176.

Salapatek, P. (1969, December). *The visual investigation of geometric patterns by the one– and two–month–old infant.* Paper presented at the meeting of the American Association for the Advancement of Science, Boston.

Sameroff, A. J. (1975). Early influences on development: Fact or fancy? *Merrill–Palmer Quarterly, 21*, 267–294.

Sameroff, A. J., & Chandler, M. J. (1984). Reproductive risk and the continuum of caretaking casualty. In L. Grinspoon (Ed.), *Psychiatry Update: Vol. 3.* (pp. 197–244). Washington, DC: American Psychiatric Press.

Sander, L. W. (1969). The longitudinal course of early mother–child interaction: Cross case comparison in a sample of mother–child pairs. In B. M. Foss (Ed.), *Determinants of infant behavior: Vol. IV* (pp 198–227). London: Methuen.

Sandler, J. (1986). Comments on the self and its object. In R. F. Lax, S. Bach, & J. A. Burland (Eds.), *Self and object constancy* (pp. 97–106). New York: Guilford Press.

Sandler, J., & Rosenblatt, B. (1962). The concept of the representational world. *Psychoanalytic Study of the Child, 17,* 128–145.

Scaife, M., & Bruner, J.S. (1975). The capacity for joint visual attention in the infant. *Nature, 253,* 265–266.

Scarr, S. (1969). Social introversion–extroversion as a heritable response. *Child Development, 40,* 823–832.

Schachter, S., & Singer, J. E. (1962). Cognitive, social and physiological determinants of emotional state. *Psychological Review, 69,* 179–399.

Schally, A. V., Arimura, A., & Kastin, A. J. (1973). Hypothalmic regulatory hormones. *Science, 179,* 341–350.

Schatzberg, A. F., Orsulak, P. J., Rosenblaum, A. H., Maruta, T., Kruger, E. R., Cole, J. O., & Schildkraut, J. J. (1982). Toward a biochemical classification of depressive disorders, V: Heterogeneity of unipolar depressions. *American Journal of Psychiatry, 139,* 471–475.

Schatzberg, A. F., Rosenbaum, A. H., Orsulak, P. J., Rohde, W. A., Maruta, T., Kruger, E. R., Cole, J. O., & Schildkraut, J. J. (1981). Toward a biochemical classification of depressive disorders: III Pretreatment urinary MHPG levels as predictors of response to treatment with maprotiline. *Psychopharmacology, 73,* 34–38.

Schildkraut, J. J. (1965). The catecholamine hypothesis of affective disorders: A review of supporting evidence. *American Journal of Psychiatry, 122,* 509–522.

Schildkraut, J. J. (1970). *Neuropsychopharmacology and the affective disorders.* Boston: Little, Brown and Company.

Schildkraut, J. J. (1978). Current status of the catecholamine hypothesis of affective disorders. In M. A. Lipton, A. DiMasacio, & K. F. Killam (Eds.), *Psychopharmacology: A generation of progress* (pp. 1223–1234). New York: Raven Press.

Schneider–Rosen, K., & Cicchetti, D. (1984). The relationship between affect and cognition in maltreated infants: Quality of attachment and the development of visual self–recognition. *Child Development, 55,* 648–658.

Schulman, A. H., & Kaplowitz, C. (1977). Mirror–image response during the first two years of life. *Developmental Psychobiology, 10,* 133–142.

Secord, P. F., & Peevers, B. H. (1974). The development and attribution of person concepts. In T. Mischel (Ed.), *Understanding other persons* (pp. 117–142). Oxford: Blackwell.

Seegmiller, B., & King, W. (1974). Relations between behavioral characteristics of infants, their mothers' behavior and performance on the Bayley mental and motor scales. *Journal of Psychology, 90,* 99–111.

Seligman, M. E. P. (1972). Learned helplessness. *Annual Review of Medicine, 23,* 407–412.

Seligman, M. E. P. (1975). *Helplessness: On depression, development and death.* San Francisco: Freeman.

Seligman, M. E. P., & Maier, S. F. (1967). Failure to escape traumatic shock. *Journal of Experimental Psychology, 74,* 1–9.

Seligman, M. E. P., Maier, S. F., & Geer, J. (1968). Alleviation of learned helplessness in the depressed. *Journal of Abnormal Sociology and Psychology, 73,* 256–262.

Seligman, M. E. P., Maier, S. F., & Soloman, R. L. (1971). Unpredictable and uncontrollable aversive events. In F. R. Brush (Ed.), *Aversive conditioning and learning* (pp. 347–400). New York: Academic Press.

Selman, R. (1980). *The growth of interpersonal understanding.* New York: Academic Press.

Sette, M., Raisman, R., Briley, M., & Langer, S. Z. (1981) Localisation of tricyclic anti-depressant binding sites of serotonin nerver terminals. *Journal of Neurochemistry, 37,* 40–42.

Sheldon, R. E., Peeters, L. I. H., Jones, M. D., Makowski, E. L., & Meschia, J. (1979). Redistribution of the cardiac output and oxygen delivery in the hypoxemic fetal lamb. *American Journal of Obstetrics and Gynecology, 135,* 1071–1078.

Shields, J. (1981). Genetics and mental development. In M. Rutter (Ed.), *Scientific foundations of developmental psychiatry* (pp. 8–24). Baltimore, MD: Park Press.

Shirley, M. (1933). *The first two years: A study of twenty–five babies: Vol. 2. Personality manifestations.* Minneapolis, MN: University of Minnesota Press.

Siever, L. J., & Davis, K. L. (1985). Overview: Toward a dysregulation hypothesis of depression. *American Journal of Psychiatry, 142,* 1017–1031.

Sigman, M., & Parmelee, A. (1974). Visual preferences of four–month–old premature and full–term infants. *Child Development, 45,* 959–965.

Simner, M. L. (1971). Newborn's response to the cry of another infant. *Developmental Psychology, 5,* 136–150.

Sjöström, R., & Roos, B.–E. (1972). 5–Hydroxyindoleacetic acid and homovanillic acid in cerebrospinal fluid in manic-depressive psychosis. *European Journal of Clinical Pharmacology, 4.* 170–176.

Slee, P. T. (1984). The nature of mother–infant gaze patterns during interaction as a function of emotional expression. *Journal of the Academy of Child Psychiatry, 21,* 385–391.

Slusher, M. A., & Hyde, J. E. (1969). Influence of limbic system and related structures on the pituitary adrenal axis. *Modern Trends in Physiological Science, 27,* 146–170.

Solnit, A. J. (1980). Three homes in two years. *Zero to Three, 1,* 4–5, 9.

Solnit, A. J. (1982). Developmental perspectives on self and object constancy. *Psychoanalytic Study of the Child, 32,* 201–217.

Solomon, R. L., & Corbitt, J. D. (1974). An opponent–process theory of motivation: 1. Temporal dynamics of affect. *Psychological Review, 81,* 119–145.

Spelke, E. (1979). Percieving bimodally specified events in infancy. *Developmental Psychology, 15,* 626–636.

Spielberger, C. D., Gorsuch, R. L., & Lushene, R. E. (1970). *The State–Trait Anxiety Inventory.* Palo Alto: Consulting Psychologists Press.

Spitz, R. A., & Wolf, K. M. (1946). Anaclitic Depression: An inquiry into the genesis of psychiatric conditions on early conditions, II. *Psychoanalitic Study of the Child, 2,* 313–342.

Spitz, R. A. (1965). *The first year of life.* New York: International Universities Press.

Spitz, R. A. (1966). Metapsychological implications of my research on infantile development. *Revue Francaise de Psychanalyse, 30*(5–6), 535–568.

Spitz, R. A., & Wolf, K. M. (1949). Autoerotism: Some empirical findings and hypotheses on three of its manifestations in the first year of life. *Psychoanalytic Study of the Child, 3/4*, 85–119.

Squires, P. L. (1927). "Wolf children" of India. *American Journal of Psychology, 38*, 313–335.

Sroufe, L. A. (1979). The coherence of individual development. *American Psychologist, 34*, 834–841.

Sroufe, L. A. (1983). Infant–caregiver attachment and patterns of adaptation in preschool: The roots of maladaptation and competence. *Minnesota Symposia on Child Psychology, 16*, 14–83.

Sroufe, L. A., Fox, N. E., & Pancake, V. R. (1983). Attachment and dependency in developmental perspective. *Child Development, 54*, 1615–1627.

Sroufe, L. A. & Rutter, M. (1984). The domain of developmental psychology. *Child Development, 55*, 17–29.

Sroufe, L.A., Schork, E., Motti, E., Lawroski, N., & LaFreniere, P. (1984). The role of affect in emerging social competence. In C. Izard, J. Kagan, & R. Zajonc (Eds.), *Emotion, cognition and behavior* (pp. 289–319). New York: Cambridge University Press.

Sroufe, L. A., & Waters, E. (1977). Attachment as an organizational construct. *Child Development, 48*, 1184–1199.

Sroufe, L. A., Waters, E., & Matas, L. (1974). Contextual determinants of infant affective response. In L. M. Rosenblum (Ed.), *The origins of behavior: Vol. II. Fear* (pp. 49–72). New York: John Wiley.

Starkman M. J., & Schteingart, D. E. (1981). Neuropsychiatric manifestations of patients with Cushing's Syndrome. Relationship to cortisol and adrenocorticotropic hormone levels. *Archives of Internal Medicine, 141*, 215–219.

Stechler, G. (1964). Newborn attention as affected by medication during labor. *Science, 114*, 315–317.

Stern, D. N. (1974a). General issues in the study of fear, Section III. In L. M. Rosenblum (Ed.), *The origins of fear*. New York: John Wiley.

Stern, D. N. (1974b). Mother and infant at play: The dyadic interaction involving facial, vocal and gaze behaviors. In M. Lewis & L. A. Rosenblum (Eds.), *The effect of the infant on its caregiver* (pp. 187–215). New York: John Wiley.

Stern, D. N. (1985). *The interpersonal worlds of the infant*. New York: Basic Books.

Stern D. N., Beebe, B., Jaffe, J., & Bennett, S. L. (1977). The infant's stimulus world during social interaction: A study of caregiver behaviours with particular reference to repetition and timing. In H.R. Schaffer (Ed.) *Studies in mother–infant interaction*. London: Academic Press.

Stern, D. N., & Gibbon, J. (1978). Temporal expectancies of social behaviors in mother–infant play. In E. Thoman (Ed.), *Origins of the infant's social responsiveness* (pp. 409–429). New York: Erlbaum Press.

Stern, D. N., Hofer, L., Haft, W., & Dore, J. (1985). Affect attunement: The sharing of feeling states between mother and infant by means of inter–modal fluency. In T. Field and N. Fox (Eds.), *Social perception in infants* (pp. 1–35). Norwood, NJ: Ablex.

Stipek, D. (1981a). Social–motivational development in first–grade. *Contemporary Educational Psychology, 6*, 33–45.

Stipek, D. (1981b). Children's perceptions of their own and their classmates' ability. *Journal of Educational Psychology, 3*, 404–410.

Stipek, D., & Hoffman, J.M. (1980). Development of children's performance–related judgments. *Child Development, 51*, 912–914.

Stipek, D., Roberts, T. A., & Sanborn, M. E. (1984). Preschool–age children's performance expectations for themselves and another child as a function of the incentive value of success and the salience of past performance. *Child Development, 55*, 1983–1989.

Stirnimann, F. (1944) Uber das Farbempfinden neugoborener. *Annales Paediatrici, 163*, 1–25.

Strayer, J. (1980). A naturalistic study of empathic behaviors and their relation to affective states and perspective–taking skills in preschool children. *Child Development, 51*, 815–822.

Suomi, S. J., Seaman, S. F., Lewis, J. K., Delizio, R. D., & McKinney, W. T. (1978). Effects of imipramine treatment on separation–induced social disorders in rhesus monkeys. *Archives of General Psychiatry, 35*, 321–325.

Surber, C. F. (1980). The development of reversible operations in judgments of ability, effort and performance. *Child Development, 51*, 1018–1029.

Surber, C. F. (1981). Effects of information reliability in predicting task performance using ability and effort. *Journal of Personality and Social Psychology, 40*, 977–989.

Talbert, L. M., Kraybill, E. N., & Potter., H. D. (1976). Adrenal cortical response to circumcision in the neonate. *Obstetrics and Gynecology, 48*(2), 208–210.

Tanguay, P. E. (1984). Toward a new classification of serious psychopathology in children. *Journal of the American Academy of Child Psychiatry, 23*, 373–384.

Tanner, J. M. (1973). Resistance to exogenous growth hormone in psychosocial short stature (emotional deprivation). (Letter to the editor). *Journal of Pediatrics, 82*, 171–172.

Tennes, K., & Carter, D. (1973). Plama cortisol levels and behavioral states in early infancy. *Psychsomatic Medicine, 35*, 121–128.

Tennes, K., Downey, K., & Vernadakis, A. (1977). Urinary cortisol excretion rates and anxiety in normal 1–year–old infants. *Psychosomatic Medicine, 39*, 178–187.

Tennes, K. H., & Mason, J. W. (1982). Developmental psychoendocrinology: An approach to the study of emotions. In C.E. Izard (Ed.), *Measuring emotions in infants and children* (pp. 21–37). Cambridge, MA: Cambridge University Press.

Thoman, E. B. (1975). How a rejecting baby affects mother–infant synchrony. In R. Porter & M. O'Connor (Eds.), *Parent–infant interaction, Ciba Foundation Symposium No. 33*. New York: American Elsevier.

Thomas, A., & Chess, S. (1977). *Temperament and development*. New York: Bruner/Mazel.

Thomas, A., & Chess, S. (1980). *The dynamics of psychological development*. New York: Brunner/Mazel.

Thomas, A., & Chess, S. (1984). Genesis and evolution of behavior disorders: From infancy to early adult life. *American Journal of Psychiatry, 141*, 1–9.

Thomas, A., Chess, S., & Birch, H. G. (1968). *Temperament and behavior disorders in children*. New York: New York University Press.

Thomas, A., Chess, S., & Birch, H. G. (1970). The origin of personality. *Scientific American, 223*, 102–109.

Thomas, A., Chess, S., Birch, H.G., Hertzig, M.E., & Korn, S. (1963). *Behavioral individuality in early childhood*. New York: New York University Press.

Tinbergen, N., & Moynihan, M. (1952). Head flagging in the black–headed gull: Its function and origin. *British Birds, 45,* 19–22.

Toolan, J. M. (1962). Depression in children and adolescents. *American Journal of Orthopsychiatry, 32,* 404–414.

Torgensen, A. M., & Kringlen, E. (1978). Genetic aspects of temperamental differences in twins. *Journal of the American Academy of Child Psychiatry, 17,* 433–444.

Tracy, R. L., Lamb, M. E., & Ainsworth, M. D. S. (1976). Infant approach behavior as related to attachment. *Child Development, 47,* 571–578.

Trevarthen, C., & Hubley, P. (1978). Secondary intersubjectivity: Confidence, confiding and acts of meaning in the first year. In A. Lock (Ed.), *Action, gesture and symbol* (pp. 183–229). New York: Academic Press.

Tronick, E. (Ed.). (1982). *Social interchange in infancy: affect, cognition, and communication*. Baltimore: University Park Press.

Tronick, E., Als, H., Adamson, L., Wise, S., & Brazelton, T. B. (1978). The infant's response to entrapment between contradictory messages in face–to–face interaction. *Journal of American Academy of Child Psychiatry, 17,* 1–13.

Tronick, E., Als, H., & Brazelton, T. B. (1977). Mutuality in mother–infant interaction. *Journal of Communication, 27,* 74–79.

Tronick, E. Z., Ricks, M., & Cohn, J. F. (1982). Maternal and infant affective exchange: patterns of adaptation. In T. Field & A. Fogel (Eds.), *Emotion and early interaction* (pp. 83–100). Hillsdale, NJ: Erlbaum.

Trulson, M. E., & Jacobs, B. L. (1979). Chronic amphetamine administration to cats: Behavioral and neurological evidence for decreased central serotinergic function. *Journal of Pharmacology and Experimental Therapeutics, 2,* 375–384.

Tyson, P. (1984). Developmental lines and infant assessment. In J. D. Call, E. Galenson, & R. L. Tyson (Eds.), *Frontiers in infant psychiatry: Vol. 2.* (pp. 121–125). New York: Basic Books.

Underwood, B., Froming, W. J., & Moore, B. S. (1977). Mood, attention and altruism: A search for mediating variables. *Developmental Psychology, 13,* 541–542.

Underwood, B., Moore, B. S., & Rosenhan, D. L. (1973). Affect and self–gratification. *Developmental Psychology, 8,* 209–214.

Uzgiris, I. E., & Hunt, J. M. (1966). *An instrument for assessing infant psychological development*. Unpublished manuscript, University of Illinois.

Uzgiris, I. E., & Hunt, J. M. (1975). *Assessment in infacy: ordinal scales of psychologic development*. Urbana, IL: University of Illinois Press.

Van den Brande, J. L., Van Buul, S., Heinrich, U., Van Roon, F., Zurcher, T., & Van Steirtegem, A. C. (1975). Further observations on plasma somatomedin activity in children. In R. Luft & K. Hall (Eds.), *Advances in metabolic disorders, 8,* 171–181.

Vandenberg, S. G. (1966). Hereditary factors in normal personality traits (as measured by inventories). *Recent Advances in Biological Psychiatry, 9,* 65–104.

Van der Kolk, B., Greenberg, M., Boyd, H., & Krystal, J. (1985). Inescapable shock, neurotransmitters, and addition to trauma: Toward a psychology of post traumatic stress. *Biological Psychiatry, 20,* 314–325.

van Praag, H. M. (1976). *Depression and Schizophrenia: A contribution on their chemical pathology*. New York: Spectrum.

van Praag, H. M. (1977). Significance of biochemical parameters in the diagnosis, treatment, and prevention of depressive disorders. *Biological Psychiatry, 12*, 101–131.

van Praag, H. M. (1978). Amine hypothesis of affective disorders, in L. Iversen, S. Iversen, & S. Snyder (Eds.), *Handbook of psychopharmacology: Vol. 13. Biology of mood and antianxiety drugs* (pp. 187–297). New York: Plenum Press.

van Praag, H. M. (1982). Neurotransmitters and CNS disease. *Lancet*, 1259–1264.

van Praag, H. M., & de Haan, S. (1980). Depression vulnerability and 5–hydroxotryptophan prophylaxis. *Psychiatry Research, 3*, 75–83.

Vaughn, B., & Sroufe, L. (1979). The temporal relationship between infant heart rate acceleration and crying in an aversive situation. *Child Development, 50*, 565–567.

Velten, E. A. (1968). A laboratory task for induction of mood states. *Behaviour Research and Therapy, 6*, 473–482.

Veroff, J. (1969). Social comparison and the development of achievement motivation. In C. P. Smith (Ed.), *Achievement–related motives in children* (pp. 46–101). New York: Russell Sage.

Vietze, P. H., McCarthy, M., McQuiston, S., MacTurk, R. H., & Yarrow, L. J. (1983). Attention and exploratory behavior in infants with Down's syndrome. In T. Field & A. Sostek (Eds.), *Infants born at risk: Physiological, perceptual and cognitive processes* (pp. 251–278). New York: Grune & Stratton.

Vogt, J. L., & Levine, S. (1980). Response of mother and infant squirrel monkeys to separation and disturbance. *Physiology and Behavior, 24*, 829–832.

Wachs, T. D. (1975). Relation of infants' performance on Piaget scales between twelve and twenty–four months and their Stanford–Binet performance at thirty-one months. *Child Development, 46*, 929–935.

Waters, E. (1978). The reliability and stability of individual differences in infant–mother attachment. *Child Development, 49*, 483–494.

Waters, E., Matas, L., & Sroufe, L. A. (1975). Infants' reactions to an approaching stranger: Description, validation and functional significance of wariness. *Child Development, 46*, 348–356.

Waters, E., Vaughn, B. E., & Engeland, B. R. (1980). Individual differences in infant–mother attachment relationships at age one: Antecedents in neonatal behavior in an urban, economically disadvantaged sample. *Child Development, 51*, 208–216.

Waters, E., Wippman, J., & Sroufe, L.A. (1979). Attachment, positive affect, and competence in the peer group: Two studies in construct validation. *Child Development, 50*, 821–829.

Watson, J. S. (1966). The development of and generalization of "contingency awareness" in early infancy. *Merrill Palmer Quarterly, 12*, 123–125.

Watson, J. S. (1971). Cognitive–perceptual development in infancy: Setting for the seventies. *Merrill Palmer Quarterly, 17*, 139–152.

Watson, J. S. (1972). Smiling, cooing and "the game." *Merrill Palmer Quarterly, 18*, 323–339.

Watson, J. S., & Ramey, C. T. (1969). *Reactions to response–contingent stimulation in early infancy*. Revision of paper presented at biennial meeting of the Society for Research in Child Development, Santa Monica, CA.

Watson, J. S., & Ramey, C. T. (1972). Reactions to response-contingent stimulation in early infancy. *Merrill-Palmer Quarterly, 18*, 219–227.

Weinberg, W. A., Rutman, J., Sullivan, L., Penick, E. C., & Dietz, S. G. (1973). Depression in children referred to an educational diagnostic center: Diagnosis and treatment. *Journal of Pediatrics, 836*, 1065–1072.

Weiner, B. (Ed.). (1974). *Achievement motivation and attribution theory*. Morristown, NJ: General Learning Press.

Weiner, B., Graham, S., Stern, P., & Lawson, M. E. (1982). Using affective cues to infer causal thoughts. *Developmental Psychology, 18*, 278–232.

Weiner, G., Rowland, V. R., Oppel, W. C., Fischer, L. K., & Harper, P. D. (1965). Correlates of low birth weight: Psychological status at six to seven years of age. *Pediatrics, 35*, 434–444.

Weiner, B., Russell, D. & Lerman, D. (1978). Affective consequences of causal ascriptions. In J. H. Harvey, W. J. Ickes, & R. F. Kidd (Eds.), *New directions in attribution research: Vol. 2.* (pp. 59–90). Hillsdale, NJ: Erlbaum.

Weiss, J. M., & Glazer, H. I. (1975). Effects of acute exposure to stressors on subsequent avoidance–escape behavior. *Psychosomatic Medicine, 37*, 499–521.

Weiss, J. M., Glazer, H. I., & Pohorecky, L.A. (1974). Neurotransmitters and helplessness: A chemical bridge to depression? *Psychology Today, 8*, 58–62.

Weiss, J. M., Glazer, H. I., Pohorecky, L. A., Bailey, W. H., & Schneider, L. H. (1979). Coping behavior and stress–induced behavioral depression: Studies of the role of brain catecholamines. In R.A. Depue (Ed.), *The psychobiology of the depressive disorders: Implications for the effects of stress* (pp 125–160). New York: Academic Press.

Weiss, J. M., Glazer, H. I., Pohorecky, L. A., Brick, J., & Miller, N. E. (1975). Effects of chronic exposure to stressors on avoidance escape behavior and on brain norepinephrine. *Psychosomatic Medicine, 37*, 522–533.

Weiss, J. M., Stone, E. A., & Harrell, N. (1970). Coping behavior and brain norepinephrine level in rats. *Journal of Comparative Physiological Psychology, 72*, 153–160.

Weissman, M. M., & Boyd, J. H. (1985). Affective disorders; epidemiology. In H. I. Kaplan & B. J. Sadock (Eds.), *Comprehensive textbook of psychiatry* (4th Ed., pp. 764–769). Baltimore: Williams & Wilkins.

Weisz, J. R. (1980). Developmental change in perceived control: Recognizing noncontingency in the laboratory and perceiving it in the world. *Developmental Psychology, 16*, 385–390.

Weisz, J. R. (1981). Illusory contingency in children at the state fair. *Developmental Psychology, 17*, 481–489.

Weisz, J. R., Yeates, K. O., Robertson, D., & Beckham, J. C. (1982). Perceived contingency of skill and chance events: A developmental analysis. *Developmental Psychology, 18*, 898–905.

Weller, E. B., Weller, R. A., Fristad, M. A., & Preskorn, S. H. (1984). The dexamethasone suppression test in hospitalized prepubertal depressed children. *American Journal of Psychiatry, 141*, 290–291.

Werner, H. (1957). The concept of development from a comparative and organismic point of view. In D.B. Harris (Ed.), *The concept of development*. Minneapolis: University of Minnesota Press.

White, R. W. (1959). Motivation reconsidered: The concept of competence. *Psychological Review, 66*, 297–333.

White, R. W. (1963). Ego and reality in psychoanalytic theory. *Psychological Issues, 3*, 1–210.

Whiteside, M., Busch, F., & Horner, T. (1976). From egocentric to cooperative play in young children. *Journal of the American Academy of Child Psychiatry, 15*, 294–313.

Wilk, S., & Watson, W. (1973). VMA in spinal fluid: Evaluation of the pathways of cerebral catecholamine metabolism in man. In E. Usdin & S. Snyder (Eds.), *Frontiers in catecholamine research* (pp. 1067–1069). New York: Pergamon Press.

Willer, J. C., Boureau, F., Dauthier, C., & Banora, M. (1979). Study of naloxone in normal awake man: effects of heart rate and respiration. *Neuropharmacology, 18*, 469–472.

Willerman, L. (1973). Activity level and hyperactivity in twins. *Child Development, 44*, 283–293.

Wolff, P. H. (1963). Observations on the early development of smiling. In B. M. Foss (Ed.), *Determinants of infant behavior: Vol. 2.* (pp. 113–138). London: Methuen.

Wolff, P. H. (1969). Observations on the early development of smiling. In B. M. Foss (Ed.), *Determinants of infant behavior: Vol. 4.* (pp. 113–138.). London: Methuen.

Wylie, R. C. (1974). *The self–concept: A review of methodological considerations and measuring instruments: Vol. 1.* (Rev. Ed.). Lincoln: University of Nebraska Press.

Wylie, R. C. (1979). *The self–concept: Theory and research on selected topics: Vol. 2.* (Rev. Ed.). Lincoln: University of Nebraska Press.

Yanaihara, T., & Arai, K. (1981). In vitro release of steroids from the fetal adrenal tissue. *Acta Obstetricia et Gynocologica Scandinavica, 60*, 225–228.

Yarrow, L. J. (1961). Maternal deprivation: Toward an empirical and conceptual re–evaluation. *Psychological Bulletin, 58*, 459–490.

Yarrow, L. (1964). Separation from parents during early childhood. *Review of Child Development Research, 1*, 89–136.

Yarrow, L. J., McQuiston, S., MacTurk, R. H., McCarthy, M. E., Klein, R. P., & Vietze, P. M. (1983). Assessment of mastery motivation during the first year of life: Contemporaneous and cross– age relationships. *Developmental Psychology, 159*, 159–171.

Yates, F. E., & Maran, J. W. (1974). Stimulation and inhibition of adrenocorticotropin release. In E. Knobil & W. Sawyer (Eds.), *Handbook of Physiology: Sec. 7. Endocrinology: Vol. 4. The Pituitary Gland (Part 2).* (pp. 367–404). Washington, DC: American Physiological Society.

Young–Browne, G., Rosenfeld, H. M., & Horowitz, F. D. (1977). Infant discriminations of facial expressions. *Child Development, 48*, 555–562.

Zahn–Waxler, C., Cummings, E. M., McKnew, D. H., Jr., Davenport, Y. B., & Radke–Yarrow, M. (1984). Altruism, aggression, and social interactions in young children with a manic–depressive parent. *Child Development, 55*, 112–122.

Zahn–Waxler, C., Radke–Yarrow, M., & King, R. A. (1979). Child rearing and children's prosocial initiations toward victims of distress. *Child Development, 50*, 319–330.

Zeller, E. A., Barsky, J., Berman, E. R., & Fouts, J. R. (1952). Action of isonicotinic acid hydrazine and related compounds on enzymes involved in the autonomic nervous system. *Journal of Pharmacology and Experimental Theraputics, 106*, 427–428.

Zingg, R. M. (1940). Feral man: extreme cases of isolation. *American Journal of Psychology, 53*, 487–517.

Zwerling, I., Titchner, J., Gottschalk, L., Levine, M., Culbertson, W., Cohen, S., & Silver, H. (1955). Personality disorder and the relationships of emotion to surgical illness in 200 surgical patients. *American Journal of Psychiatry, 112*, 270–277.

Index